Klaney B

A Clinical Manual of Emergency Pediatrics

* Does the history
Fit the crime *

Appleton Clinical Manuals

Ayres, et al.: Medical Resident's Manual, 4th edition
Chung: A Clinical Manual of Cardiovascular Medicine
Crain and Gershel: A Clinical Manual of Emergency Pediatrics
Ellis and Beckmann: A Clinical Manual of Gynecology
Ellis and Beckmann: A Clinical Manual of Obstetrics
Gomella, et al.: Clinician's Pocket Reference, 4th edition
Hanno and Wein: A Clinical Manual of Urology
Matthews, et al.: A Clinical Manual of Adverse Drug Reactions
Steele: A Clinical Manual of Pediatric Infectious Disease
Walker and Margouleff: A Clinical Manual of Nuclear Medicine

A Clinical Manual of Emergency Pediatrics

EDITORS

Ellen F. Crain, M.D., Ph.D
Assistant Professor of Pediatrics
Albert Einstein College of Medicine
Director, Pediatric Emergency Services
Bronx Municipal Hospital Center
Bronx, New York

Jeffrey C. Gershel, M.D.
Assistant Clinical Professor of Pediatrics
Albert Einstein College of Medicine
Bronx, New York
Attending Pediatrician
Northern Westchester Hospital Center
Mount Kisco, New York

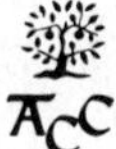

APPLETON-CENTURY-CROFTS/Norwalk, Connecticut

0-8385-1126-0

Notice: Our knowledge in clinical sciences is constantly changing. As new information becomes available, changes in treatment and in the use of drugs become necessary. The author(s) and the publisher of this volume have taken care to make certain that the doses of drugs and schedules of treatment are correct and compatible with the standards generally accepted at the time of publication. The reader is advised to consult carefully the instruction and information material included in the package insert of each drug or therapeutic agent before administration. This advice is especially important when using new or infrequently used drugs.

86 87 88 89 / 10 9 8 7 6 5 4 3 2

Prentice-Hall of Australia, Pty. Ltd., Sydney
Prentice-Hall Canada, Inc.
Prentice-Hall Hispanoamericana, S.A., Mexico
Prentice-Hall of India Private Limited, New Delhi
Prentice-Hall International (UK) Limited, London
Prentice-Hall of Japan, Inc., Tokyo
Prentice-Hall of Southeast Asia (Pte.) Ltd., Singapore
Whitehall Books Ltd., Wellington, New Zealand
Editora Prentice-Hall do Brasil Ltda., Rio de Janeiro

Library of Congress Cataloging in Publication Data
Main entry under title:

A Clinical manual of emergency pediatrics

(Appleton clinical manuals)
Includes index.
1. Pediatric emergencies. I. Crain, Ellen F.
II. Gershel, Jeffrey C. III. Series. [DNLM:
1. Emergencies—in infancy & childhood. 2. Emergency
Medicine—in infancy & childhood. WS 200 C641]
RJ370.C55 1986 618.92′0025 85–22976
ISBN 0–8385–1126–0

PRINTED IN THE UNITED STATES OF AMERICA

To Bill and Jodi
and to our children

Contributors

Henry Adam, M.D.
Assistant Professor of Pediatrics
Albert Einstein College of Medicine
Bronx, New York

Sophie J. Balk, M.D.
Assistant Professor of Pediatrics
Albert Einstein College of Medicine
Bronx, New York

Marjorie A. Boeck, M.D., Ph.D.
Assistant Professor of Pediatrics
Albert Einstein College of Medicine
Bronx, New York

Francine H. Brooks, M.D.
Instructor in Ambulatory Care
Albert Einstein College of Medicine
Bronx, New York

William B. Caspe, M.D.
Associate Professor of Pediatrics
Albert Einstein College of Medicine
Bronx, New York

Robert J. Coffey, M.D.
Assistant Attending Pediatrician
Saint Vincent's Hospital and Medical Center
New York, New York

Ellen F. Crain, M.D., Ph.D.
Assistant Professor of Pediatrics
Albert Einstein College of Medicine
New York, New York

Thomas J. Daley, M.D.
Associate Professor of Pediatrics
Albert Einstein College of Medicine
Bronx, New York

Gabriel Dinari, M.D.
Director, Pediatric Gastroenterology Unit
Beilinson Medical Center
Tel Aviv, Israel

Sheila M. Fallon, M.D.
Fellow in Infectious Disease
Albert Einstein College of Medicine
Bronx, New York

David L. Fenner, M.D.
Instructor in Pediatrics
Albert Einstein College of Medicine
Bronx, New York

Paul Gennis, M.D.
Assistant Professor of Medicine
Albert Einstein College of Medicine
Bronx, New York

Jeffrey C. Gershel, M.D.
Assistant Clinical Professor of Pediatrics
Albert Einstein College of Medicine
Bronx, New York

J. Martin Gewirtz, M.D.
Assistant Clinical Professor of Pediatrics
Albert Einstein College of Medicine
Bronx, New York

Joy Glaser, M.D.
Associate Professor of Pediatrics
Albert Einstein College of Medicine
Bronx, New York

Dario Gonzalez, M.D.
Director, Emergency Services
Queens Hospital Center
Queens, New York

Sue Y. E. Hahm, M.D.
Assistant Professor of Pediatrics
Albert Einstein College of Medicine
Bronx, New York

Gregg Husk, M.D.
Assistant Professor of Clinical Medicine
Columbia University College of Physicians and Surgeons
New York, New York

Theodore Kastner, M.D.
Fellow in Child Development
Albert Einstein College of Medicine
Bronx, New York

Stanley J. Kogan, M.D.
Adjunct Professor of Urology
New York Medical College
Valhalla, New York

Alan Kulberg, M.D.
Associate Professor of Clinical Pediatrics
New York University School of Medicine
New York, New York

Selwyn B. Levitt, M.D.
Adjunct Professor of Urology
New York Medical College
Valhalla, New York

Ross S. Levy, M.D.
Associate Professor of Medicine
Albert Einstein College of Medicine
Bronx, New York

Neil J. Macy, M.D.
Instructor in Orthopedic Surgery
Albert Einstein College of Medicine
Bronx, New York

Robert Marion, M.D.
Assistant Professor of Pediatrics
Albert Einstein College of Medicine
Bronx, New York

Dan M. Mayer, M.D.
Attending Physician, Emergency Department
Booth Memorial Hospital Center
Queens, New York

Andrew P. Mezey, M.D.
Associate Professor of Pediatrics
Albert Einstein College of Medicine
Bronx, New York

Peter Moyer, M.D.
Director, Emergency Services
Boston City Hospital Center
Boston, Massachusetts

Gerald Novak, M.D.
Assistant Professor of Neurology and Pediatrics
Albert Einstein College of Medicine
Bronx, New York

Jane A. Petro, M.D.
Associate Professor of Surgery
New York Medical College
Valhalla, New York

Samuel B. Ritter, M.D.
Assistant Professor of Pediatrics
The Mount Sinai School of Medicine
New York, New York

Deborah S. Saunders, M.D.
Assistant Professor of Pediatrics
Albert Einstein College of Medicine
Bronx, New York

Jay E. Selman, M.D.
Attending Pediatric Neurologist
Westchester County Medical Center
Valhalla, New York

Steven P. Shelov, M.D.
Associate Professor of Pediatrics
Albert Einstein College of Medicine
Bronx, New York

Marc J. Sicklick, M.D.
Associate Clinical Professor of Pediatrics
Albert Einstein College of Medicine
Bronx, New York

Barry J. Silverman, D.M.D.
Assistant Professor of Dentistry
Albert Einstein College of Medicine
Bronx, New York

Arthur J. Smerling, M.D.
Department of Anesthesiology
Columbia University College of Physicians and Surgeons
New York, New York

Paul Smey, M.D.
Associate Professor of Surgery
The Milton S. Hershey Medical Center
New York, New York

Ruth E. K. Stein, M.D.
Professor of Pediatrics
Albert Einstein College of Medicine
Bronx, New York

Jodi Sutton, M.D.
Attending Obstetrician
Northern Westchester Hospital Center
Mount Kisco, New York

Howard Trachtman, M.D.
Assistant Professor of Pediatrics
State University of New York at Stony Brook
Stony Brook, New York

Jerome V. Vaccaro, M.D.
Assistant Professor of Psychiatry
University of Hawaii John A. Burns School of Medicine
Honolulu, Hawaii

Steven B. VanDonsellar, R.P.A.
Physician Assistant, Department of Ambulatory Care
Albert Einstein College of Medicine
Bronx, New York

Frederick M. Wang, M.D.
Associate Clinical Professor of Ophthalmology and Pediatrics
Albert Einstein College of Medicine
Bronx, New York

Marc Weinblatt, M.D.
Assistant Professor of Pediatrics
Cornell University Medical College
New York, New York

Contents

Preface

Physicians caring for children in an emergency room must be able to recognize and treat a great variety of conditions. Moreover, they must identify the minority of patients who are seriously ill and know when urgent management is necessary. We believe that all of us who work in emergency room settings could use a portable handbook which summarizes most of the conditions that we see. This manual is an attempt to meet that need. It includes the essential points and priorities for diagnosis, management, and follow-up care, as well as indications for hospitalization. Physicians who work in other settings, such as a private office or clinic, may also be faced with potential or real emergencies; we hope this manual will be of use to them also.

There is no end to the topics that could be included in an emergency manual. Any selection is influenced by the experiences of the editors, which in our case has been caring for children in a large medical center in New York City. As a result, we have emphasized some areas more than others might have. However, we have made an effort to be representative and discuss most problems faced by those working in an emergency room.

A word of caution is in order. Although a manual for emergency care can be very useful, it also presents a danger, especially for those who are still in training. The physician may be tempted to look for instructions and automatic solutions, using the manual as a "how to" book with all the answers, rather than developing his or her own cognitive processes and interpersonal skills. No manual can substitute for careful thought and sensitivity to children and their families.

Many individuals have helped us on this project, and we are grateful to them. For all that they have taught us, we would like to give special thanks to Drs. Lewis M. Fraad, Andrew P. Mezey, and Steven P. Shelov, as well as to Lynda Levy, R.N., Patricia Donovan, R.N., P.N.P., and all the pediatric emergency room nursing staff of Jacobi hospital. Finally, we are indebted to the pediatric housestaff and to the medical students of the Albert Einstein College of Medicine who we have had the privilege of teaching and learning from over the years. Their thoughtful questions provided the impetus for this manual.

E.F.C.
J.C.G.
September, 1985

CT indicat-

1 ↓LOC at time of arrival in ER

2 Focal Neuro signs

3. Penetrating skull injury OR palp depression

4 H/O prog H/A

5 unreliable h/o injury

6. Basilar skull Fx

7. mult trauma + head

8. <2 yo consider

1

Resuscitation

Cardiopulmonary Resuscitation in Infants and Children

INTRODUCTION

Cardiopulmonary arrest in children is most often pulmonary in origin. Foreign body aspiration, suffocation, carbon monoxide poisoning, drowning, upper airway infection, drug ingestion, or head trauma can all be antecedent events. However, cardiac arrest as a primary event does occur. Causes include abnormalities of the heart and its conduction system (particularly following cardiac surgery), metabolic acidosis, drug ingestion, trauma to the chest, and electrocution.

When oxygen is no longer available, the body shifts to anaerobic metabolism, with the development of a metabolic acidosis. This is augmented by a respiratory acidosis as the pCO_2 level rises. Hypoxia, acidosis, and hypercarbia depress the myocardium, causing dysrhythmias that can lead to fatal arrest or fibrillation. Many young children and infants, however, can tolerate a pH as low as 7.10 for extended periods without cardiovascular dysfunction, and an occasional patient may tolerate a pH as low as 6.90.

ER MANAGEMENT

The Team Approach

In order for any resuscitation to be successful, participants must have clearly understood responsibilities. Ideally, each member of the team has a preassigned specific task to perform (team leader, airway/head, chest, intravenous access/meds, messenger, history-taker). Alternatively, designate a "team leader" to coordinate the resuscitation, assign tasks as indicated, order all medications, and be responsible for deciding to terminate the effort. This "team leader" should arrive on the scene early and not be involved in performing any of the procedures so that he or she can maintain an overview of the entire resuscitation effort.

Priorities

The ABCs of resuscitation, Airway, Breathing and Circulation, must be adhered to in all situations. Exercise caution when dealing with patients with possible cervical spine or internal injuries, but the priorities are the establishment of adequate ventilation and the generation of palpable pulses. Everything else is secondary.

Airway. Clear the airway using a large diameter suction catheter or by turning the patient's head to the side (unless a C-spine injury is suspected) and scooping material out with gauze-covered fingers. Insert an oropharyngeal airway.

Breathing. Establish adequate ventilation using bag-valve-mask apparatus appropriate for the child's size, connected to humidified flow O_2 at 10–15 L/min. To deliver close to 100% O_2, an extension adapter must cover the intake valves of the bag. Assess the adequacy of ventilation by auscultating both sides of the chest and noting the movement of the chest wall.

Straighten the head and place the infant or small child in the "sniffing position," ie, chin elevated slightly toward the ceiling. Hyperextension of the neck, necessary in adolescents and adults, may actually interfere with ventilation (and intubation) in younger patients. If these maneuvers do not provide adequate ventilation, consider the possibility of an aspirated foreign body (p 107) and the need for intubation.

Circulation. Once adequate ventilation is achieved, palpate the pulses. In the larger child, the carotid pulse is ideal, while in the smaller patient, femoral or brachial pulses may be preferable. Palpation of an apical pulse can be misleading as apical activity may be discernible without generation of an adequate pulse pressure. If no pulses are palpable, begin external cardiac compression immediately.

For an infant, the chest encircling technique has proven to be more effective than two-finger sternal compression. Surround the infant's chest with both hands so that both thumbs are over the midsternum and the fingers are supporting the back. For an older patient, place the heel of one hand over the midsternum with the fingers of both hands interlocking, as in adult cardiopulmonary resuscitation (CPR).

Compressing too low on the sternum can cause the xiphoid to lacerate the liver, while compressing laterally to the sternum can result in a rib fracture. The duration of relaxation equals the time of compression, so that the heart has time to refill. Do not allow the heel of the hand (or fingers or thumbs) to leave the chest wall. Compressions of 1½ cm in infants and 1½ inches in older children generate palpable pulses.

The rate and timing of external cardiac massage is age dependent, as shown in Table 1-1. In all infants and in the two-rescuer technique for children and adolescents, the ratio of compression to ventilation is always 5:1. In older patients when only one rescuer is present, a ratio of 15:2 is necessary. Recent evidence suggests that simultaneous ventilation and compression (SVC) causes increased cerebral blood flow when compared to the traditional method of ventilating between compressions. This seems particularly true after catecholamines have been administered. This technique, however, might not be appropriate for patients with suspected increased intracranial pressure (head trauma, stroke).

Airway Obstruction

Consider the possibility of a foreign body or anatomical airway obstruction if there is resistance to ventilation or no movement of air in the thorax despite vigorous suctioning and clearing of the oral cavity. Frequently the tongue slides backward and occludes the airway. Techniques for relieving this obstruction include:

Head Tilt, Chin Lift. Place one hand on the forehead tilting the head back, while the other hand grasps the mandible to elevate the chin.

TABLE 1-1. COMPRESSION AND VENTILATION RATES BY AGE

Age	Compression/min	Ratio	Breaths/min
Infants	100	5:1	20
Children	80	5:1	16
Adolescents	60	5:1	12

Head Tilt, Neck Lift. Place one hand over the forehead, and the other behind the neck. Lift the neck while gently pushing the forehead back.

Jaw Thrust. Push upward on the rami of the mandible to lift the jaw upward and forward.

Consider a foreign body (p 107) obstructing the airway if there is a positive history or if ventilation is not achieved after adequate clearing of the airway and positioning of the head. Abdominal thrusts (Heimlich maneuver) are recommended in children over 1 year old, as a sharp increase in the intrathoracic pressure can expel the object. Back blows loosen the object, but may change partial airway obstruction into total occlusion. Chest thrusts are effective, but rib fractures can occur, with subsequent injuries such as pneumothorax and liver or spleen laceration. Alternatively, the object can be extracted under direct visualization using a laryngoscope and Magill forceps.

Secondary Steps

Intubation. This may be attempted by the rescuer ventilating the patient or an anesthesiologist skilled in the intubation of children. The choice of an appropriately-sized laryngoscope blade and endotracheal (ET) tube is based on the age and size of the patient (see Table 1-2). As soon as the ET tube is in place, assess and frequently reassess the adequacy of ventilation by auscultating both sides of the chest.

Intravenous (IV) Access. A cutdown, usually in the groin, is often required in infants and small children, although a large-bore peripheral vein angiocath is acceptable. An internal jugular or subclavian line provides direct access to the heart. Placement is difficult, however, and intubation is required prior to internal jugular puncture. Once access is achieved, obtain blood for spun hematocrit, complete blood count (CBC), type and cross-match, and appropriate chemistries and drug levels. In addition, an arterial blood gas (ABG) is

TABLE 1-2. METHODS FOR CORRECT ENDOTRACHEAL TUBE SELECTION

1. Diameter of child's little finger or nostril.
2. $\frac{16 + \text{patient's age in years}}{4}$

necessary to assess the adequacy of ventilation and the degree of acidosis.

Electrocardiographic Monitoring. Obtain an electrocardiogram (ECG) as soon as possible using standard lead II. When the patient initially arrives in the ER, or when rapid placement of the limb leads is hampered by other procedures taking place, use the "quick look" paddles of the Life Pak Monitor.

Nasogastric Tube. Insert a nasogastric (NG) tube as soon as practical in order to decompress the stomach. This lessens the risk of aspiration of gastric contents and improves ventilation by relieving pressure on the diaphragm. Use an orogastric tube if there is severe nasal trauma or cerebrospinal fluid (CSF) rhinorrhea.

Foley Catheter. Since monitoring of the patient's urine output is critical for determining the required fluid volumes, insert a Foley catheter as soon as possible.

History Taking. Designate a member of the team to speak with family members or witnesses of the event. Obtain a detailed account of the circumstances surrounding the child's illness or accident and inform the family of the patient's status. Whenever possible, have an emergency department staff member remain with the family to answer questions and provide emotional support.

Physical Examination. Perform a complete physical as soon as possible. Important considerations include:

Skin:	Color, temperature, dependent lividity
Head:	Palpate for fractures, hematomas
Eyes:	Pupil size, reactivity (hypoxia causes dilated, fixed pupils) and extraocular movements, which are asymmetric in structural coma. Check for corneal clouding
Neck:	Subcutaneous air (pneumomediastinum), position of the trachea (tension pneumothorax if not midline)
Chest:	Breath sounds, obvious chest wall trauma
Heart:	Distant heart sounds can be secondary to pericardial effusion; displaced sounds may indicate a tension pneumothorax
Abdomen:	Distention, rigidity
Extremities:	Palpate for fractures

Medication and Fluid Administration

All decisions regarding the dosage and timing of administration of medication and fluids are the responsibility of the team leader. To avoid unnecessary confusion, all orders should emanate from the team leader to a member of the nursing staff designated to prepare the medication.

If difficulty is encountered in achieving intravenous access, epinephrine, lidocaine, and atropine can be given via the endotracheal tube. Suction the tube, ventilate with 100% O_2, instill the medication, then continue ventilation.

Intracardiac administration of medication may be considered, although it is not the route of choice. Among the many risks of this procedure are laceration of the myocardium, pericardial tamponade, pneumo- or hemothorax, and instillation of medication directly into a coronary artery or the myocardium leading to irreversible fibrillation or myocardial necrosis. The anterior approach is preferred, using a 22-gauge, 3- or 4-inch needle directed perpendicular to the chest wall, one finger-breadth lateral to the left sternal border in the 4th intercostal space (nipple line). The subxiphoid approach is the alternative, inserting the needle to the left of the xiphoid tip directed toward the left scapular acromion process. In either approach, never change the direction of the needle once it is past the skin surface. The intracardiac route is used only if the patient is asystolic, and cardiac massage must cease while the needle is in the heart.

Bicarbonate. Myocardial contractility is significantly weakened at an acidotic pH (<7.20). Bicarbonate causes a rapid increase in serum pH. However, excessive sodium bicarbonate can lead to overcorrection of the acidosis with a shift of the oxygen-hemoglobin dissociation curve to the left, hyperosmolality, and hypernatremia. Give 1 mEq/kg as an initial bolus. Give half this dose every 5–10 minutes or calculate subsequent doses if the base deficit value is available:

$$\text{mEq NaHCO}_3 = 0.3 \times \text{body weight (kg)} \times \text{base deficit (mEq/L)}$$

The base deficit is equal to the difference between the normal and measured serum bicabonate.

Whatever the route of administration, circulate the bicarbonate for 3–5 minutes using external cardiac massage before giving more. Usually by that time the initial blood gas results are available and can be used to determine the need for further bicarbonate.

Epinephrine. Epinephrine is a potent beta-adrenergic stimulator with alpha-adrenergic effects as well. It increases myocardial contractility and stimulates contractions in the asystolic heart. The dose is 0.1 cc/kg of a 1:10,000 dilution. If venous access has not been established, intratracheal instillation is preferable to intracardiac injection, but the patient must be intubated. Simultaneous administration of intratracheal epinephrine and intracardiac bicarbonate is the optimal method of administering these two drugs in the absence of an intravenous line. If these drugs are given intravenously, flush the IV line with normal saline prior to administering the epinephrine.

Calcium. With inadequate tissue perfusion the ionized calcium decreases rapidly, adversely affecting myocardial contractility. Since calcium is a positive inotrope and facilitates the response of the heart to catecholamines, it may be effective in reestablishing adequate, coordinated cardiac activity. It is especially useful in electromechanical dissociation (EMD). Calcium is indicated only when hypocalcemia has been documented. Calcium chloride (0.1–0.3 cc/kg intravenously only) is preferred over calcium gluconate because the ion is readily available without the need for hepatic metabolism of the solution. Intracardiac administration must never be attempted, and intravenous calcium and bicarbonate must not be given closely together as a precipitate of calcium carbonate will form.

Glucose. Give glucose as soon as feasible. Because of the risk of intraventricular hemorrhage, use a 25% (2 cc/kg) solution in neonates and infants up to 3 months of age. In older patients, 1 cc/kg of a 50% solution is equivalent to a 0.5 g/kg bolus.

Fluids. Normal saline, Ringer's lactate and plasmanate are good choices for the initial expansion of the intravascular volume and reestablishment of adequate perfusion pressure. Establishing an adequate blood pressure overrides the usual recommendations on fluid restriction in patients with severe head injuries or suspected anoxic renal insult.

Dopamine. Dopamine is both an alpha- and beta-adrenergic stimulant in addition to having independent dopaminergic action. It is useful in treating congestive heart failure and shock after intravascular volume has been restored. The major side effects are tachycardia and tachyarrhythmias. The relative degrees of dopamine's various actions are dose dependent, with some overlap:

2–4 μg/kg/min:	Dopaminergic action (dilation of renal and mesenteric vessels
4–10 μg/kg/min:	Beta adrenergic action (positive inotropic and chronotropic effects)
10–20 μg/kg/min:	Alpha stimulation (peripheral vasoconstriction)

> To make a dopamine solution, multiply the patient's weight in kg times 30. Add this number of milligrams of dopamine to 500 cc D5W. The IV rate in cc/hr is the same as the infusion rate in μg/kg/min.

Dobutamine. Dobutamine is chemically similar to isoproterenol, but it is an inotropic drug with little chronotropic effects. This potential advantage over dopamine must be weighed against the absence of any dopaminergic action. The drug is useful in refractory heart failure at a dose of 5 to 10 μg/kg/min.

Isoproterenol. Isoproterenol is a pure beta-adrenergic receptor stimulator with potent inotropic and chronotropic effects. It increases cardiac output at the expense of an increased myocardial oxygen requirement. It is useful in atropine-resistant bradycardia once a sinus rhythm has been established and for shock unresponsive to dopamine or dobutamine. Since peripheral vasodilation also results, isoproterenol is not indicated if significant hypotension or volume depletion is present.

> Add 6 mg of isoproterenol to 500 cc D5W, so 1 cc/kg/hr = 0.2 μg/kg/min. The initial dose of 0.1 μg/kg/min (0.5 cc/kg/hr) can be increased in 0.1 μg/kg/min increments until the desired effect is achieved.

Atropine. Atropine is a parasympatholytic drug that reduces cardiac vagal tone, thus enhancing the rate of discharge of the sinus node and improving atrioventricular (A-V) conduction. Atropine is extremely useful in early bradycardia once a normal sinus rhythm has been reestablished. It can be given via the ET tube, as well as by the IV route (0.1 cc/kg up to 2 mg).

The airway must always be reassessed in patients who become bradycardic after a normal sinus rhythm has been established. Occlusion of the ET tube is the most frequent cause of bradycardia and this, of course, does not respond to atropine.

Lidocaine. Lidocaine is indicated for all ventricular arrhythmias, including frequent venticular premature contractions (VPCs) ($>$3/min), multiform VPCs, bigeminy, ventricular tachycardia (V-tach), or ventricular fibrilation (V-fib) resistant to defibrillation. After an initial bolus of 1 mg/kg, which can be given via the ET tube, use a continuous intravenous infusion of 10–20 μg/kg/min to maintain serum levels.

Prepare the lidocaine infusion by adding 600 mg of lidocaine to 500 cc D5W. Then, 1 cc/kg/hr = 20 μg/kg/min.

Bretylium. Bretylium is useful in the treatment of V-tach or V-fib resistant to defibrillation and lidocaine. The usual dose is 5 mg/kg IV bolus followed by electrical defibrillation. The dose may be doubled and repeated every 15–30 minutes until a maximum total of 30 mg/kg has been given.

Defibrillation. Treat pulseless V-tach or V-fib with immediate defibrillation, using an initial charge of 1–2 watt-sec/kg. If the rhythm does not convert to normal, double the dose of current and immediately repeat the defibrillation attempt. If there is no response, administer bicarbonate and epinephrine and try defibrillation again. A bolus (1 mg/kg) of lidocaine may be useful in this situation as an adjunctive measure.

REFERENCES

1. Rosenberg N: Emerg Clin North Am 1:609–617, 1983.
2. Singer J: JACEP 6:198, 1977.
3. Galvis AG: Topics in Emerg Med 1:87–94, 1979.
4. JAMA, 255:2961–2973, 1986.

Anaphylaxis

INTRODUCTION

Anaphylaxis is a complex of signs and symptoms, often life threatening, secondary to exposure to a foreign substance. Most often the causative agent is administered parenterally, although cases are reported after oral exposure and rarely after inhalation. The most common antigens are the penicillins, hymenoptera venom, and allergenic extracts, but the cephalosporins, gamma globulin, tetanus toxoid, aspirin, insulin, and certain foods (nuts, eggs, milk, milk products, shellfish) have also been implicated.

CLINICAL PRESENTATION AND DIAGNOSIS

Most reactions occur within minutes of exposure to the antigen and, in general, the sooner the symptoms develop, the more severe the findings. Symptoms include severe anxiety, generalized warmth, tingling of the mouth and face, chest tightness, difficulty swallowing, hoarseness, and ocular pruritis. Some patients immediately lose consciousness. On examination, urticaria, flushing, angioedema, wheezing, and hypotension are seen. Fatal reactions are secondary to laryngeal edema and shock and generally occur in patients over 20 years old.

ER MANAGEMENT

Successful treatment requires early recognition and prompt action.

1. Determine the etiology of the reaction and the mechanism of exposure.
2. Rapidly evaluate the patency of the airway and the cardiorespiratory status.
3. If the source of the antigen is on an extremity, place a *tourniquet* proximally to occlude venous return and lymphatic drainage.
4. Inject 1:1000 *epinephrine* (0.01 cc/kg up to 0.3 cc) subcutaneously. If the reaction is due to a sting or an injection, infiltrate an equal amount around the site to limit absorption. Repeat the doses every 15 minutes, if necessary. If the patient is in shock, give 0.1 cc/kg of 1:10,000 epinephrine intravenously as well.

5. Give *oxygen* for the hypoxemia caused by bronchospasm and laryngeal edema.
6. Give *intravenous fluids,* as normal saline or lactated Ringer's, to maintain an adequate blood pressure. If the patient is in shock, use volume expanders such as plasmanate.
7. Treat bronchospasm with an IV *aminophylline* bolus (7 mg/kg, 300 mg maximum), followed by an IV drip (0.9–1.3 mg/kg/hr) if the bronchospasm persists.
8. *Diphenhydramine* (Benadryl) therapy is a secondary measure. The initial dose is 2 mg/kg (50 mg maximum) intramuscularly (IM) or slowly IV, followed by 5 mg/kg/day PO, divided q 6h.
9. *Hydrocortisone* has no effect on the acute symptoms, but may aid the recovery phase. Given an initial intravenous dose of 10 mg/kg, followed by 10 mg/kg/day PO, for a maximum of 3 days.

INDICATION FOR ADMISSION

- Any anaphylactic reaction

REFERENCE

1. Barach EM, Nowak RM, Lee TG: JAMA 251:2112–2118, 1984

Shock

INTRODUCTION

Shock occurs when the metabolic demands of the tissues are not met by the supply of nutrients. In children, shock is most commonly caused by hypovolemia. Other types of shock (Table 1-3) include cardiogenic shock (pump failure) and distributive shock.

CLINICAL PRESENTATION

The signs of shock (Table 1-4) result from the effects of both direct tissue starvation and compensatory mechanisms, although the blood pressure may be normal until very late. Other findings are an ileus,

TABLE 1-3. ETIOLOGIES OF SHOCK

Hypovolemic Shock	Cardiogenic Shock
Trauma (bleeding)	Myocarditis
Vomiting	Supraventricular tachycardia
Diarrhea	Congenital heart disease
Burns	Pericardial tamponade
Excessive sweating	Tension pneumothorax
Diabetes	Distributive Shock
Third space losses (sepsis, peritonitis)	Anaphylaxis
	Sepsis
Central nervous system bleeds (infants)	Spinal injury
	Drug overdose

decreased urine output, and an increased anion gap (lactic acid) acidosis.

DIAGNOSIS

Maintain a high index of suspicion, since the signs of early shock are subtle, while the late stages are difficult to treat. Obtain a complete set of vital signs, assess capillary refill and mental status, and observe the respiratory pattern.

In patients who do not appear seriously ill, look for orthostatic pulse and blood pressure changes. These are assessed by obtaining a supine pulse and blood pressure, then counting the heart rate 2 minutes after the patient stands, followed by a standing blood pressure.

TABLE 1-4. SIGNS OF SHOCK

Early	Late
Narrowed pulse pressure	Confusion and lethargy
Tachycardia	Decreased systolic pressure
Orthostatic changes	Decreased peripheral pulses
Hyperventilation	Diaphoresis
Delayed capillary filling of nailbeds, forehead, or lips	Cold, pale skin

An increase in pulse by 20 or more beats per minute or a fall in systolic pressure by more than 20 mm Hg are indicative of impending shock.

Inquire about a history of fever, lethargy, vomiting, diarrhea, abdominal pain, trauma (especially abdominal), or flu. A history of diabetes, cystic fibrosis, or heart disease may be important. On examination, check for scalp hematomas in infants, obvious bleeding or hematomas, cutaneous burns, a heart murmur, and a rigid or distended abdomen.

ER MANAGEMENT

Resuscitation is discussed on pp 1–9; the goal is to increase the delivery of oxygen to the tissues. This requires maximizing both the O_2 content of the blood and the cardiac output.

Cardiac output is determined by heart rate × stroke volume; stroke volume, in turn, depends on preload, contractility, and afterload. Since hypovolemia is the cause of most cases of shock in children, increasing the preload is often the easiest and most effective way to improve cardiac output.

1. The *airway* is the first priority. Intubate and mechanically ventilate all obtunded or hypoventilating (↑ pCO_2) patients with warm, humidified, 100% O_2.
2. Start two *large bore IV* (abdominal trauma victims require at least one line in an upper extremity).
3. Obtain the following *blood tests*:
   - Arterial blood gas
   - Spun hematocrit
   - CBC with differential
   - Type and cross-match
   - Electrolytes
   - Glucose
   - Calcium
   - PT and PTT
   - Blood culture (septic shock)
   - BUN and creatinine
4. Attach a *blood pressure cuff* and *ECG monitor*.
5. Apply the military antishock trousers (*MAST pants*).
6. Give a 20 cc/kg push of *crystalloid isotonic fluid* (NS, lactated Ringer). Repeat the 20 cc/kg bolus if there has been no improve-

TABLE 1-5. 5-2 RULE FOR INTRAVENOUS FLUID

Change in CVP		Therapy
Increase by >5 cm H_2O	→	Change to D5 1/2NS at maintenance
Increase by 2–5 cm H_2O	→	Wait 10 minutes and recheck CVP or Slowly give another 20 cc/kg bolus
Increase by <2 cm H_2O	→	Repeat the bolus

ment in the vital signs or urine output. No response to a second push is an indication for placement of a CVP line to follow the central pressure while a third 20 cc/kg bolus is administered over 10 minutes. Follow the "5–2 rule" to determine further therapy (Table 1-5).

A high CVP (>15 cm H_2O) implies faulty placement of the line, cardiac tamponade (p 479), tension pneumothorax (p 493), or heart failure (p 35).

For patients in shock because of blood loss, change to packed red cells or whole blood after the initial two crystalloid boluses.

7. Insert a *Foley catheter* and a *nasogastric tube*. If the patient is a trauma victim, perform a rectal examination prior to inserting the Foley. Contraindications to insertion include blood at the meatus or in the scrotum or a high-riding prostate. Use an orogastric tube instead of an NG tube if there are *any* signs of a basilar skull fracture (CSF rhino- or otorrhea, hemotympanum, raccoon eyes, Battle sign).
8. Once the patient is no longer volume depleted, cardiac output may be improved with *pressors*. *Dopamine*, at a rate of 5–10 μg/kg/min, is a good inotrope (see p 7 to prepare a dopamine infusion).

   If the etiology of the shock is pump failure or sepsis, *dobutamine* at 5 μg/kg/min may be preferred.

   Isoproterenol has positive inotropic and chronotropic actions, but it is also a potent peripheral vasodilator. Therefore, it is contraindicated if the patient's volume status is in question.
9. Give *glucose* (1 cc/kg of D50).
10. If sepsis is likely, give *methylprednisolone* (30 mg/kg IV) and start doses of *antibiotics*. For infants under 4 weeks, use am-

picillin (150 mg/kg) and cefotaxime (50 mg/kg); for older patients use ampicillin, chloramphenicol (20 mg/kg) and gentamicin (2 mg/kg).

11. If the etiology of the shock is sepsis, and the blood pressure does not respond to volume and pressors, give *naloxone* (0.05 mg/kg IV). If there is no improvement, double the dose and repeat.

INDICATION FOR ADMISSION

- Shock, sepsis, or heart failure

REFERENCES:

1. Perkin RM, Levin DL: J Pediatr 101:163–169, 319–332, 1982
2. Peters WPL: Lancet 1:529–531, 1981

2

Cardiac Emergencies

Arrhythmias

Atrial Fibrillation

INTRODUCTION

Atrial fibrillation is usually associated with a dilated left atrium, most commonly secondary to rheumatic heart disease. Other etiologies include hyperthyroidism, atrial septal defects, Ebstein anomaly, status postcardiac surgery, and atrial tumors.

CLINICAL PRESENTATION AND DIAGNOSIS

Suspect atrial fibrillation when the pulse is noted to be "irregularly irregular." There is also variation in the intensity of the heart sounds and the cardiac impulse and pulse. Electrocardiographically, atrial fibrillation causes a distorted baseline and chaotic atrial deflections that vary markedly in timing, amplitude, and contour (Fig. 2-1). The atrial rate is generally over 350 beats/min, which is considerably faster than *supraventricular tachycardia* (SVT) (180–240 beats/min). The ventricular response is irregular, secondary to varying atrioventricular (A-V) conduction, with a rate between 50 and 240 beats/min.

ER MANAGEMENT

In general, treatment can be delayed until the patient is admitted to an intensive care setting. The goals are slowing of the ventricular rate (if rapid) and restoration of a normal sinus rhythm. If the ventricular rate is acceptable (60–100 beats/min), therapy is not urgently indicated. If there is underlying myocardial dysfunction or congenital heart dis-

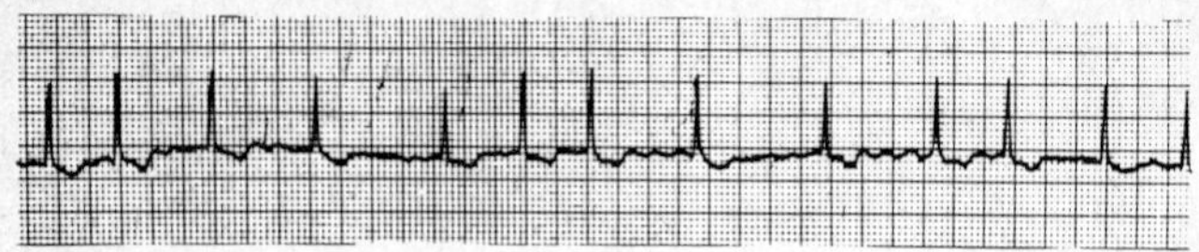

Figure 2-1. Atrial fibrillation.

ease, however, treatment is necessary to maintain adequate cardiac output.

Digitalis, as discussed later under SVT, is the drug of choice, unless there is associated Wolff-Parkinson-White (WPW) syndrome. In that case, digitalis may facilitate conduction in the aberrant pathway and lead to serious ventricular dysrhythmias.

Quinidine (see p 19) may convert fibrillation to normal sinus rhythm *after* digitalization.

DC cardioversion, 1–2 watt-sec/kg, can also be used. However, it is usually unsuccessful in patients with chronic left atrial enlargement (ie, long-standing rheumatic mitral disease), heart failure, and long-standing fibrillation.

INDICATION FOR ADMISSION

- All patients who require acute treatment of atrial fibrillation, including children with newly diagnosed fibrillation or chronic fibrillation with an increase in ventricular rate

REFERENCE

1. Redford DJ, Izukawa T: Pediatr 59:250–256, 1977

Atrial Flutter

INTRODUCTION

Atrial flutter, a rare dysrhythmia in children, is secondary to either a low ectopic atrial focus or impulse reentry. In contrast to adults, associated organic heart disease is unusual in children with flutter. However, occasionally there may be coexistent rheumatic heart disease, cardiomyopathy, Wolff-Parkinson-White syndrome, coronary artery disease, or pulmonary embolism.

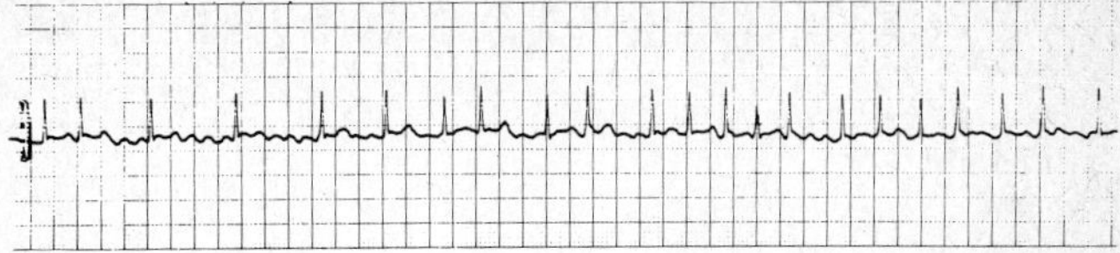

Figure 2-2. Atrial flutter.

DIAGNOSIS

Atrial flutter is characterized by an atrial tachycardia between 220 and 350 beats/min. The associated ventricular response is one-half to one-quarter of the atrial rate, depending on the degree of A-V block. Electrocardiographically, rapid atrial deflections replace the normal P-waves. Identical in timing and contour, they have a characteristic "sawtooth" configuration without intervening isoelectric intervals (Fig. 2-2).

In *SVT*, the atrial rate is 180–240 beats/min with 1:1 conduction and a fixed R-R interval. Flutter may slow during carotid massage, but SVT usually terminates abruptly.

ER MANAGEMENT

Cardioversion. Synchronized DC cardioversion is the treatment of choice, provided the patient is not taking digoxin. In such a case, well-appearing patients should have the drug discontinued for at least 24–48 hours. If the patient is hypotensive or lethargic, cardioversion is indicated, regardless of the medication history. A dose of 1–2 watt-sec/kg is almost always successful in converting atrial flutter to a normal sinus rhythm. If there is no response, double the dose of energy and repeat the cardioversion once. Follow cardioversion with digitalis maintenance therapy.

Digitalis. Give a digitalizing dose of 40–60 μg/kg PO in infants (see supraventricular tachycardia, p 26).

Propranolol. The beta-blocking effect may help slow the ventricular rate. Use a dose of 0.05–0.10 mg/kg, given slowly IV (p 26).

Quinidine and Procainamide. Either of these agents may be effective in slowing the atrial rate. However, the A-V junction must be blocked beforehand with digitalis to avoid 1:1 conduction at a very rapid ventricular rate. The dose of quinidine is 15–60 mg/kg/day orally divided qid; procainamide is 15–50 mg/kg/day, divided 6 times a day.

INDICATION FOR ADMISSION

- All patients treated for atrial flutter, for overnight observation

REFERENCES

1. Martin TC, Hernandez J: J Pediatr 100:239–242, 1982
2. Dunningan A, Benson W Jr, Benditti DG: Pediatrics 75:725–729, 1985

Heart Block

INTRODUCTION

Heart block, secondary to abnormal A-V conduction, is uncommon in childhood.

CLINICAL PRESENTATION AND DIAGNOSIS

First-degree Block. First-degree block is a rate-related prolongation of the P-R interval (Fig. 2-3) that is usually asymptomatic. It occurs most commonly with acute rheumatic fever, digoxin administration, myocarditis, and diptheria.

Second-degree Block. Second-degree block is usually secondary to acute or chronic heart disease. Although many patients are asymptomatic, syncope can occur. It may be *Mobitz type I* (Wenckebach) in which there is progressive lengthening of the P-R interval in successive cycles, until the impulse is not conducted and a ventricular beat is dropped (Fig. 2-4). In *Mobitz type II,* ventricular beats are dropped without previous P-R prolongation (Fig. 2-5). Generally, the site of block is more proximal in type I and more distal in type II; the more distal the block, the more worrisome the arrhythmia. Rarely type I can progress to type II and type II to third-degree block.

Third-degree Block. Third-degree (complete) heart block represents an absolute failure of conduction of the atrial impulses to the ventricles. Therefore, the atria and ventricles beat completely independently (Fig. 2-6). Generally, the lower the location of the pacemaker

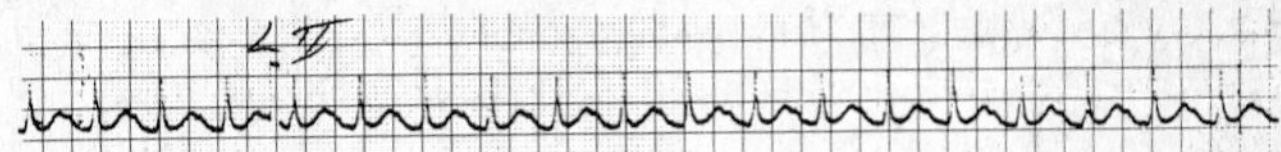

Figure 2-3. First-degree A-V block with prolonged P-R interval. The P-wave is buried in the T-wave.

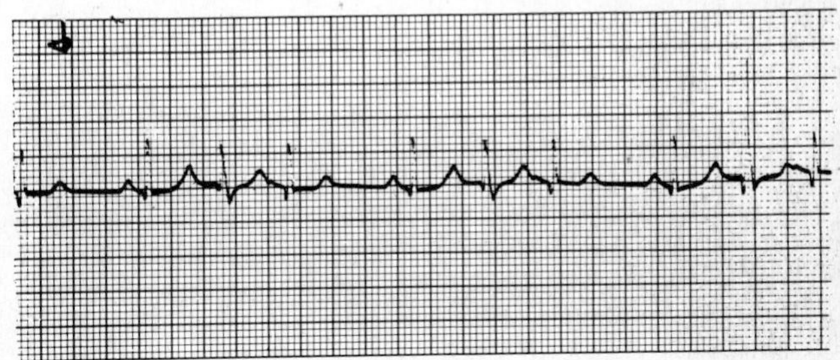

Figure 2-4. Second-degree A-V block: Wenckebach (Mobitz type I).

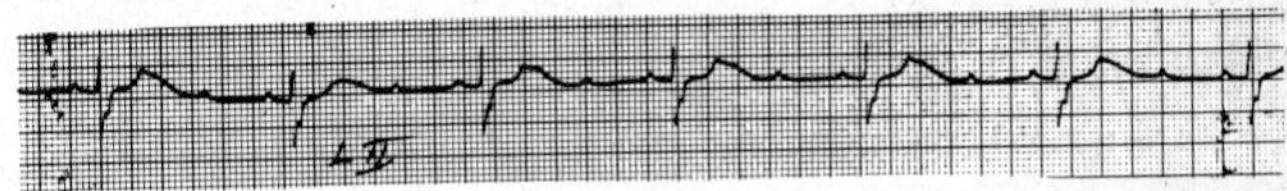

Figure 2-5. Second-degree A-V block: 3:1.

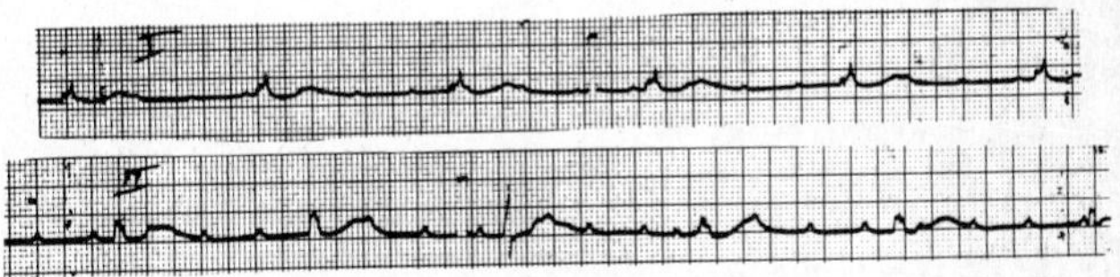

Figure 2-6. Third-degree A-V block.

within the ventricular conduction system, the slower the idioventricular rate and the wider the QRS complexes. The etiology may be congenital (either isolated or associated with congenital heart disease) or acquired (postoperative, acute rheumatic fever, streptococcal infection, digoxin toxicity, hyper- and hypocalcemia).

Most patients with third-degree heart block are asymptomatic. In unusual cases there may be syncopal episodes or, if there are associated structural defects, congestive heart failure. Bounding pulses, systolic hypertension, and varying intensity of S2 are other features. Infants with congenital block might also have electrocardiographic evidence of ventricular hypertrophy.

ER MANAGEMENT

In general, *first-degree* and *second-degree* blocks require no treatment other than monitoring the cardiogram for possible deterioration. Patients with postoperative second-degree blocks and those with syncopal episodes require inpatient monitoring and, possibly, pacing.

Congenital *complete heart block* rarely requires treatment if the infant can weather the first few months with a relatively "rapid" ventricular rate. Symptomatic congenital and acquired third-degree blocks may require temporary or permanent pacing. The actions of pharmacologic agents such as beta-adrenergics are usually unsuccessful and unpredictable, and ventricular tachycardia may ensue.

INDICATIONS FOR ADMISSION

- First-degree: Serious underlying disease
- Second-degree: Newly diagnosed, postoperative, or associated with syncope
- Third-degree: Congestive failure, newly diagnosed, or change in rate or morphology of QRS complex

REFERENCE

1. Pinsky WW, Gilette PC, Garson A Jr, et al: Pediatrics 69:728–733, 1982

Sinus Tachycardia

INTRODUCTION

Sinus tachycardia (ST) is a persistently elevated heart rate relative to age, in association with P-waves of normal contour, duration, and polarity. The rate is generally 100–180 beats/min, although in infants the rate may reach 200–220 beats/min. The most common causes of ST are anxiety, anemia, hypovolemia, congestive heart failure, exercise, fever, hyperthyroidism, emotional upset, and medications (bronchodilators, decongestants).

CLINICAL PRESENTATION AND DIAGNOSIS

Since normal hemodynamics are generally maintained, ST is usually an incidental finding in a patient with some other presentation (see above). Sinus tachycardia (ST) can easily be confused with *supraventricular tachycardia* (SVT), a disease with different etiologies, treatments, and prognosis. In SVT the rate can be as rapid as 340 beats/min and the QRS complexes may not be preceded by recognizable P-waves. Also, in SVT the R-R interval is identical throughout the rhythm strip, while in ST it varies slightly.

ER MANAGEMENT

Inquire about possible precipitating causes. If none is found, check for orthostatic changes in the vital signs and obtain a complete blood count (CBC), spun hematocrit, blood urea nitrogen (BUN), electrolytes, thyroid function tests, and a chest x-ray. Treatment is directed toward the underlying cause, rather than the tachycardia itself. This may include discontinuing certain medications, giving antipyretics, or rehydration.

REFERENCE

1. Fisher DJ, Gross DM, Garson A: Am J Dis Child 137:164–166, 1983

Supraventricular Tachycardia

INTRODUCTION

Supraventricular tachycardia (SVT), the most common arrhythmia in children, is a series of rapidly repeated premature beats originating in the atria or atrioventricular junction region proximal to the bundle of His. The typical rate is 180–240 beats/min, although in infants the rate can be as fast as 340 beats/min.

SVT may be secondary to reentry pathways, an anomalous pathway, A-V node bypass, or an ectopic focus. Forty percent of cases are found to have predisposing factors (Table 2-1).

TABLE 2-1. FACTORS PREDISPOSING TO SUPRAVENTRICULAR TACHYCARDIA

Wolf-Parkinson-White syndrome	Hyperthyroidism
Fever	Drugs
Sepsis	Epinephrine
Myocarditis	Decongestants
Cardiomyopathy	Ephedrine
Ebstein anomaly	Methylphenidate
Previous cardiac surgery (Mustard or Sennig procedure for transposition of the great vessels)	

CLINICAL PRESENTATION

The presentation depends on whether there is preexisting heart disease, the duration of the tachycardia, and the age and emotional state of the patient. Common clinical findings include palpitations, irritability, pallor, lethargy, hypothermia, and cyanosis.

The occurrence of congestive heart failure (tachypnea, hepatomegaly, pulmonary rales) depends on a number of factors. Almost 50% of infants under 4 months of age present in congestive heart failure, but this rarely occurs in patients over 1 year. Although heart failure is unusual with SVT lasting less than 24 hours, it is associated with half of the episodes of more than 48 hours' duration. Finally, patients with rates less than 200 beats/min rarely present in congestive heart failure.

DIAGNOSIS

The electrocardiogram is diagnostic in SVT. Generally, there is a rapid rate of 180–240 beats/min with 1:1 conduction. Ventricular complexes are usually normal in contour, although aberrant conduction can cause slight widening. P-waves are often buried in the T-waves, ST-T changes are common, and the R-R interval is fixed (Fig. 2-7).

SVT can resemble *ST*. In the latter, however, the rate is usually less than 180 beats/min (220 beats/min in infants), a P-wave precedes the QRS complex, and there is some variation in the R-R interval from one segment of the electrocardiogram to another.

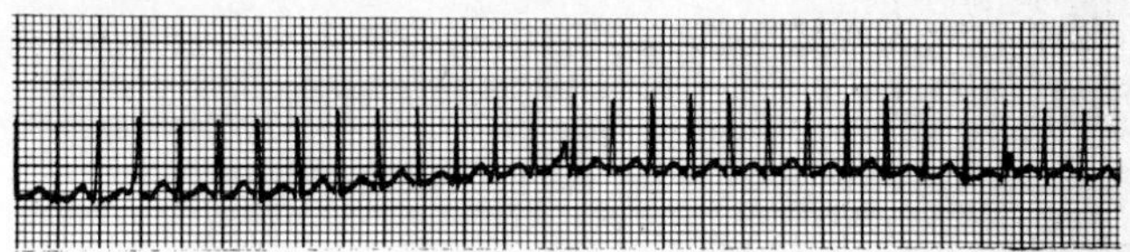

Figure 2-7. Supraventricular tachycardia.

Ventricular tachycardia may be extremely difficult to differentiate from SVT with aberrancy and widened QRS complexes. The sicker clinical condition of the patient, slower rate of the tachycardia, varying R-R interval, and isolated premature ventricular contractions found elsewhere in the ECG suggest ventricular tachycardia (V-tach).

ER MANAGEMENT

Perform a careful history and physical examination, looking for an underlying treatable etiology. If the patient is under 4 months of age, has had the tachycardia for more than 24 hours, or is already in congestive heart failure, urgent treatment is often necessary to terminate the episode. A number of therapeutic modalities are available.

Vagal Maneuvers

Vagal nerve stimulation causes a slowing of the spontaneous rate of the sinus pacemaker and potential atrial and junctional pacemakers and increases the effective refractory period of the A-V node. Continuously monitor the ECG when vagal maneuvers are attempted. If successful, the tachycardia breaks abruptly and is replaced by a normal sinus rhythm (Fig. 2-8). Gradual slowing suggests that either sinus tachycardia or atrial flutter was misdiagnosed as SVT. Commonly employed vagal techniques include:

1. *Unilateral* carotid massage at the junction of the carotid artery and the mandible.
2. A *Valsalva maneuver,* performed by asking the patient to "bear down" or "strain" as if he is attempting to move his bowels.
3. *Submersion of the face* for 10–20 seconds in ice-cold water or application of an ice bag, filled with equal volumes of ice and water, to the patient's face converts up to 90% of episodes of SVT.

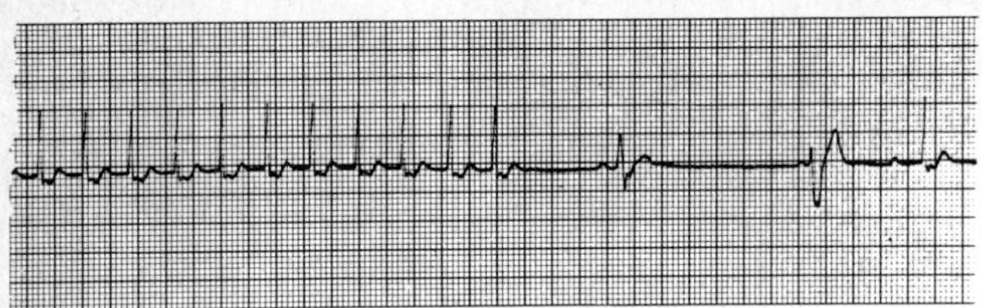

Figure 2-8. Supraventricular tachycardia: response to ice bag over face.

Combined carotid massage and submersion may be efficacious when either alone is unsuccessful.

4. Eyeball pressure is NOT recommended as retinal detachment can occur.
5. Gagging and inducing vomiting may be effective but are not recommended in agitated patients and infants who might aspirate.

Pharmacotherapy

Verapamil. Verapamil is a potent calcium channel blocker that converts 90% of SVT episodes within 60 seconds. The dose is 0.1 mg/kg, to a maximum of 5 mg, by slow intravenous push over 1–2 minutes. This can be repeated once, after 5–10 minutes. Monitor the blood pressure, as significant hypotension can ensue, especially when it is used in newborns and young infants. Also, do not use verapamil in conjunction with other negative inotropes such as propanolol.

Digoxin. Digoxin, through its vagal effect, has been the mainstay of SVT therapy and is indicated if verapamil fails. The major drawback is that an average of 6 hours may be required to terminate an episode after oral or intravenous digitalization. The total oral digitalizing dose in infants is 40–60 μg/kg. Give one-half of the dose immediately, with additional quarters at 6- to 8-hour intervals. Consult with a cardiologist before using digoxin for patients with known WPW syndrome, since it may shorten the refractory period of the accessory or bypass tract.

Propranolol. Propranolol is a beta sympathetic blocker that slows impulse conduction. Give a dose of 0.05–0.1 mg/kg, to a maximum of 2 mg, slowly IV. Do not give propranolol to patients with underlying myocardial dysfunction or asthma. If verapamil has previously been tried, allow 6–8 hours to elapse before propranolol is employed.

Phenylephrine. Phenylephrine (Neo-Synephrine) is an alpha agonist that increases peripheral vascular resistance, thereby increasing the blood pressure, and causing a reflex vagal stimulation. Start an infusion of 0.1 μg/kg/min and titrate the rate against the patient's blood pressure (end point is a diastolic pressure of 90 mm Hg). Phenylephrine often succeeds when other modalities have failed, but restrict its use to an intensive care setting.

Edrophonium. Edrophonium (Tensilon) is a cholinesterase inhibitor that causes increased vagal stimulation. The dose is 0.5–2 mg by slow IV push.

Cardioversion

DC cardioversion is indicated when there are signs of heart failure, shock, or acidosis, or if other treatment modalities have failed. A dose of 1–2 watt-sec/kg of synchronous current causes total electrical fibrillation and allows the most stable pacemaker (sinus node) to resume functioning. Cardioversion may be repeated at double the initial dose (to a maximum of 2 watt-sec/kg) if the first attempt is unsuccessful. Sedate older patients with diazepam (0.1–0.3 mg/kg) prior to cardioversion and always have isoproterenol available.

Overdrive Pacing

Insertion of a pacemaker into the atrium and overdriving the atrial rate (pacemaker rate exceeds SVT rate), performed by a pediatric cardiologist, is effective in over 80% of refractory cases.

OUTPATIENT MANAGEMENT

Refer all patients to a pediatric cardiologist. Maintenance digoxin therapy for 6–12 months is recommended after the first episode of SVT in infants under 1 year of age. In older patients, generally no therapy is needed until the second episode, unless symptoms other than palpitations have occurred. Refer patients with repeated attacks to a pediatric cardiologist for combination drug therapy and invasive evaluation (electrophysiologic studies).

Recurrences occur in only 20% of patients who present prior to 4 months of age, but 80% of children presenting after 4 months have subsequent episodes. Most recurrences (80%) are within the first year after presentation.

INDICATIONS FOR ADMISSION

- First episode of SVT
- SVT causing heart failure

REFERENCES

1. Lundberg A: Pediatrics 70:638–642, 1982
2. Garson A, Gilette PC, McNamara DG: J Pediatr 98:875–882, 1981

Ventricular Premature Contractions

INTRODUCTION

Ventricular premature contractions (VPCs) are most commonly seen in normal, asymptomatic adolescents, although they can occur secondary to ingestion of digoxin, sympathomimetic agents, tricyclic antidepressants, tobacco, and caffeine. Other causes include electrolyte imbalances, anesthesia, and underlying heart disease (coronary artery disease, mitral valve prolapse, cardiomyopathy, myocarditis). With some VPCs, palpitations, syncope, or chest pain are reported and the peripheral pulses can be either weaker than normal, or not palpable. The majority of cases, however, are discovered during routine physical examination, when an irregular heart rhythm is appreciated.

DIAGNOSIS

VPCs are characterized by bizarre, widened QRS complexes which are not preceded by a P-wave (Fig. 2-9). They may occur in a fixed ratio with normal beats (bigeminy, trigeminy) (Fig. 2-10). They are

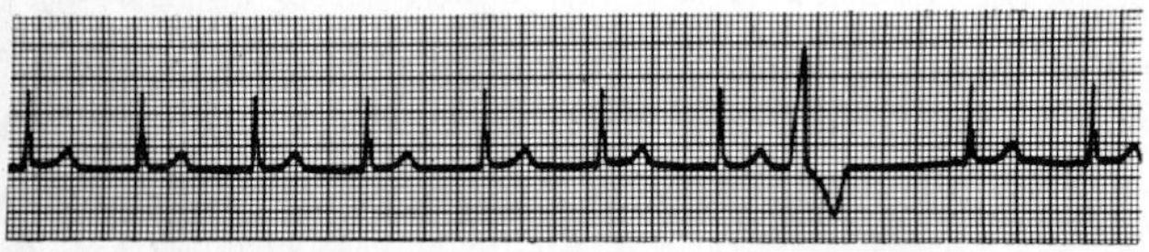

Figure 2-9. Ventricular premature contraction (VPC).

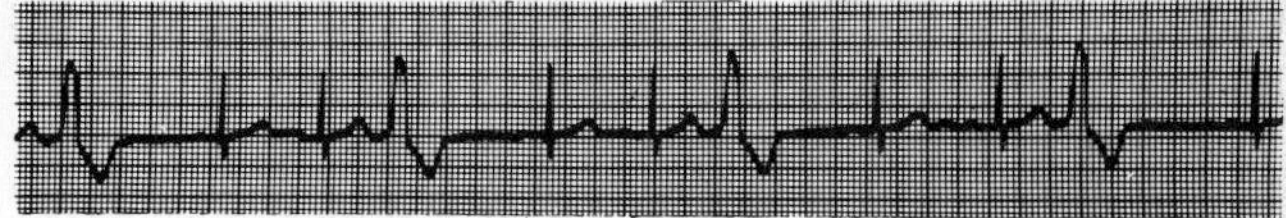

Figure 2-10. VPC in trigeminal pattern.

usually designated as unifocal (identical electrocardiographic appearance, and consistent interval from the preceding QRS) or multifocal (dissimilar morphologic electrocardiographic appearances and varying coupling intervals with the preceding QRS). With a short coupling interval, it is possible for the ectopic beat to fall on the T-wave of the preceding normal QRS complex (R-on-T phenomenon), and initiate or precipitate ventricular tachycardia.

Dividing ventricular extrasystoles into benign and serious categories is helpful for determining treatment and follow-up. Benign VPCs are unifocal, single, infrequent, with a fixed coupling interval, no R-on-T phenomenon, and a normal resting QT interval. There is no underlying heart disease and they decrease in frequency with exercise (10–20 sit-ups while being monitored). Serious VPCs are multifocal, with a varying coupling interval, R-on-T phemonenon, and a prolonged resting QT interval; 2–3 (or more) consecutive VPCs or runs of ventricular tachycardia (≥3 consecutive VPCs) are seen. Associated heart disease is common and exercise either has no effect or increases the frequency of the VPCs.

TREATMENT

Patients in the benign group generally do not require any treatment. In the serious category, symptomatic patients (hypotension, lethargy) require ER treatment (see p 31), while all others can be treated electively after admission to the hospital. Quinidine (15–60 mg/kg/day PO divided q 6h) is commonly used, although gastrointestinal irritation is frequent. Procainamide (15–50 mg/kg/day PO, IV) is better tolerated, but has a shorter half-life, so that it must be given q 4h. Diphenylhydantoin (2–5 mg/kg/day PO, IV divided q 12h) is the drug of choice for digoxin-induced or postoperative (tet repair) VPCs, and propranolol (0.05–0.10 mg/kg slowly IV) is indicated in cases of catecholamine excess.

INDICATIONS FOR ADMISSION

- Newly diagnosed VPCs
- Serious VPCs
- Benign-appearing VPCs in association with cardiac symptoms (syncope, palpitations, chest pain)
- Change in the pattern of previously known VPCs

REFERENCE

1. Jacobsen JR, Garson A Jr, Gilette PC, et al: J Pediatr 92:36–38, 1978

Ventricular Tachycardia and Fibrillation

INTRODUCTION

Ventricular tachycardia (V-tach) is defined as three or more consecutive ventricular premature contractions (VPCs). They usually occure in long runs and are most often a sequela of VPCs, so that the etiologies, clinical presentations, and electrocardiographic findings of ventricular tachycardia and VPCs are similar.

Occasional patients are asymptomatic, although chest pain, syncope, and palpitations are common, and lethargy, disorientation, and hypotension can occur. Ventricular tachycardia can degenerate into ventricular fibrillation, either as a terminal event or when there is a prolonged QT interval or R-on-T phenomenon. Patients with ventricular fibrillation are generally pulseless.

DIAGNOSIS

Ventricular tachycardia (Fig. 2-11) must be differentiated from *supraventricular tachycardia with aberrant conduction*. The former is con-

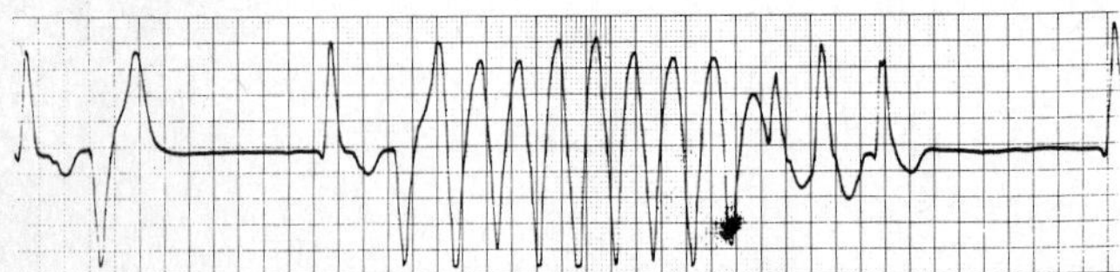

Figure 2-11. Ventricular tachycardia.

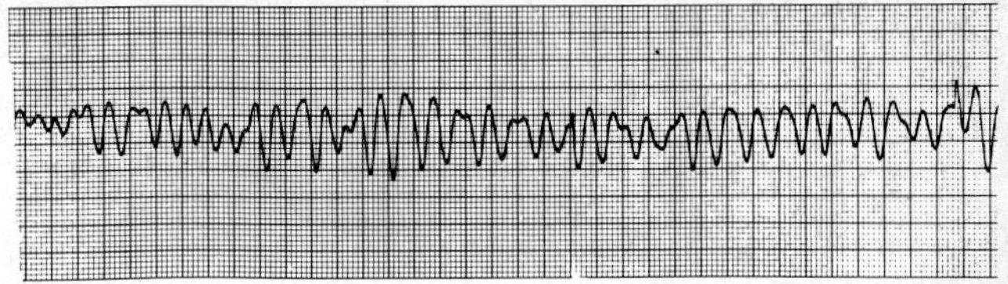

Figure 2-12. Ventricular fibrillation.

firmed if single VPCs appear elsewhere and are morphologically similar, or if fusion beats are seen. Fusion beats are complexes that appear between normal and VPC-like, caused by the VPC occurring just after a P-wave. Also, A-V dissociation is often seen, with variation in the T-waves due to P-wave superimposition.

In ventricular fibrillation (Fig. 2-12) there is a wavy, sinusoidal line, without any true QRS complexes.

ER MANAGEMENT

Although occasional patients are asymptomatic, most are disoriented or hypotensive and require emergency therapy. The treatment of choice is cardioversion at an initial dose of 1–2 watt-sec/kg. If successful, give a lidocaine bolus (1 mg/kg), followed by a continuous infusion (15 to 40 μg/kg/min). Treat continued ventricular tachycardia with another attempt at cardioversion at twice the initial dose. If the patient does not convert, give a lidocaine bolus (1 mg/kg IV), followed by a third and final attempt at cardioversion. If these measures are ineffective, try intravenous procainamide (3–6 mg/kg/min over 5 minutes) or bretylium (5 mg/kg). Bretylium is contraindicated in patients with arrhythmias secondary to digoxin toxicity.

If the ventricular tachycardia degenerates into ventricular fibrillation, immediate defibrillation (1–2 watt-sec/kg), followed by lidocaine, is indicated. Treat continued fibrillation with procainamide or bretylium, as above.

Admit the alert, normotensive patient to an intensive care setting for elective treatment.

INDICATION FOR ADMISSION

- Ventricular tachycardia or fibrillation

REFERENCE

1. Pedersen E, Zipes DP, Foster PR, et al: Circulation 60:988–997, 1979

Chest Pain

INTRODUCTION

Chest pain is a common complaint in late childhood and adolescence. Although it is often a manifestation of underlying disease in the adult population, in children it is only infrequently associated with significant organic illness.

CLINICAL PRESENTATION AND DIAGNOSIS

Note the characteristics of the pain, including position in which it is greatest, quality, radiation, duration, and alleviating or exacerbating factors. Associated symptoms may be especially useful in determining the etiology of the pain.

Musculoskeletal Problems. Musculoskeletal problems are the most common cause of chest pain in the pediatric population. Tietze syndrome (costochondritis) is characterized by anterior chest pain and tenderness to palpation over the costosternal or costochondral junctions. Reproduction of the patient's pain on palpation is the most helpful sign. Intercostal muscle cramping (precordial catch syndrome) in the left substernal area may mimic this condition.

Psychogenic Causes. Although psychogenic causes are the second most frequent, always consider them to be diagnoses of exclusion. Adolescents with hyperventilation or anxiety can present with chest pain. The history may reveal repeated episodes of hysterical behavior, recent personal or family stresses, or a relative with severe heart disease. Typical complaints include shortness of breath, palpitations, or tingling of the extremities. The pain often mimics one or more organic conditions but usually it suggests several conditions in the differential diagnosis (classic symptoms of pericardial chest pain with the physical findings of pain of musculoskeletal origin).

Pleuritic Chest Pain. Chest pain can be pleuritic in nature, exacerbated by deep inspiration, swallowing, and coughing, and improved by sitting up. It is caused by inflammation or irritation of the pleura, and is seen most commonly in pneumonia, pleurodynia (Coxsackie virus) or pneumothorax, although pulmonary embolism or infarction can present similarly. Associated history (fever, cough, preceding upper respiratory infection [URI], birth control pill use, underlying chronic disease such as sickle cell anemia, cystic fibrosis, asthma, or lupus) is useful for differentiating among these etiologies.

Pericarditis. Pericarditis can also present with pleuritic-type chest pain. Patients are often unable to assume the supine position, and the pain is usually referred to the neck and shoulders. On physical examination, a pericardial friction rub may be noted during systole in the midprecordial area with the patient supine or in the left lateral decubitus position. ECG, chest x-ray, and echocardiography assist in making this diagnosis.

Prolapse of the Mitral Valve. Vague anterior chest pain has been described in patients found to have prolapse of the mitral valve and may be part of a constellation of symptoms in this condition (dyspnea, palpitations, near syncope, and fatigue). The diagnosis is suggested by auscultation (late systolic click or clicks and late systolic murmur) and confirmed by M-mode and two-dimensional echocardiography.

Gastrointestinal Reflux. Gastrointestinal reflux can cause esophagitis and gastrointestinal spasm. The substernal ''burning'' or ''crushing'' pain may mimic angina pectoris, which is distinctly uncommon in the pediatric age group. The discomfort is usually associated with eating (between meals or in the early morning before breakfast), accentuated in the recumbent position and with straining, and relieved with antacids or cold milk.

Aortic Dissection. Although aortic dissection is extremely rare in childhood, consider it in patients with connective tissue disorders (Marfan syndrome, Ehlers-Danlos syndrome). The pain is typically ''tearing'' in quality, sudden in onset and debilitating. Radiation is from the anterior chest to the neck and lower back.

Coronary Artery Disease. Coronary artery disease (myocardial ischemia, angina pectoris, myocardial infarction) is extremely rare in the pediatric population. Patients with arteritis may present with the pain of myocardial ischemia or infarction. Severe persistent irritability has been noted in infants with aberrant origin of the left coronary artery from the pulmonary artery. Patients with a history of mucocutaneous lymph node syndrome, at risk for coronary artery thrombosis and aneurysm, may present with pallor, diaphoresis, or irritability.

ER MANAGEMENT

Since most cases of chest pain are either psychogenic or musculoskeletal in origin, a careful history, palpation of the chest wall, and pulmonary and cardiac auscultation usually suffice to determine the etiology.

Obtain an ECG if a musculoskeletal or psychogenic etiology is not clearly evident. Except in cases of myocardial involvement, coronary artery disease, or severe pericarditis, the ECG is normal; many patients with noncardiac chest pain are concerned about the possibility of heart disease and are reassured by a normal recording.

Further evaluation is dictated by the history and physical findings. A chest x-ray is indicated for patients with pleuritic chest pain, dyspnea, or cyanosis. Place a 5 TU PPD on the forearm of all patients with pneumonia or effusion. Also obtain a CBC, erythrocyte sedimentation rate (ESR), and echocardiogram if pericarditis is suspected.

INDICATIONS FOR ADMISSION

- Coronary artery disease, pleural effusion, pericarditis, or aortic dissection
- Severe chest pain of unknown etiology

REFERENCES

1. Pantell RH, Goodman BW Jr: Pediatrics 71:881–887, 1983
2. Driscoll BJ, Blickloch LB, Gallen WJ: Pediatrics 57:648, 1976
3. Selbst SM: Pediatrics 75:1068–1070, 1985

Congestive Heart Failure

INTRODUCTION

Congestive heart failure (CHF) occurs when the heart is unable to deliver blood at a rate adequate to meet basal metabolic requirements.

Four principal factors regulate stroke volume and cardiac output: preload (ventricular end diastolic volume), contractility (force of ventricular contraction independent of preload), afterload (intraventricular systolic tension during ejection), and heart rate. Changes in heart rate (bradyarrhythmias, heart block) or stroke volume (myocardial contractility) directly affect cardiac output, which, in turn, is a major determinant of blood pressure.

CHF in children usually results from arrhythmias or congenital structural heart defects. Over 90% of the cases of heart failure occur within the first year of life, with most occurring in the first few months.

CLINICAL PRESENTATION AND DIAGNOSIS

Pulmonary congestion causes tachypnea, wheezing (cardiac asthma), and a chronic, persistent, nonparoxysmal and nonproductive cough. Infants present with progressive tiring and sweating during feeding. The hypermetabolic state combined with poor caloric intake leads to poor weight gain and eventually to growth failure. Hepatomegaly is the most common sign of systemic venous congestion; generally, the liver is palpable approximately 3–4 cm below the right costal margin. Neck vein distention and peripheral edema are uncommon in infancy but may be noted in children and adolescents. Tachycardia is caused by increased sympathoadrenal activity. A protodiastolic gallop (ventricular filling) suggests impaired ventricular function and is a common finding, along with bibasilar rales and tachypnea. Weak pulses, mottled extremities, and lowered blood pressure, if present, are all signs of decreased perfusion. Cardiomegaly is also present (point of maximal impulse [PMI] left of the midclavicular line) since the response to congestive heart failure is left ventricular hypertrophy or dilation.

The chest x-ray usually reveals cardiomegaly and pulmonary vascular congestion (increased pulmonary vascular markings, butterfly pattern). A pleural or pericardial effusion may also be seen.

The ECG is of little help in the diagnosis and subsequent treatment of congestive heart failure. The classic ECG finding is left ventricular hypertrophy, while combined ventricular hypertrophy is present in one-third of cases.

Usually a patient with CHF presents with a combination of wheezing, respiratory distress, bibasilar rales, and hepatomegaly. However, wheezing is most often secondary to *asthma*. There may be a history of asthma or allergies, a family history of allergies or physical evidence of eczema or prolonged expiration. *Bronchiolitis* occurs during seasonal epidemics; the patient may have fever, rhonchi and rales in addition to the wheezing. Other causes of tachypnea, respiratory distress and cough are *pneumonia* (fever, localized fine end expiratory rales, no hepatomegaly), *croup* (fever, inspiratory stridor), and *foreign body aspiration* (sudden onset of inspiratory stridor).

Most etiologies of hepatomegaly (see p 192) do not lead to tachypnea or respiratory distress.

When the diagnosis is in doubt, obtain a chest x-ray to look for cardiomegaly and pulmonary vascular congestion (CHF).

ER MANAGEMENT

If possible, evaluate the patient in a semisitting position that permits pooling of blood in the dependent areas and thus decreases the work of breathing.

Give all patients supplemental oxygen (40% by face mask or head box).

Start an IV and give furosemide (1 mg/kg) if no pericardial effusion is suspected.

Obtain an arterial blood gas and a hemoglobin/hematocrit to rule out severe anemia (ie, sickle cell anemia) which can result in a high output state secondary to the decreased oxygen carrying capacity of the blood. Anemia may also exacerbate preexisting congestive heart failure.

Rarely, endotracheal intubation and positive end expiratory pressure (PEEP) may be required if the above measures do not lead to an improvement in clinical status and oxygenation. Finally, the management of severe refractory congestive heart failure associated with decreased cardiac output may require the use of sympathomimetic amines, particular dopamine or dobutamine (see CPR, pp 7–9). Reserve digitalization for inhospital management, since its onset of action is too slow to be of use in the emergency situation.

Once the patient is stable, two-dimensional echocardiography may help to identify the cause of the failure and document the magnitude of the decrease in ventricular function (ejection fraction) as well as the extent of left ventricular dilation.

INDICATION FOR ADMISSION

- Newly diagnosed or worsening congestive heart failure

REFERENCE

1. Fowler REL: PIR 1:321–327, 1980

Cyanosis

INTRODUCTION

Central cyanosis occurs when at least 5 g/dl of reduced or abnormal hemoglobin is present in the capillary blood. This is usually secondary to the entrance of unsaturated blood from the systemic venous return into the systemic arterial circulation via intracardiac or intrapulmonary shunting.

Cardiac lesions can cause either decreased pulmonary blood flow (tetralogy of Fallot, Ebstein anomaly, pulmonic stenosis or atresia, tricuspid atresia) or pulmonary plethora (transposition, truncus arteriosus, total anomalous pulmonary venous drainage). Pulmonary causes include upper airway obstruction (croup, epiglottitis, subglottic stenosis, aspiration), infections (pneumonia, bronchiolitis), asthma, and atelectasis. Alternatively, normal hemoglobin may be replaced by significant amounts of an abnormal hemoglobin (methemoglobin) that cannot combine with oxygen. Finally, central nervous system depression of any etiology can lead to hypoventilation and cyanosis.

CLINICAL PRESENTATION AND DIAGNOSIS

The initial evaluation of the cyanotic patient includes careful observation of the respiratory pattern. In general, hypoxia on a central nervous system (CNS) basis is associated with weak, irregular respirations. The infant may have a weak suck, and patients of any age may have convulsions. Hypoxia and cyanosis on a cardiopulmonary basis are usually associated with rapid, vigorous, labored respirations. Associated findings may include grunting, retractions (suprasternal, intercostal, subcostal), and nasal flaring.

The differential diagnosis between pulmonary and cardiac etiologies can be difficult, but a careful clinical evaluation, an arterial blood gas (ABG), and a chest x-ray usually provide sufficient information. In general, with cardiac lesions, the cyanosis deepens with crying, the lungs are clear, and there is often a murmur. In contrast, with pulmonary etiologies, the infant becomes pinker when crying and, while there is usually no murmur, there may be rhonchi, rales, or wheezes. The ABG reveals CO_2 retention in pulmonary, but not cardiac, disease. However, a repeat ABG after 10–15 minutes of breathing 100% O_2 usually documents an improved pO_2 in pulmonary diseases, but little change with cardiac lesions. Finally, the chest x-ray may show cardiomegaly and variable pulmonary vascularity with cardiac etiologies, but atelectasis, hyperinflation, infiltrates, or an effusion in pulmonary diseases.

If methemoglobinemia is suspected (chocolate brown arterial blood with normal pO_2), inquire about a history of nitrite, sulfonamide, or phenacetin ingestion and contact with aniline dyes.

Occasionally, a well-appearing infant is brought to the ER by parents who report witnessing a cyanotic episode at home. The baby may have been found limp and apneic, but responded to mouth-to-mouth resuscitation. Alternatively, he may have turned blue after feeding (with or without choking). It may be difficult to obtain an accurate history of the event because of parental anxiety and fear. The essential fact to determine is whether the patient in fact turned blue (true cyanotic episode) rather than red.

If the history seems reliable, ask about sudden infant death syndrome (SIDS, p 442) in a sibling, perform a complete physical examination, and obtain a CBC and blood culture. Also obtain a chest x-ray and ABG if the patient is febrile, tachycardic, tachypneic, or coughing, since pneumonia can present with apnea or cyanosis in an infant. If the patient has fever, or if meningitis is suspected (toxic appearance, bulging fontanelle, meningeal signs), perform a lumbar puncture at once.

ER MANAGEMENT

Persistent Cyanosis. The keystones of therapy are supplemental oxygen (head box or face mask with 40–50% O_2) and intubation and mechanical ventilation, if necessary. Antibiotics may be indicated for pulmonary infections.

If cyanotic congenital heart disease is suspected, immediately perform an electrocardiogram and consult with a pediatric cardiologist. In addition to oxygen and ventilation, give sodium bicarbonate (1–2 mEq/kg IV) for severe acidosis (pH $\leq$ 7.10). The management of Tet spells is detailed on p 46.

For suspected methemoglobinemia, obtain a methemoglobin level. If it is greater than 40% or if the patient is unconscious or complaining of chest pain, infuse 1–2 mg/kg of methylene blue intravenously over 5 minutes as a 1% solution in normal saline. In severe cases, give 200–500 mg/day of ascorbic acid and 3–5 mg/kg/day of methylene blue orally.

History of Cyanosis. Admit an infant with a reliable history of a cyanotic episode at home, regardless of appearance in the ER.

INDICATION FOR ADMISSION

- All patients with cyanosis or history of a cyanotic episode

REFERENCES

1. Shannon DC, Lusser M, Goldblatt A, et al: N Engl J Med 287:951–953, 1972
2. Nudel DB, Berman MA, Talner MS: Pediatrics 58:248–251, 1976

Heart Murmurs

INTRODUCTION

Although congenital heart disease is present in approximately only 0.8% of the general population, the incidence of heart murmurs in children approaches 50–60%. Most murmurs, therefore, are innocent or functional in nature.

CLINICAL PRESENTATION AND DIAGNOSIS

An innocent murmur is any *systolic ejection murmur* produced by the turbulent forward flow of blood across a normal right or left ventricular outflow tract. It is short in duration, stops well before the second heart sound, and is midfrequency in quality. The intensity is less than or equal to grade 3/6 and decreases with upright position or a Valsalva maneuver. It is usually best heard in the second or third left intercostal space and is not associated with other findings suggestive of cardiovascular disease (wide splitting of S2, ejection click, diastolic murmur). Still's murmur and pulmonic ejection murmurs meet most of these criteria.

Still's Murmur. Still's murmur occurs in over 50% of children between the ages of 3 and 8 years. It is described as vibratory, musical, or squeaking, is heard best in the midprecordium between the lower left sternal border and the apex, and is generally grade 2–3 in intensity. It is probably secondary to vibrations caused by the impact of blood on the ventricular wall. There is a normal S2 and no click, and good pulses are palpated in both upper and lower extremities.

Pulmonic Ejection Murmur. The pulmonic ejection murmur is noted most frequently in young adolescents and older children and is thought to result from an exaggeration of normal turbulence or flow in the right ventricular outflow tract and pulmonary artery. It is early to midsystolic, diamond shaped, grade 1–3 in intensity, and blowing rather than vibratory in quality. It is best detected in the second left intercostal space. There is a normal S2, no thrill, no click, no parasternal heave, and no diastolic murmur.

Venous Hum. A venous hum is detectable in over 60% of children between the ages of 3 and 6 years. It arises from blood flow at the confluence of the jugular and subclavian venous streams. It is heard best in the supraclavicular area, especially on the right. It is systolic-diastolic in nature with diastolic accentuation and generally grade 1–3/6 in intensity. However, the intensity may change with rotation of the head and generally diminishes with compression of the jugular vein; release of pressure causes accentuation of the murmur for a few seconds. There is no thrill, systolic accentuation, or increased peripheral pulsation.

Functional murmurs, like innocent murmurs, occur in association with normal cardiac anatomy but are generally associated with altered states in which stroke volume is increased (fever, anemia, hyperthyroidism).

In contrast to the conditions described above, organic murmurs are the result of turbulent blood flow through abnormal cardiac structures or communications. They are classified as systolic or diastolic and subdivided according to their timing in the cardiac cycle.

Left-sided Midsystolic Ejection Murmurs

Midsystolic ejection murmurs (crescendo–decrescendo) from left-sided structures are caused by aortic stenosis and idiopathic hypertrophic subaortic stenosis/asymmetric septal hypertrophy (IHSS/ASH).

Aortic Stenosis. The murmur of aortic stenosis is short in duration and either soft or harsh, depending on the severity of the stenosis. It is best heard at the upper right sternal border (second right intercostal space) and the fourth left intercostal space. It is transmitted into the carotid vessels and to the lower left sternal border and apex. The second heart sound is normal, but the murmur may be associated with an ejection click heard at the third to fourth left intercostal space. There also may be a systolic thrill at the second right intercostal space or the suprasternal notch.

IHSS/ASH. The murmur of IHSS/ASH is heard best at the mid to lower left sternal boder and is transmitted well over the apex and to the right base. A systolic thrill is often felt over the area of maximal intensity, the apex, and the right base. The Valsalva maneuver enhances the murmur by reducing ventricular volume and thereby increasing the gradient in the left ventricular outflow tract.

Right-sided Midsystolic Ejection Murmurs

Midsystolic ejection murmurs from right-sided structures are secondary to atrial septal defect, pulmonic stenosis, and the tetralogy of Fallot.

Atrial Septal Defect. The murmur of atrial septal defect (ASD) is heard best in the second left intercostal space and is generally grade 2–3/6 in intensity. It is associated with a wide, fixed split S2, and there often is a middiastolic rumble at the lower left sternal border.

Pulmonic Stenosis. Pulmonic stenosis is heard best in the second left intercostal space and the duration of the murmur is directly proportional to the severity of the stenosis. There may be an associated ejection click heard in the same place, and there is wide splitting of the second heart sound that increases on inspiration.

Tetralogy of Fallot. The murmur of tetralogy of Fallot is a harsh midsystolic ejection murmur heard best between the third to fourth left intercostal space and the left base and is caused by turbulent blood flow across the narrowed infundibulum of the right ventricular outflow tract (not across the ventricular septal defect [VSD]). Associated findings on physical examination (cyanosis and clubbing) help to differentiate this from other conditions.

Holosystolic Murmurs

Holosystolic murmurs are caused by ventricular septal defect and mitral and tricuspid regurgitation.

Ventricular Septal Defect. The harsh VSD murmur is heard best along the lower left sternal border and radiates well over the precordium and to the back. The second heart sound may have a loud P2 component due to pulmonary hypertension. There may be a thrill over the area of maximum murmur intensity and a middiastolic rumble at the lower left sternal border/apex which is due to increased diastolic flow across the mitral valve (increased pulmonary venous return).

Mitral Regurgitation. Mitral regurgitation is often associated with rheumatic heart disease in children. The murmur is blowing in nature, heard best at the apex, and transmits well into the axilla.

Tricuspid Regurgitation. Tricuspid regurgitation may be caused by severe pulmonary hypertension and is often present in newborns with persistent fetal circulation. It may present after open heart surgery that involves manipulation of the septal leaflet of the tricuspid valve (closure of a membranous VSD via the right atrium) and is often found in Ebstein anomaly of the tricuspid valve. The murmur is heard best along the lower left sternal border and over the tricuspid valve (fifth interspace).

Late Systolic Murmurs

The most common late systolic murmur is *prolapse of the mitral valve*. It is ejective in nature, heard best with the patient in the left lateral decubitus position, and often associated with or preceded by a late systolic click or series of clicks. Echocardiography is diagnostic.

Diastolic Murmurs

Diastolic murmurs are almost always organic and include aortic and pulmonic regurgitation, and tricuspid and mitral stenosis.

Aortic and Pulmonary Insufficiency. These conditions produce a high pitched blowing murmur heard best at the upper to midleft sternal border at expiration, with the patient sitting up and leaning slightly forward. Aortic insufficiency may be a component of either acquired (rheumatic) or congenital aortic valvular disease. Pulmonary insufficiency is uncommon but may be noted postoperatively after repair of congenital heart disease (tetralogy of Fallot repair with right ventricular outflow tract patch, pulmonary valvotomy).

Atrioventricular Valve Stenosis. The murmur of atrioventricular valve stenosis is harsh, rumbling, and middiastolic in nature and is heard best either in the tricuspid area (lower left sternal border) or the mitral area (midprecordium-lower left sternal border-apex). The murmur may be due to an absolute stenosis with a narrowed A-V valve or "relative" stenosis with a normal valve, as in ASD (flow murmur across the tricuspid valve secondary to the left to right shunt) or VSD (flow murmur across the mitral valve secondary to increased pulmonary venous return).

ER MANAGEMENT

A murmur does not require acute management. Rather, the underlying disease causing the murmur may require intervention, depending on the clinical condition of the patient. Refer all patients with murmurs that do not meet the strict criteria of an innocent or functional murmur to a pediatric cardiologist. These include holosystolic murmurs, systolic ejection murmurs associated with a click or a diastolic murmur, late systolic ejection murmurs with or without a click, all diastolic murmurs, and any murmur associated with "unusual" signs: cyanosis, clubbing, signs and symptoms of congestive heart failure or low cardiac output, a thrill, absent lower extremity pulses, or a wide, fixed second heart sound.

All children with organic murmurs require subacute bacterial endocarditis (SBE) prophylaxis prior to undergoing dental or genitourinary manipulation (see pp 291–293). Those children whose murmurs are secondary to rheumatic heart disease require rheumatic fever prophylaxis. The fact that a child is receiving the latter does not obviate the need for the former.

INDICATIONS FOR ADMISSION

- A murmur with signs of congestive heart failure
- Fever and a murmur that does not seem to be functional or innocent

REFERENCE
1. Liebman J: PIR 3:321–329, 1982

Syncope

INTRODUCTION

Syncope is loss of consciousness accompanied by muscular weakness. It is caused by decreased perfusion of the brain, most often vasovagal, orthostatic, or hysterical, in origin. Syncope must always be differentiated from breathholding spells and seizures, common causes of nonsyncopal loss of consciousness in children.

CLINICAL PRESENTATION AND DIAGNOSIS

An acute fall in peripheral vascular resistance accounts for most cases of syncope.

Vasovagal Syncope. Vasovagal syncope is the most common form and may be precipitated by strong emotions or fatigue.

Orthostatic Syncope. Orthostatic syncope can occur when assuming an erect posture, in patients who are dehydrated or taking vasodilatory drugs, and occasionally, in healthy young males immediately after voiding (micturition syncope).

Respiratory Causes. Respiratory causes of syncope include *hyperventilation* in adolescents and *breathholding spells* in infants and toddlers (see p 380). The infant or child with a breathholding spell becomes pallid or cyanotic before losing consciousness, while hyperventilating adolescents may have paresthesias or carpopedal spasm. In both, there is usually a history of emotional upset.

Hysterical Fainting. Hysterical fainting occurs primarily in patients with a histrionic (theatrical) personality style. Typically, these are adolescent females who present with a history of fainting in front of others.

Hypolglycemia. *Fasting hypoglycemia* is the major metabolic cause of syncope. Ascertain whether there is a history of diabetes or insulin use. Weakness, diaphoresis, confusion, and palpitations may occur prior to the actual syncopal episode, which is gradual in onset. With *reactive hypoglycemia,* (tumor of the islets of Langerhans), syncope generally occurs 2–4 hours after meals. Certain *ingestions* are associated with hypoglycemia (aspirin, ethanol), so inquire about the possibility of an overdose.

Arrhythmias. Rule out alterations in heart rate and rhythm by physical examination (pulse) and by reviewing the ECG for *SVT, v-tach, tachycardia-bradycardia syndrome,* or *complete heart block.* If these are not found, 24-hour ambulatory monitoring may be indicated, particularly when the history does not suggest another etiology for the syncope.

Valvular Aortic Stenosis. There is a frequent association between right or left ventricular outflow tract obstruction and syncope. Patients with valvular aortic stenosis exhibit excessive reduction of peripheral vascular resistance with exertion. Congenital heart disease, especially *tetralogy of Fallot* (p 46) may cause syncope when acute peripheral vasodilation (fever, warm bath, exercise) increases right to left shunting and decreases pulmonary blood flow. The syncope is usually abrupt in onset and may occasionally be associated with chest pain in the immediate presyncopal period. There may be a family history of syncope, particularly in patients with asymmetric hypertrophy (IHSS).

Seizures. Consider seizures in the differential diagnosis, although true syncope lacks convulsive movements, an aura, or a postictal state. Frequent episodes of loss of consciousness suggest epilepsy.

ER MANAGEMENT

Inquire about the frequency of the attacks, the nature of the onset of the loss of consciousness, any sequelae after the episode, possible drug ingestion, and family history of syncope.

Perform a careful evaluation, including orthostatic vital signs and auscultation for murmurs, and obtain an ECG with a long rhythm strip. The smell of ethanol or ketones on the breath may suggest the etiology.

Obtain a hematocrit, dextrostix, and serum glucose to rule out anemia and persistent hypoglycemia. If an ingestion is suspected, other specific tests may be indicated (pp 334–338).

Instruct patients with *orthostatic syncope* to get up slowly after lying or sitting and discontinue any offending medications. Treat documented *hypoglycemia* with 0.5–1 g/kg (1–2 cc/kg IV) of 50% dextrose. Reassurance and close follow-up are all that are usually needed for *hyperventilation* or *breathholding*.

INDICATIONS FOR ADMISSION

- Syncope on any basis other than vasovagal or hysterical, especially if associated with severe anemia (hemoglobin <7 mg/dl), an arrhythmia, or hypoglycemia in a nondiabetic

REFERENCE

1. Noble RS: JAMA 237:1372–1376, 1977

Tet Spells

INTRODUCTION

The essential features of tetrology of Fallot are a VSD and pulmonic stenosis. The amount of right to left shunting across the VSD (and thus the degree of cyanosis) depends on the relationship between the systemic vascular resistance and the degree of right ventricular outflow tract obstruction. A tet spell is caused by diminished pulmonary blood flow, secondary to a precipitous fall in arterial blood pressure, or increased right outflow obstruction (infundibular spasm).

CLINICAL PRESENTATION AND DIAGNOSIS

A child having a tet spell will usually present after a crying episode with increased cyanosis, tachypnea, and severe respiratory distress. The more agitated the child, the worse the cyanosis and dyspnea. An ABG reveals hypercapnea, hypoxia, and a metabolic acidosis, while right ventricular hypertrophy (RVH) and right axis deviation are seen on the electrocardiogram. The chest radiograph shows a *coeur en sabot* (boot-shaped) heart with diminished pulmonary vasculature and, in 25% of cases, a right-sided aortic arch.

ER MANAGEMENT

If the child is crying or arousable, increase the systemic vascular resistance by placing him or her in a squatting or knee-chest position. Give oxygen (100%) to further increase systemic vascular resistance while decreasing pulmonary vascular resistance and increasing peripheral oxygen delivery. Give morphine sulfate, 0.1 mg/kg intravenously or subcutaneously, to calm the patient.

If the child is obtunded or fails to respond to the above conservative measures, establish an IV and give 20 cc/kg of normal saline to increase the systemic vascular resistance. Follow this with $NaHCO_3$, 1–2 mEq/kg IV over 30–60 minutes, and propranolol, 0.1–0.2 mg/kg IV slowly. Treat continuing respiratory failure and hypotension with intubation and dopamine (p 7).

A patient with a history of brief, mild spells may be treated under close observation with oral propranolol, 0.05–2 mg/kg/day divided q 6h. If the spells are not adequately controlled, refer the patient to a cardiac surgeon.

INDICATION FOR ADMISSION

- A history of tet spells or any spell that lasts long enough to be witnessed by the ER physician

REFERENCES

1. Nadas AS: Hospital Practice 103–111, 1977
2. Bonchek LI, Starr A, Sunderland CO, et al: Circulation 48:392, 1973

3

Dental Emergencies

Caries and Dental Infections

INTRODUCTION

Dental caries (cavities) result from the interaction of normal oral flora (*Streptococcus mutans*) and dietary sugars, particularly sucrose. Dental infections are common during childhood and are caused by pulp necrosis secondary to caries or tooth trauma. Infection then spreads through the root canal into the periodontal tissue, causing an acute dentoalveolar abscess. The usual organisms are streptococci and anaerobes.

CLINICAL PRESENTATION

Cavity. A dental cavity is usually evident on careful examination of the teeth. Cavities can be asymptomatic or accompanied by local or diffuse pain, gingival swelling, and percussion sensitivity, without excessive mobility.

Dental Abscess. A dental abscess usually causes gingival erythema and pain, particularly upon percussion of the tooth. The tooth may be mobile and extruded from the socket. Sometimes a fistulous tract develops and opens onto the buccal or lingual gingival mucosa, forming a parulis (gum boil). Drainage may occur spontaneously or upon palpation of the tooth or gingiva.

Occasionally a dentoalveolar abscess extends into the skin, causing *facial cellulitis,* with fever and regional lymphadenopathy. In adolescents, a similar picture can result from severe gingivitis around an erupting third molar (*pericoronitis*). The erupting tooth may be palpable and there is associated dysphagia, trismus, oral pain, and swelling of the occlusional surface.

DIAGNOSIS

Inquire about a history of recent dental trauma or dental work. Inspect the oral cavity for obvious caries, gingival swelling and erythema, or a gum boil. Palpate the gums and molar occlusional surfaces for swelling and tenderness, tap each tooth with a tongue blade (percussion sensitivity), and check for tooth mobility.

Dental trauma (p 51) can cause pain, swelling, percussion sensitivity, and tooth mobility. Look for associated injuries.

Facial cellulitis may also be secondary to either a break in the skin integrity (associated *insect bite, impetigo, trauma*) or *Haemophilus influenzae type B* bacteremia (1- to 5-year-old, violaceous color, high fever, toxicity). Always examine the gingiva and teeth of a patient with facial cellulitis.

ER MANAGEMENT

Refer all patients with *caries* to a dentist within a few days.

Treat *dental abscesses* with penicillin, 500 mg q 6h (≥30 kg) or 500 mg initially, then 250 mg q 6h (<30 kg). Erythromycin (40 mg/kg/day) is the alternative for patients allergic to penicillin. Refer these patients to a dentist either immediately (temperature over 103°F, unable to drink) or within 24 hours (afebrile, relatively painless).

Treat *facial cellulitis* secondary to a dental infection with intravenous penicillin, 100,000 units/kg/day, warm oral rinses, and parenteral hydration, if necessary.

INDICATIONS FOR ADMISSION

- High fever (>103°F) or inability to take fluids orally
- Facial cellulitis accompanied by fever

REFERENCE

1. Chow AW, Roser SM, Brady FM: Ann Int Med 88:392–400, 1978

Dental Trauma

INTRODUCTION

Dental trauma represents a true emergency, since injured teeth can suffer permanent damage if not treated expiditiously.

CLINICAL PRESENTATION

Concussion. A concussion is minor injury to a tooth's supporting structures (periodontal ligaments) without displacement or excessive mobility. The tooth is sensitive if percussed or when the patient chews.

Subluxation. Subluxation reflects a more serious injury to the periodontal ligaments. There is excessive horizontal mobility and percussion sensitivity, but no displacement.

Displaced Teeth. Displaced teeth may be intruded into the socket (more common in primary teeth), extruded lingually (permanent teeth), or completely *avulsed.* At times, an intruded tooth may be misdiagnosed as avulsed.

Tooth Fractures. Tooth fractures can involve the crown or the root. *Crown infractions* (craze lines) appear as cracks in the enamel, without any abnormal color reflecting involvement of the dentin. Similarly, in fractures involving the *enamel* only, the tooth is normal color with a small piece of the edge missing. Fractures of the *dentin* appear yellow, while pulp exposure, which is nearly always painful, is suggested by a pink or red color. *Root fractures* are difficult to diagnose, but may present with mobility and crown fractures of adjacent teeth. Combined crown–root fractures can also occur.

Mandibular Fractures. Mandibular fractures are uncommon, but may occur in the area of the condyles (below the temporomandibular joints) or along the ramus where the teeth are developing. With unilateral fractures, the mandible will deviate toward the ipsilateral side when the patient opens his mouth; with bilateral fractures, the mouth may remain slightly open at all times. There is malocclusion along with the usual signs of a fracture (local swelling, ecchymoses, pain, and tenderness).

Alveolar bone fractures involve the bony processes into which the teeth are imbedded and typically affect the maxillary incisors. There is displacement and mobility of the involved tooth and alveolar process, mobility of adjacent teeth, and bleeding from the surrounding gingiva.

DIAGNOSIS

A systematic approach is necessary so that subtle injuries are not missed. First, examine the face and lips for lacerations, abrasions, asymmetry, and ecchymoses. Have the patient open and close his mouth, or observe the young patient when crying, to check for asymmetry and deviation. Palpate along the mandible, looking for tenderness. Then, palpate both the mandible and temporomandibular joints for asymmetry and instability while the patient opens and closes his mouth.

The intraoral examination is next. Look inside the mouth for bleeding points, swelling, and avulsed or fractured teeth. Have the patient bite down, check the occlusion and ask if biting feels normal. Then, have him bite down on a tongue depressor. A patient with a mandibular fracture is unable to prevent the examiner from pulling the blade from his mouth. Assess horizontal and vertical mobility of each tooth. Suspect an alveolar process fracture if several adjacent teeth move when one tooth is being checked. Finally, tap each tooth with a fingernail or tongue blade. Percussion sensitivity in the absence of mobility is a concussion and not a serious injury.

ER MANAGEMENT

While elective dental referral is all that is necessary for concussions, crown infractions, and fractures of the enamel, immediate dental consultation is required for subluxations, intrusions, extrusions, and fractures of the dentin or root, or when the pulp is exposed. Immediately consult an oral surgeon for mandibular and alveolar bone fractures.

Reimplant avulsed permanent teeth if less than 1 hour has elapsed since the injury. Rinse the tooth in water or saline, reimplant it using a gentle rotating motion, then maintain firm finger pressure for 5 minutes. Once the tooth has been reimplanted, have the patient bite down firmly on a piece of folded gauze and immediately consult an oral surgeon so the tooth can be stabilized. If the tooth cannot be reimplanted immediately, store it under the patient's tongue or in the buccal fold, if he can cooperate without risk of aspiration. Alternatives are the parent's mouth, a cup of milk, saliva, or a clean moistened towel. Do not reimplant primary teeth.

INDICATION FOR ADMISSION

- Mandibular or alveolar bone fracture

REFERENCE

1. Josell SD, Abrams RG: Pediatr Clin North Am 29:717–741, 1982

Gingivostomatitis and Oral Ulcers

INTRODUCTION

Although generally not serious disorders, gingivostomatitis and oral ulcers are frustrating management problems. There are a number of distinct disease entities, but for most no specific treatment exists. Therefore, determining the exact etiology is usually not crucial to choosing therapy.

CLINICAL PRESENTATION AND DIAGNOSIS

Herpes Simplex. Herpes simplex (p 77) is the most common cause of gingivostomatitis in 1–3 year olds. After a 1- or 2-day prodrome of fever, malaise and vomiting, small vesicles appear anywhere on the oral mucosa, lips, tongue, perioral skin, or cheeks. These rapidly rupture, forming 2–10 mm lesions that are covered by a yellowish membrane. The membrane then sloughs, leaving a shallow ulcer on an erythematous base. Healing begins within 4–5 days, and is usually completed within 1–2 weeks. Fever up to 105°F, excessive salivation, diminished oral intake leading to dehydration, and submental and submaxillary lymphadenopathy can also occur.

Recurrent Herpes. Recurrent herpes ("cold sores") usually is secondary to some stress (fever, menses, sunlight exposure). Small vesicles appear limited to the outer aspect of the lips and adjacent skin, then rupture, coalesce, and become crusted. Healing takes 1–2 weeks.

Aphthous Ulcers. Aphthous ulcers, or canker sores, are solitary or multiple (≤5), painful lesions involving any site of the oral mucosa. They begin as erythematous papules that become well-circumscribed ulcers with a gray fibrinous exudate on an erythematous base. Their appearance is related to stress (allergies, infections, drugs, trauma, emotional upset). Fever is less common than with herpes. The ulcers usually last 10–14 days, but recurrent episodes are the rule.

Herpangina. Herpangina is a summertime infection caused by type A Coxsackie virus. The lesions are found only in the posterior oral cavity which distinguishes them from herpes or apthous ulcers. The soft palate, uvula, tonsils, and anterior tonsillar pillars are the sites of multiple, superficial, painful ulcers. Once again, fever, drooling, and severe dysphagia can lead to dehydration.

Hand-Foot-Mouth Disease. Hand-foot-mouth disease is also caused by type A Coxsackie virus. Vesicles and ulcers occurring anywhere in the oral cavity are accompanied by fever, malaise, and abdominal pain. Many patients also have a characteristic exanthem consisting of vesicles on an erythematous base located in one or more of the following sites: the palms and soles, dorsum of the hands and feet, and dorsal aspects of the fingers and toes.

Candidal Thrush. Candidal thrush (moniliasis, p 66) is a common problem in the first year of life. The complaint is diminished oral intake or white spots in the oral cavity. On inspection, the oral mucosa is beefy red with a curd-like white exudate on the tongue, gingiva, hard palate or buccal mucosa. This can resemble milk, but it is not easily removed by scraping with a tongue depressor. On occasion, cracking or fissuring at the angle of the mouth, or cheilitis, is seen. Many infants simultaneously have a typical Candida diaper dermatitis.

Acute Necrotizing Ulcerative Gingivostomatitis. Acute necrotizing ulcerative gingivostomatitis (Vincent angina, trench mouth) is an uncommon infectious disease of adolescents and young adults probably caused by *Fusobacterium* and spirochetes. Characteristic findings are painful gingiva that bleed easily, ulcerated interdental papillae covered by a grayish membrane, foul-smelling breath, and fever. In some cases there is underlying malnutrition or an immune deficiency.

ER MANAGEMENT

Whether the etiology is herpes, Coxsackie, or apthous ulceration, the major therapeutic goals are oral hygiene and pain relief, so that adequate oral intake can continue. For older children, recommend oral rinsing with mouthwash (Cepacol or Chloraseptic) or Gly-Oxide (carbamide peroxide) to clean the ulcers. For pain, swab either 2% viscous lidocaine or a 1:1 diphenhydramine-Maalox solution onto the lesions. Do not use viscous lidocaine as an oral rinse or gargle, since if it is accidentally swallowed it can cause seizures. In addition, give aspirin or acetaminophen for pain relief and fever. If, after these measures, the child still refuses to take fluids by mouth, admit him for intravenous hydration.

The treatment of *thrush* is specific: instill 1 cc of nystatin suspension (100,000 units/cc) into each side of the mouth four times a day. Give the doses after feedings to prolong contact between the medication and the areas of involvement. For persistent lesions, ask the parent to rub the area with a gauze pad soaked in nystatin. Also, look for a source of reinfection such as an old pacifier.

Treat *trench mouth* with penicillin or erythromycin (250 mg qid) and rinsing with a 1:1 solution of 3% hydrogen peroxide and water. Treat the underlying condition, if any, and refer the patient to a dentist.

INDICATION FOR ADMISSION

- Dehydration or inability to take adequate amounts of fluids by mouth

REFERENCE

1. Wright JM, Taylor PP, Allen EP, et al: Ped Infect Dis 3:80–88, 1984

4

Dermatology

Acne

INTRODUCTION

Acne vulgaris, a disorder involving the pilosebaceous follicles, is the most common skin disease of the second and third decades. The onset is at puberty, with an incidence approaching 100% between the ages of 14–17 in females and 16–19 in males. Drug acne is a folliculitis most commonly caused by the prolonged use of topical or systemic corticosteroids or adrenocorticotropic hormone (ACTH). Other implicated agents include diphenylhydantoin, isoniazid, iodides and bromides, and lithium. Neonatal acne is probably secondary to hormonal stimulation of sebaceous glands that have not yet involuted to a prepubertal immature state.

CLINICAL PRESENTATION

Acne vulgaris primarily involves sites where pilosebaceous glands are most numerous (face, chest, upper back). The initial lesions are the pathognomonic open comedones (blackheads) and closed comedones (whiteheads). As the disease progresses, papules, pustules, nodules, and cysts are seen. The resolution phase is characterized by postinflammatory hyperpigmentation and scarring.

The typical lesions of drug acne are small erythematous papules and pustules, without comedones, primarily located on the back and chest.

Neonatal acne causes erythematous papules and pustules, rather than comedones, on the nose and cheeks.

DIAGNOSIS

Adenoma sebaceum manifests as pink papules on the face of prepubertal patients with *tuberous sclerosis*. Other cutaneous manifestations (ash leaf spots, shagreen patch, periungual fibromas) can be present. *Verrucae* (warts) and *molluscum contagiosum* cause flesh-colored papules without comedones or an inflammatory response. *Hidradenitis,* or apocrine acne, is a chronic suppurative disease of the sweat glands of the axilla and inguinal regions. These are sites where acne vulgaris does not occur.

ER MANAGEMENT

Acne vulgaris is a chronic disease, so while treatment may be started in the ER, refer the patient to a primary care setting for ongoing care. The therapeutic measures that are appropriate for ER use are summarized below.

Successful topical therapy is possible in almost all cases of acne without resorting to dietary restrictions, abrasive cleansers, or exfoliants (sulfur, salicylic acid). Benzoyl peroxide (5 or 10%) is an effective keratolytic and antibacterial agent that is useful for comedones and mild inflammatory lesions. Common side effects are redness, drying, and scaling of the skin. Retinoic acid (tretinoin), or vitamin A, is extremely useful for treating comedonal acne. Severe skin irritation, peeling, and photosensitization can result; start treatment on an every other day basis, usually at night. Instruct patients to limit face washing and to be sure the face is dry prior to applying retinoic acid in order to minimize these effects. Do not use in females who may be pregnant.

Topical antibiotics are a useful adjunct in mild to moderate inflammatory acne. Clindamycin (1%), erythromycin (2%), and tetracycline (2%) are all effective without the same risk of side effects as with oral administration. Systemic antibiotics are valuable in inflammatory acne, although usually 4 weeks or more are required before any improvement occurs. Tetracycline is most frequently used, provided the patient is over 12 years of age and not pregnant. Side effects include gastrointestinal upset, photosensitization, and monilial vaginitis.

Mild Comedonal Acne. Use benzoyl peroxide cream or gel (5%), every other morning, increasing to every morning, if necessary. If more treatment is required, first try 10% benzoyl peroxide. Then add retinoic acid to the regimen (tretinoin cream or gel 0.05%) every other day, increasing to every day, generally at night. This combination is particularly effective, as the tretinoin facilitates absorption of the benzoyl peroxide.

Mild-to-Moderate Inflammatory Acne. To the above regimen, add topical clindamycin or erythromycin, twice each day. Instruct the patient to apply the antibiotic first, followed by the benzoyl peroxide. If there is no improvement, give oral tetracycline, starting with 250 mg four times a day. Once there is a response (4 or more weeks), taper the dose to the minimum required, usually 250 mg every day or every other day.

Severe Inflammatory Acne. Refer the patient to a dermatologist, rather than instituting therapy in the ER.

For *drug acne,* either discontinue the agent or treat with a topical antibiotic (as above). No therapy is required for *neonatal acne.*

REFERENCE

1. Matsuoka LY: J Pediatr 103:849–854, 1983

Alopecia

INTRODUCTION

Alopecia, or hair loss, primarily involves the scalp in children, and is usually localized. Etiologies include alopecia areata, a presumed autoimmune disorder; tinea capitis (fungal infection); trauma or traction secondary to hair care techniques (braiding, straightening, blow drying) or friction; trichotillomania (self-induced hair loss); and male pattern baldness.

Diffuse hair loss is far less common. In most instances, within the previous few months the patient has suffered a significant stress (high fever, crash diet, parturition, or convulsion). Cancer chemotherapeutic agents (cyclophosphamide, vincristine), drugs (propranolol, coumadin), radiation, toxins (lead, boric acid), endocrinopathies (hyper- and hypothyroidism, hypoparathyroidism), nutritional deficiencies (zinc, vitamin A), secondary syphilis, and systemic lupus erythematosus are other etiologies.

CLINICAL PRESENTATION

Alopecia Areata. Alopecia areata is characterized by the sudden (possibly overnight) appearance of sharply demarcated round or oval patches of hair loss without associated scalp inflammation or scarring. Regrowth may occur in some areas while the disease progresses elsewhere. In 5–10% of cases, the lesions may expand to involve the entire scalp (alopecia totalis) or all the body hair (alopecia universalis). At the margin of active lesions, there are loose, easily plucked, "exclamation mark" hairs with shortened bulbs and small stumps. The course is variable, but up to 95% of children have complete regrowth within 1 year. Younger patients and those with extensive involvement have a poorer prognosis.

Tinea Capitis. Tinea capitis causes patchy alopecia with scaling and erythema similar to seborrheic dermatitis. Within the patch, "black dots," infected hairs which are broken off at the scalp level, may be seen. An allergic vesicular and pustular reaction (kerion) can develop acutely and be associated with fever, leukocytosis, and lymphadenopathy. A minority of cases fluoresce under Wood's lamp exposure.

Traumatic and Traction Alopecia. Traumatic and traction alopecia occur where the hair is being pulled, as from braiding, or on the occiput of a young infant who remains supine all day. Characteristically, hair loss is incomplete; short (1–2 cm) hairs are found at the margins or within the affected area. These hairs are firmly rooted in normal-appearing scalp.

Trichotillomania. Trichotillomania primarily occurs in school-age girls and in some cases the eyebrows and eyelashes are affected as well. The patches of alopecia are not well demarcated and there are well-rooted residual hairs of varying length.

Male Pattern Baldness. Male pattern baldness presents as a bilateral frontoparietal recession with thinning over the vertex. It is genetically determined but also can occur in females taking oral contraceptives.

With diffuse hair loss, the scalp generally has a normal appearance and hairs are easily plucked from the periphery of areas of alopecia.

DIAGNOSIS

For localized conditions, a careful examination of the scalp facilitates making the correct diagnosis. Well-demarcated hair loss with normal-appearing scalp suggests alopecia areata. Inflammation and scaling, black dots, fluorescence under Wood lamp examination, or a kerion are typical of tinea capitis. Hair loss in areas of possible trauma with no scalp inflammation is characteristic of traumatic or traction alopecia. The patient may be an infant; there may be a history of hair braiding or straightening, or the child may have been observed pulling at his or her hair. In addition, the remaining hairs are firmly rooted in the scalp.

When the diagnosis is in doubt, pluck a few hairs from the periphery of the lesion, and examine them under a microscope, after mixing with 10–20% potassium hydroxide and gently heating. In tinea infections, chains of spores within or surrounding the hair shaft are seen. If "exclamation point" hairs are noted, alopecia areata is confirmed. Placing the hairs on either Sabouraud agar or Dermatophyte Test Medium (DTM) facilitates the growth of fungi. Obtaining a positive culture is absolutely necessary prior to treating tinea capitis.

A careful history may confirm the stressful incident which caused a diffuse alopecia. If a previously undiagnosed systemic disorder such as syphilis, thyroid disease, lupus, or hypoparathyroidism is suspected, obtain blood for VDRL, thyroid function tests, FANA, or calcium.

ER MANAGEMENT

Most cases of *alopecia areata* require no treatment other than reassurance. If the lesions persist or become particularly widespread, refer the patient to a dermatologist. A change of hair care techniques or reassuring an infant's mother is usually all that is necessary for *traction* or *traumatic alopecia*. Refer the patient with *trichotillomania* to a primary care setting for further psychosocial evaluation.

After obtaining specimens for culture, treat *tinea capitis* with oral griseofulvin, 10 mg/kg/day of the microsize or 5 mg/kg/day of the ultramicrosize preparation. A 6- to 8-week course is usually necessary. Leukopenia, neutropenia, and hepatotoxicity have been reported, so obtain pretreatment and then biweekly liver function tests and complete blood counts. If liver transaminases exceed two and one-half times normal or the absolute neutrophil count is less than

$1000/mm^3$, discontinue the drug. Abnormalities then usually correct spontaneously. Topical antifungal agents (clotrimazole, miconazole) or selenium sulfide shampoo (Selsun) may reduce infectivity, but they do not adequately treat the infection.

Manage *diffuse alopecia* by avoiding the offending agent, drug, or toxin (if possible), or by treating the primary condition (lupus, thyroid disease, etc). If the hair loss is stress-related, then complete regrowth usually occurs without any specific treatment.

REFERENCE

1. Rasmussen JE: PIR 3:85–90, 1981

Atopic Dermatitis

INTRODUCTION

Atopic dermatitis is a disease that predisposes the skin to excessive dryness and pruritis. Up to 75% of patients have a family history of allergy, asthma, hay fever, or eczema, and about half of affected children will develop one of these other diseases.

CLINICAL PRESENTATION

Atopic dermatitis can be categorized into three different age-dependent phases, that may or may not follow one another. Pruritis and dry skin are the hallmarks at all ages. The infantile stage occurs between 2 months and 3 years and is characterized by erythema, papules, and vesicles on the face, neck, chest, and extensor surfaces of the extremities. In children 4–10 years of age, subacute and chronic papular and scaly lichenified lesions occur on the flexor aspects of the neck, arms, and legs. The antecubital and popliteal fossae are particularly involved. The adolescent and adult forms blend into the childhood phase with marked lichenification and flexural, hand, and foot involvement.

Other manifestations may include numular eczema (well-demarcated papular coin lesions) in young children and pityriasis alba (discrete hypopigmented macules) in children and adolescents.

At any age the severe pruritis causes scratching which can lead to secondary bacterial infection. The superimposed pyoderma can confuse the clinical picture.

Atopic individuals have a number of associated findings, including accentuated palmar creases, white dermographism (blanching of the skin when stroked), and Dennie pleat (an extra groove of the lower eyelid).

DIAGNOSIS

The diagnosis of atopic dermatitis is suggested by a family history of atopy, a personal history of allergies or asthma, dry and pruritic skin, and the typical location of the lesions that blend into the surrounding normal skin. In infants, *seborrheic dermatitis* causes a salmon-colored, greasy eruption of the face and scalp that is not pruritic. The eruption of a *contact dermatitis* has a sharp border with the uninvolved skin and the patient history may suggest the offending agent. *Bacterial infections* are not preceded by pruritis and are generally more localized than atopic rashes. *Psoriatic* lesions are usually well demarcated with a silvery scale. The lesions of *scabies* do not follow the usual sites of predilection that eczema does, and the family or personal history of atopy may be negative.

ER MANAGEMENT

Atopic dermatitis is a chronic disease that is best managed in the clinic or office setting. Therapy can be initiated at an episodic ER visit, but ongoing follow-up must be arranged.

The goals of therapy are to hydrate the skin, prevent itching, and treat the inflammation. Instruct the patient to use bath oils (Alpha-Keri) or soap substitutes (Cetophil, Aveeno), avoid excessive bathing, and use emollients after bathing (Eucerin, Aquaphor). Hydroxyzine (2 mg/kg/day divided qid) is an effective antipruritic agent. Finally, use a moderate potency topical corticosteroid (0.1% triamcinalone) on the body and extremities, but use only 1% hydrocortisone on the face. Do not use oral steroids without consultation with a dermatologist.

Treat acute, oozing lesions with Burow solution or tap water open dressings for 20 minutes, qid. Oatmeal baths (Aveeno) may also be soothing. If there is a secondary bacterial infection, use dicloxacillin (50 mg/kg/day) or erythromycin (40 mg/kg/day) divided q 6h.

INDICATION FOR ADMISSION

- Severe involvement in a patient who cannot be adequately treated at home

REFERENCE

1. Oakes RC, Cox AD, Burgdorf WHC: Clin Pediatr 22:467–475, 1983

Bacterial Skin Infections

INTRODUCTION

Bacterial skin infections, or pyodermas, are most commonly caused by group A *Streptococcus* and *Staphylococcus aureus*. Impetigo, folliculitis, furunculosis, and cellulitis are the usual forms of infection.

CLINICAL PRESENTATION AND DIAGNOSIS

Impetigo. The most common type is *impetigo contagiosum* caused by group A *Streptococcus*. The eruption usually appears on the face and extremities. Small erythematous macules develop into vesicles that rupture, leaving a typical honey-colored crust that is easily removed, but recurs. Fever and regional lymphadenopathy may also occur. Some cases of impetigo are caused by nephritogenic strains of *Streptococcus,* so that subsequent acute glomerulonephritis occasionally occurs. Impetigo is extremely contagious, spreading by autoinoculation (satellite lesions), close contact, and fomites (towels).

Bullous Impetigo. Bullous impetigo is caused by phage group II staphylococci. Yellowish vesicles on the face, extremities, and trunk rupture, leaving well-demarcated, erythematous, circular macules with a "collarette of scale." Once again, the infection is highly contagious, and fever and lymphadenopathy can occur.

Folliculitis. Folliculitis is a pyoderma involving the hair follicles. Painless, round-topped, yellow pustules with a hair shaft in the middle occur on the scalp, face, thighs, and buttocks. Coagulase-positive *Staphylococcus* is the most common etiologic agent.

Furunculosis. Furunculosis is a deep follicular infection, usually arising from a preceding folliculitis. Furuncles (boils) are tender, erythematous 1–5 cm nodules that become fluctuant, then suppurate. They are seen in hair-bearing areas that are subject to perspiration and friction, including the face, thighs, buttocks, and scalp. Consider associated conditions, including diabetes mellitus, obesity, corticosteroid treatment, immunoglobulin deficiency, and defective or absent neutrophils in patients with recurrent furuncles.

Cellulitis. Cellulitis, an infection involving the subcutaneous tissues, causes poorly demarcated, tender, erythematous swelling. It is often associated with fever, local lymphadenopathy, and lymphangitic streaking. Sites of infection are areas subjected to superficial trauma, such as the face and extremities. Most common pathogens are coagulase-positive *Staphylococcus* and group A *Streptococcus,* although children under 5 years of age may develop a violaceous cellulitis in association with systemic toxicity caused by *Hemophilus influenzae type B*.

Erysipelas. Erysipelas is a superficial cellulitis caused by group A *Streptococcus*. A tense, erythematous, tender, well-demarcated, rapidly spreading swelling results.

ER MANAGEMENT

Treat *impetigo* with honey-colored crusts with intramuscular (IM) benzathine penicillin (600,000 units <6 years old; 1.2 million units >6 years old); or oral penicillin (250 mg qid) or erythromycin (40 mg/kg/day) for 10 days. Staph *impetigo, furunculosis,* and *cellulitis* require antistaphylococcal antibiotics (dicloxacillin 50 mg/kg/day; erythromycin 40 mg/kg/day; cephradine 25 mg/kg/day). Warm soaks every 2 hours are an essential component of the therapy for *furunculosis* and *cellulitis*. In addition, antistaphylococcal skin cleansers (phisohex, hibiclens) are useful for impetigo, and bacitracin ointment may be applied after crusts are removed.

Give patients with *erysipelas* penicillin (250 mg qid) for 10 days.

Folliculitis often responds to topical antibiotics (bacitracin, erythromycin, tetracycline) only.

If *Hemophilus cellulitis* is suspected, obtain a complete blood count (CBC) with differential and blood culture and consider a lumbar puncture for the irritable patient. Admit the child for intravenous therapy with both ampicillin and chloramphenicol (100 mg/kg/day).

Any child with an *immune deficiency* and furunculosis or cellulitis should receive intravenous nafcillin, with chloramphenicol added if *Hemophilus* infection is suspected.

INDICATIONS FOR ADMISSION

- Suspected *Hemophilus influenza* cellulitis
- Furunculosis or cellulitis in a patient with an immune deficiency
- Fever, proximal lymphadenopathy, lymphangitic streaking in association with cellulitis or other deep skin infection

REFERENCE

1. Tunnessen WW Jr: Pediatr Clin North Am 30:515–532, 1983

Candida

INTRODUCTION

Candidiasis is caused by the fungus *Candida albicans,* which inhabits the gastrointestinal tract of young infants and the vaginal vault of mature females. Factors that predispose to candidiasis include local heat or moisture, systemic antibiotics, diabetes mellitus, and corticosteroids.

CLINICAL PRESENTATION

Cutaneous Candidiasis. Cutaneous candidiasis is most frequently found in the intertriginous areas. It is characterized by moist, beefy red, well-demarcated macules with raised, scaly edges with satellite vesicles and pustules near the borders. Primary infection in the diaper region causes a perianal rash, and secondary infection of a diaper rash of any other etiology is very common.

Oral Candidiasis. Oral candidiasis (thrush) presents in the first weeks of life with loosely adherent, cheesy white plaques on the tongue, soft and hard palates, and buccal mucosa. The mucosal surfaces are beefy red and the lesions bleed when scraped lightly with a tongue blade. These lesions are often painful, and a marked decrease in oral intake can occur in young infants. Thrush in older patients is usually associated with some underlying condition (immunosuppression, broad-spectrum antibiotics), but can occur occasionally in otherwise healthy infants.

Perlèche. Perlèche (angular chelitis) presents as erythema and fissuring at the corners of the mouth and may be associated with overbite, braces, poor mouth closure, or lip smacking.

DIAGNOSIS

The typical intense erythema, scaly border, and satellite lesions usually confirm the diagnosis of cutaneous candidiasis. *Contact diaper rashes* do not involve the intertriginous areas, while *seborrheic* diaper eruptions are usually associated with cradle cap and postauricular scaling. When the diagnosis is in doubt, scrape the border of the eruption and examine the scale under a microscope after mixing with 10–20% potassium hydroxide and gently heating. Budding yeasts and pseudohyphae are seen with Candida.

Thrush is often confused with *milk,* but the latter is easily scraped from the oral mucosa without any bleeding.

Chelitis can resemble *impetigo,* but the characteristic honey-colored crust is not present.

ER MANAGEMENT

Nystatin is the treatment of choice. This is available as a topical cream which is applied three or four times a day to cutaneous eruptions and perlèche. Avoid combination products, as those containing steroids can worsen the eruption, while neomycin can be sensitizing. If the eruption is particularly inflamed, use 5% Burow solution soaks three or four times a day. Treat macerated or wet-looking areas with nystatin powder and frequent diaper changes. For thrush, instill 1 cc of a nystatin oral suspension in each side of the mouth four times each day, after feedings, until 5 days after the lesions have resolved. Advise the mother to rub persistent lesions with a gauze pad soaked with nystatin suspension and to discard any old pacifiers and nipples.

REFERENCE

1. Stein DR: Pediatr Clin North Am 30:545–561, 1983

Contact Dermatitis

INTRODUCTION

There are two forms of contact dermatitis: primary irritant dermatitis and allergic contact dermatitis.

Primary Irritant Dermatitis. Primary irritant dermatitis is a nonallergic reaction caused by soaps, detergents, acids, alkalis, saliva, urine, and feces. It usually occurs in infants and young children and the strength of the irritant and duration of exposure determine the severity of the eruption.

Allergic Contact Dermatitis. Allergic contact dermatitis is secondary to a delayed hypersensitivity response that depends upon a genetic predisposition, site and duration of the contact, as well as previous exposure and sensitization. Common causes include clothing, shoes, nickel, cosmetics, and poison ivy, oak, and sumac.

CLINICAL PRESENTATION

Contact dermatitis usually presents as an acute eczematous reaction, with erythema, swelling, vesicles, and pustules. Usually the eruption is seen within a few (primary irritant) or 8–12 (allergic) hours of the contact and there is a sharp demarcation between the involved and uninvolved skin. Chronic lesions resemble chronic eczema, with thickening and lichenification of the skin.

DIAGNOSIS

Inquire about exposure to possible offending agents (new soap, detergent, shoes, or foods, or playing in the woods) and whether there have been previous similar episodes or known sensitivity to a substance. On examination, the presence of an eczematoid eruption either in nontypical locations or in a linear pattern is highly suggestive of the diagnosis, as are the sharp borders of the rash (true eczema blends into neighboring normal skin).

ER MANAGEMENT

The need to avoid further contact is obvious. Treat an acute dermatitis with open wet dressings (tap water, normal saline, 5% Burow's solution) qid, soothing baths (Aveeno, Aveeno oilated oatmeal) qd, and antihistamines (hydroxyzine 2 mg/kg/day or diphenhydramine 5 mg/kg/day, divided q 6h). For severely edematous and vesicular dermatitis, if the diagnosis is certain, give prednisone (0.5–1.5 mg/kg/day) and taper over 1 week.

For a chronic dermatitis, a moderate potency topical corticosteroid (0.1% triamcinolone) tid is helpful, along with soothing baths. Tar preparations (Estar gel, Zetar emulsion) may also be effective.

INDICATION FOR ADMISSION

- Severe disease with extensive involvement

REFERENCE

1. Esterly NB: PIR 1:85–90, 1979

Diaper Dermatitis

INTRODUCTION

Diaper rashes can begin as early as the first month of life and may persist or wax and wane over the next 2 years. *Candida* superinfection commonly occurs with a diaper rash of any other etiology.

CLINICAL PRESENTATION

Irritant and Contact Dermatitis. Irritant and contact dermatitis is usually located on the convex surfaces of the buttocks, genitalia, and lower abdomen, sparing the intertriginous folds. Secondary candidal infection is common.

Candida. *Candida* infections may be primary, with perianal erythema, or secondary. Beefy red erythema with well-demarcated, raised scaly borders and satellite papules and vesicles are seen. Involvement of the intertriginous creases and associated oral thrush are common. The eruption can spread both up the abdomen and down the thighs. Consider secondary candidiasis if a diaper rash does not respond to the usual therapeutic measures.

Seborrheic Dermatitis. Seborrheic dermatitis presents as nonpruritic, salmon-red, greasy scales on a well-demarcated erythematous base. Characteristically, a similar eruption occurs on the face, as well as scaling of the scalp and retroauricular areas. Once again, secondary candidiasis can occur.

Atopic Dermatitis. Atopic dermatitis causes a moist, erythematous diaper rash in association with a similar eruption on the face, trunk, and extensor surfaces of the extremities. These infants are extremely unhappy because of the intense pruritis. The onset is between 2 and 6 months of age and usually the family history is positive for allergies, eczema, hayfever, or asthma.

DIAGNOSIS

In general, the clinical presentations are sufficiently different so that there are no problems in making the diagnosis. When the picture is not typical, secondary *candidial* infection of an irritant, contact, or seborrheic dermatitis has probably occurred. This can be confirmed, if necessary, by microscopic examination of some scales which have been mixed with 10–20% potassium hydroxide and heated gently. Budding yeasts and pseudohyphae are seen in *Candida* infections. Pruritis is the key to diagnosing *atopic dermatitis.*

ER MANAGEMENT

Meticulous diaper care is the cornerstone of therapy. Instruct the parents to keep the diaper area dry (with frequent changes and air-drying), to use loose-fitting diapers, and to avoid rubber pants. Recommend mild cleansers such as Cetaphil or Aveeno instead of soap. Discontinue talcum powder, which may be irritating. Inflammation secondary to *irritants, seborrhea,* or *atopic dermatitis* responds to 1% hydrocortisone cream, tid after diaper changing. If the eruption is particularly moist, tap water or Burow's solution soaks are helpful.

Treat *Candida* infections with nystatin cream, applied after every diaper change. Oral nystatin (1 cc each side of the mouth tid after feeding) may be added if there is oral thrush or a recurrent candidal diaper rash.

A diaper eruption may be the presenting sign of an underlying systemic disorder (immunodeficiency, phenylketonuria, Letterer-Siwe disease, psoriasis). Therefore, referral to a dermatologist is indicated if the rash does not respond to these routine measures or the infant is either not thriving or has recurrent infections.

REFERENCE

1. Weston WL, Lane AT, Weston JA: Pediatrics 66:532–536, 1980

Drug Eruptions

INTRODUCTION

Potentially any drug can cause a rash. The most common offending agents are the penicillins and sulfonamides, while acetaminophen, antihistamines, digoxin, steroids, theophylline, and thyroid hormones rarely cause an eruption. In general, suspect that a drug which has been given within 1 week of the onset of the rash is the cause; it is unusual for medications which have been administered for long periods of time to be implicated. However, there are many exceptions to these rules, and there are no tests which can confirm that an eruption is due to a particular agent.

CLINICAL PRESENTATION

Although virtually any rash morphology can be caused by drugs, for each type of eruption there are certain agents that are most likely to be involved.

Acneiform. Acneiform eruptions are characterized by papules and pustules, without comedones. The most common agents are corticosteroids, diphenylhydantoin, isoniazid, lithium, and oral contraceptives.

Eczema. Eczema can occur after systemic administration if the patient has become sensitized to the topical form of the drug (contact dermatitis). Eczema is most commonly seen with penicillin, aminoglycosides (particularly neomycin), and sulfonamides.

Erythema Multiforme. Erythema multiforme and Stevens-Johnson syndrome (p 74) can caused by the sulfonamides, penicillins, barbiturates, diphenylhydantoin, and carbamazepine. The lesions are more common in sun exposed areas and do not always have the classic target appearance.

Erythema Nodosum. Erythema nodosum (p 76) can be caused by sulfonamides, diphenylhydantoin, and oral contraceptives.

Fixed Drug Eruptions. Fixed drug eruptions recur in the same location each time the agent is administered. The lesions are usually violaceous, round plaques that may have dusky centers with bullae. These are few in number and are most common on the extremities and genitals. Barbiturates, tetracyclines, phenolphthalein, and sulfonamides are the most frequent offenders.

Lupus-like Syndrome. A Lupus-like syndrome with cutaneous manifestations (butterfly rash) can occur with procainamide and hydralazine.

Macular Eruptions. Macular eruptions usually appear within a week of administering agents such as the sulfonamides, diphenylhydantoin, barbiturates, penicillins, gold, erythromycin, tetracyclines, isoniazid, chloramphenicol, thiazides, and salicylates. The eruption, however, might not begin until 5–7 days after the drug has been discontinued. Commonly, pink macules on the trunk coalesce into larger macular patches. The rash then spreads onto the extremities, although the palms and soles are usually spared. The eruption may be accompanied by fever, and clearing can take weeks.

Between 5 and 10% of patients taking ampicillin or amoxicillin will have an erythematous, nonpruritic, macular eruption primarily on the trunk, face, and extremities. The usual onset is between days 4 and 8, although the rash can occur after the first or last dose of a course. This is not a true allergy and does not necessitate discontinuing the drug or avoiding penicillins in the future.

Photosensitivity. Photosensitivity usually results in an exaggerated sunburn within 2–6 hours of sunlight exposure. Hyperpigmentation and desquamation follow in the exposed areas only. Etiologic agents include the tetracyclines (especially demeclocycline and doxycycline), phenothiazines, thiazides, sulfonamides, and coal-tar preparations. Soaps and detergents containing salicylanildes (hexachlorophene) can also cause these eruptions.

Purpura. Purpura (palpable), identical to Henoch-Schönlein purpura, in the absence of thrombocytopenia, can be caused by the penicillins, sulfonamides, and oral contraceptives.

Toxic Epidermal Necrolysis. Toxic epidermal necrolysis in older children and adolescents is most often caused by drugs. The eruption is clinically similar to that seen in staphylococcal scalded skin syndrome. Sandpaper-like erythema, skin tenderness, and a positive Nikolsky sign are accompanied by large flaccid bullae that rupture, leading to crusting and desquamation. The mucous membranes, palms, and soles are most frequently involved; the hairy skin is spared. Agents include the barbiturates, diphenylhydantoin, salicylates, penicillins, sulfonamides and other antibiotics, and tranquilizers.

Urticaria. Urticaria is most often caused by the penicillins, cephalosporins, sulfonamides, codeine, and salicylates. There may be accompanying angioneurotic edema, anaphylaxis, erythema multiforme, and serum sickness.

ER MANAGEMENT

Except for ampicillin/amoxicillin rash, the only requirement is discontinuation of the offending agent. Treat pruritis and *urticaria* with hydroxyzine (2 mg/kg/day divided tid).

Acne-like eruptions respond to topical or oral tetracycline, while *eczema* may require topical steroids (1% hydrocortisone or 0.1% triamcinolone). Refer severe cases of *erythema multiforme* (p 74) and *erythema nodosum* (p 76) to a dermatologist, who may recommend systemic corticosteroids (prednisone 2 mg/kg/day).

Treat *photosensitivity* reactions by avoiding sunlight and using sunscreens with a sun protection factor of 15. The management of *toxic epidermal necrolysis* (p 93) is similar to that for second-degree burns, but admit the patient and give IV antistaphylococcal antibiotics until an infectious etiology can be ruled out by examination of the skin peel.

The treatment of *anaphylactoid* reactions (p 10) includes subcutaneous epinephrine (1:1000, 0.01 cc/kg up to 0.3 cc), oxygen, and diphenhydramine (5 mg/kg/day divided qid).

INDICATIONS FOR ADMISSION

- Toxic epidermal necrolysis and Stevens-Johnson syndrome
- Anaphylactoid reactions

REFERENCE

1. Dunagin WG, Millikan LE: Med Clin North Am 64:983–1003, 1980

Erythema Multiforme

INTRODUCTION

Erythema multiforme is considered to be a hypersensitivity reaction. Infectious diseases are the most common causes, including viruses (herpes simplex, hepatitis, infectious mononucleosis, adenovirus), bacteria (tuberculosis, staphylococcus, streptococcus, gonorrhea), mycoplasma, and fungi (coccidioidomycosis, histoplasmosis). Other etiologies include drugs (penicillins, sulfonamides, tetracycline, phenytoin), collagen vascular diseases (lupus, rheumatoid arthritis), pregnancy, poison ivy, and neoplasms (leukemia, lymphoma).

CLINICAL PRESENTATION

The disease is seen in all age groups, although it is uncommon in children under 3 years. Prodromal symptoms of cough, coryza, sore throat, vomiting, and myalgias may precede the eruption by 1–10 days. The typical lesion is the erythematous iris or target-shaped lesion, occasionally with petechiae within the margins. However, macular, urticarial, and vesicular lesions can occur. In mild cases the eruption is symmetrical, predominantly on the extensor surfaces, palms, and soles. With severe disease, lesions are more generalized, with involvement of the oral, ocular, and genital mucous membranes. The association of high fever and severe constitutional symptoms with extensive, bullous involvement of the mucous membranes is termed the *Stevens-Johnson syndrome.* Superficial ulceration and hemorrhagic crusting of the mucous membranes are typically seen. Severe eye involvement can occur, with conjunctivitis, keratitis, and uveitis. Lesions appear in successive crops over 10–15 days, after which slow resolution occurs.

DIAGNOSIS

When the characteristic target lesions are present, there is little difficulty in making the diagnosis. However, erythema multiforme is most often confused with *urticaria,* in which the lesions are pruritic, but not target-like (no central clearing). In a *vasculitis,* palpable, nonblanching purpuric lesions are characteristic.

ER MANAGEMENT

If an etiology is not apparent (drug history, herpes, sore throat, etc), then obtain a throat culture, heterophile antibody, cold agglutinins, hepatitis surface antigen (HBsAg), and place a PPD. A chest x-ray may be indicated if there are lower respiratory tract symptoms.

In mild cases, all that is needed is aspirin or acetaminophen and wet compresses (normal saline or Burow solution) tid for vesicular lesions. Appropriately treat any underlying illness (erythromycin for mycoplasma, etc). In cases with mucous membrane involvement, diphenhydramine-Maalox (1:1) or viscous lidocaine rinses may ease debilitating oral pain. Consult an ophthalmologist if ocular involvement is suspected. Patients with Stevens-Johnson syndrome and those with extensive cutaneous blisters may require intravenous hydration. The use of corticosteroids is controversial for children with Stevens-Johnson syndrome. After consultation with a dermatologist, 1–2 mg/kg/day of prednisone (or equivalent) can be tried on an inpatient basis.

INDICATIONS FOR ADMISSION

- Inability to take liquids adequately
- Stevens-Johnson syndrome

REFERENCE

1. Edmond BJ, Huff JC, Weston WL: Pediatr Clin North Am 30:631–640, 1983

Erythema Nodosum

INTRODUCTION

Erythema nodosum is a delayed hypersensitivity reaction that occurs most commonly in patients with respiratory infections, particularly group A *Streptococcal* pharyngitis and primary tuberculosis. Other associations include fungal infections (coccidioidomycosis, histoplasmosis), cat scratch fever, inflammatory bowel disease, sarcoidosis, and drug reactions (penicillin, sulfonamides, oral contraceptives). Erythema nodosum is uncommon in children under 10 years of age.

CLINICAL PRESENTATION

Multiple, 1–5 cm, oval, bruise-colored, slightly elevated nodules are symmetrically distributed over the anterior tibias. Less commonly, lesions are found on the extensor surfaces of the arms, thighs, face, and neck. Nodules can be warm and extremely tender and frequently are accompanied by arthralgias.The eruption disappears without scarring within 6 weeks.

DIAGNOSIS

Usually the nodules are so characteristic that there is no difficulty in making the diagnosis. *Insect bites* are pruritic and not symmetrically distributed; *bruises* are not elevated and resolve over several days; and a *cellulitis* is hot, not well demarcated, and often associated with lymphangitic streaking or local lymphadenopathy.

Inquire about a history of upper respiratory infection, trauma, recent travel, possible tuberculosis exposure, and medication use. Obtain a throat culture, ASLO, and place a STU PPD. If tuberculosis, sarcoid, or a fungal infection is suspected, also obtain a chest x-ray.

ER MANAGEMENT

Most important is treatment of the underlying disease or discontinuation of the offending drug. Bed rest, leg elevation, and aspirin are helpful. Refer atypical, persistent, or recurrent cases to a dermatologist.

REFERENCE

1. Kibel MA: S Afr Med J Sci 44:873–876, 1970

Herpes Simplex

INTRODUCTION

Herpes simplex infections are caused by two major antigenic types, although the clinical diseases are indistinguishable. Herpes simplex I has traditionally been responsible for nongenital infections, while type II was the agent in sexually transmitted disease. With the changes in today's sexual habits, this distinction no longer holds.

After primary spread by person-to-person contact, the virus remains latent in sensory ganglia, with reactivation at a later time. Among the possible reactivating stimuli are fever, local trauma, stress, menstruation, and ultraviolet light. In general, recurrent disease is associated with fewer constitutional symptoms, smaller vesicles, closer grouping of lesions, and a shorter clinical course than the primary infection.

CLINICAL PRESENTATION

Gingivostomatitis and Labialis. Gingivostomatitis and labialis are common in infants and young children. With primary infection, fever, malaise, sore throat, salivation, and cervical adenopathy occur in association with vesicles in the oral cavity. These vesicles then ulcerate, while the gingiva become erythematous, swollen, and bleed easily. Decreased oral intake may lead to dehydration in infants. Resolution occurs in 10–14 days.

Recurrent infection is often preceded by burning or tingling for periods ranging from hours to several days in the affected area. The lesions occur on the cheeks, chin, and vermillion borders of the lips, but not in the mouth. They appear as grouped vesicles, with yellowish fluid on an erythematous base, that quickly dry and form a crust. Healing occurs in 5–14 days, but secondary impetiginization is common.

Genitalis. In females, primary vulvovaginitis is characterized by malaise, fever, vaginal burning, and exquisite dysuria. The vesicles and erosions may be superficial or deep, involve the vagina, labia, and perineum, and coalesce into large ulcers. In males, the disease affects the penile shaft, the glans, urethra, and scrotum. The lesions are painful single or multiple vesicles that rapidly erode and form a crust. Bilateral tender adenopathy is often present in both sexes. Recurrent disease affects both sexes and occurs with a prodrome of pain or tingling. Clustered vesicles on an erythematous base rupture and form ulcers. The course is 10–14 days, with pain, dysuria, and, occasionally, lymphadenopathy.

Neonatal Herpes. Neonatal disease occurs either as an ascending infection after premature rupture of the membranes or by direct spread to the neonate during passage through an infected birth canal. Herpes can be asymptomatic or present as a local infection or disseminated life-threatening disease. Generally, the baby becomes ill during the first week of life when cutaneous or oral vesicles are noted, commonly on the face and scalp. Fever, lethargy, and hepatosplenomegaly can occur, and with dissemination; there may be ocular (keratoconjunctivitis), central nervous system (encephalitis), and pulmonary (pneumonia) involvement. Dissemination can also occur in the absence of cutaneous lesions. A similar spectrum of disease can occur in older immunocompromised patients.

Keratoconjunctivitis. Primary ocular disease presents as a purulent conjunctivitis with edema, vesicles, and corneal ulcers. In contrast to other etiologies of conjunctivitis, pain and photophobia are common. With recurrent disease, keratitis or corneal ulcers occur in association with a vesicular eruption on the conjunctiva, eyelids, periocular skin, and tip of the nose.

Whitlow. Herpetic whitlow results from inoculation of the virus into the fingers, causing a painful, localized vesiculobullous eruption with swelling and erythema. It is usually found distally on the finger that the child habitually sucks. The course is 10–14 days.

Kaposi Varicelliform Eruption. This is a generalized cutaneous infection, seen primarily in infants and children with an atopic diathesis. Fever and lymphadenopathy accompany an eruption of umbilicated vesicles in areas of eczematous dermatitis. It is usually self-limited, lasting 1–2 weeks.

DIAGNOSIS

Always suspect herpes when there are grouped vesicles on an erythematous base. The presumptive diagnosis of a herpetic infection can be made by performing a Tzanck smear: open the vesicle, blot up the fluid, scrape the bottom of the lesion onto a glass slide, and stain with Wright or Giemsa stain. With herpes, multinucleated giant cells are seen. The diagnosis can be confirmed, if necessary, by culturing the virus from vesicle fluid; this requires 24–48 hours.

The differential diagnosis of mouth sores is discussed on pp 53–55, but primary gingivostomatitis causes a typical constellation of gingivitis, oral ulcers, fever, and cervical adenopathy. *Vincent angina* is an acute gingivitis, occuring in adolescents and young adults that resembles herpes without buccal involvement. *Stevens-Johnson syndrome* may be associated with cutaneous lesions, and *hand-foot-mouth disease* is often associated with vesicular lesions on the hands and feet. Recurrent herpes labialis is most often confused with *impetigo,* although the crust in impetigo has a typical honey color.

Herpes is the major cause of vesicles and ulcers of the genitalia, but confusion with *syphillis* is common. The diagnosis of sexually transmitted diseases is summarized on pp 238–250.

Neonatal herpes can resemble any of the transplacental *TORCH infections* or *bacterial sepsis,* especially when cutaneous lesions are absent. A complete sepsis work-up (including lumbar puncture) and TORCH titers are indicated for infants presenting in this manner.

Other etiologies for a "red eye" are enumerated on p 411. However, ocular pain, photophobia, and intense conjunctival involvement do not occur with a routine *viral* or *bacterial conjunctivitis*. In recurrent infection, be suspicious of ocular involvement if a vesicular eruption is noted on the tip of the nose since the innervation is the same.

A whitlow can resemble a *paronychia* or *bullous impetigo*. In the latter two, the vesicles are deep and yellowish (as opposed to whitish and superficial, as with herpes) and the pain is not as severe.

ER MANAGEMENT

Despite progress in the development of antiviral drugs, the mainstays of cutaneous herpes therapy are analgesia (acetaminophen viscous lidocaine), soaks (Sitz baths, Burow solution), and patience. On occasion, an infant with severe oral disease becomes dehydrated and requires intravenous fluids.

Acyclovir 5% ointment is effective in *initial genital infections*, only. Apply it six times a day, for 7 days, while wearing rubber gloves to prevent autoinoculation of the virus.

Refer any patient with suspected herpetic *keratoconjunctivitis* to an ophthalmologist for further evaluation and treatment (Acyclovir ophthalmic ointment). Never prescribe ocular corticosteroids, which may facilitate spread of the infection.

Acyclovir (10 mg/kg q 8h) is the treatment of choice for *neonates* or *immunocompromised patients* with herpes. Controversy exists as to the need for a brain biopsy prior to instituting therapy. Unless this can be performed without a significant delay, the consequences of delayed therapy outweigh the risks of unnecessary treatment. Attempt to culture the virus from mucocutaneous lesions, urine, saliva, and cerebrospinal fluid.

INDICATIONS FOR ADMISSION

- Herpetic infection in a neonate or immunocompromised patient
- Poor oral intake and dehydration in infants

REFERENCE

1. Whitely RJ, Alfrod, CA: PIR 1:81–84, 1982

Lice

INTRODUCTION

Three varieties of lice, the head louse, the body louse, and the pubic louse, parasitize man. The head louse is transmitted by contact with infested upholstery, and by sharing hats, combs, brushes, and towels. The body and pubic louse are acquired via bedding, clothing, and person-to-person (sexual) contact. The body louse can carry rickettsial disease (typhus and trench fever) and spirochetal disease (relapsing fever).

CLINICAL PRESENTATION

Pediculosis Capitis (Head Lice). The patient presents with pruritus of the scalp, ears, and neck, which occasionally is very severe. Nits (eggs) are oval, and yellow-white, measuring 0.3 to 0.8 mm in size; they are found firmly cemented close to the scalp on the hairs around the ears and occiput. They project from the side of the hair shaft and do not surround it. Adult lice are not usually found. Secondary pyoderma with impetigo, folliculitis, or furunculosis is common and may mask the primary problem.

Pediculosis Corporis (Body Lice). This organism lives in the lining and seams of clothing, occasionally emerging to bite its host. Erythematous macules become intensely pruritic papules and urticarial wheals, with secondary eczematization and impetiginization.

Phthirus Pubis (Pubic Lice—"Crabs"). Itching is the initial symptom, but secondary infection is uncommon. Pubic and axillary hair and the eyelashes can be affected. The organism can be identified as brownish crawling "flecks" and nits are seen attached to the hair shafts. In heavy infestations, nonblanching grey-blue macules (maculae cerulae) secondary to mite bites occur on the lower abdomen and thighs.

DIAGNOSIS

The diagnosis of lice infestation is clinical, based on the history and visualization of the lice or their ova (nits). Nits fluoresce under Wood light examination, and microscopic examination of the nit confirms the diagnosis. Body and pubic lice infestation can resemble *scabies, eczematous dermatitis,* or *bacterial pyoderma.*

ER MANAGEMENT

Pediculosis capitis. Shampoo with lindane 1% (gamma benzene hexachloride, Kwell, Scabene) and leave the lather on for 5–10 minutes. Repeat the application one week later. A fine-toothed comb is useful for removing nits, and clothing and bedding should be washed in very hot water or dry cleaned.

Pubic lice. Leave a thin layer of lindane lotion or cream on the affected areas for 12 hours. Reapplication may be necessary in 1 week, and sexual contacts should be treated.

Body lice. Frequent bathing and laundering of clothing and bedding are all that is usually necessary. If lice are seen on the body, apply lindane lotion for 8 hours; then wash it off. Boil or dry clean clothing. Systemic antipruritics (hydroxyzine 2 mg/kg/day divided qid) may be necessary for some patients.

Eyelash lice. Pediculosis of the eyelashes may be treated with petrolatum, applied twice daily for 8 days. Alternatively, a physostigmine ophthalmic preparation (Eserine) twice daily for 2 days is effective, although transient miosis can occur.

REFERENCE

1. Orkin M, Epstein F Sr, Malbach HI: JAMA 236:1136–1140, 1976

Miliaria

INTRODUCTION

Miliaria is a group of disorders caused by keratinous obstruction of the eccrine sweat ducts. It occurs at all ages, although the higher incidence in newborns may be secondary to immature sweat ducts which are more likely to plug.

CLINICAL PRESENTATION

Miliaria Crystallina. Miliaria crystallina (sudamina) is characterized by 1–2 mm, clear, thin-walled vesicles on otherwise normal skin. The lesions are asymptomatic and occur primarily in intertriginous areas. Sunburn may cause this form of miliaria.

Miliaria Rubra. Miliaria rubra (prickly heat) is the most common type and is characterized by pruritic, erythematous, 1–2 mm papules and vesicles. Generally these are grouped in clusters with surrounding erythema. Covered skin, especially where there is friction from clothing, is affected.

Miliaria Profunda. Miliaria profunda is only seen in the tropics and represents a more severe form of miliaria. It usually follows repeated attacks of miliaria rubra. Clinically, 1–3 mm firm, whitish papules, rather than vesicles, are present.

DIAGNOSIS

Under slight magnification, the lack of a hair shaft penetrating the vesicle confirms the nonfollicular nature of the eruption and rules out *folliculitis*. A history of excessive sweating in a hot, humid environment and occurrence in the newborn differentiate miliaria from *eczema*.

ER MANAGEMENT

Cool baths and the avoidance of excessive heat and humidity are all that is usually necessary. Parents often tend to overdress infants, attempting to keep their hands and feet warm. Instead, advise them that the proper amount of clothing and temperature for the child can be ascertained by feeling the child's neck or upper back, which should be comfortably warm and not hot. Talcum powder will keep intertriginous areas dry.

REFERENCE

1. Hölze E, Kligman AM: Br J Dermatol 117:99–137, 1978

Molluscum Contagiosum

INTRODUCTION

Molluscum contagiosum is an eruption caused by a virus of the pox group, spread by direct person-to-person contact and autoinoculation. The disease occurs at any age, but is most common between 3 and 15 years.

CLINICAL PRESENTATION

The lesions start as small papules that typically grow to 3–6 mm diameter, but they can be as large as 2–3 cm. They usually are flesh-colored or slightly erythematous and dome-shaped, with a central umbilication. Papules are found on the face, trunk, extremities, and pubic region, either alone or in clusters, and number from one to several hundred. The duration of the individual lesion is variable; although most resolve within 9–12 months, some may persist for 2–3 years. Chronic conjunctivitis or keratitis may occur with eyelid lesions. Particularly severe eruptions with thousands of lesions can occur in patients with atopic dermatitis or depressed cellular immunity. Although molluscum is usually an asymptomatic process, up to 10% of patients develop an eczematoid hypersensitivity reaction around the lesions.

DIAGNOSIS

Confusion with *warts, bacterial infections, papillomas,* and *acne* can occur. The diagnosis is easily proven, however, by opening the papule and smearing the contents onto a glass slide. Using either Wrights or Gram stain, the presence of microscopic round-oval smooth-walled cytoplasmic masses (''molluscum bodies'') resembling a cluster of grapes confirms the diagnosis.

ER MANAGEMENT

Treatment is not always necessary because of the tendency for spontaneous regression. If there are cosmetic concerns or lesions continue to spread, however, curettage of individual lesions is effective. It is quick but is usually not tolerated by young children. Alternatively, each papule can be pierced with a needle and the contents expressed. Removal of lesions is useful only if the eruption is limited.

If the diagnosis is in doubt or the patient has either facial lesions or multiple papules, refer the child to a dermatologist prior to the institution of any therapy.

REFERENCE

1. Rosenberg EW, Rusk JW: Arch Dermatol 101:439–441, 1970

Pityriasis Rosea

INTRODUCTION

Pityriasis rosea is a benign self-limited eruption presumed to be viral in origin because of the prodromal symptoms, seasonal clustering, and lifelong immunity that develops in 98% of patients. However, person-to-person transmission has not been confirmed.

CLINICAL PRESENTATION

Pityriasis rosea occurs predominantly in adolescents and young adults, with few cases in children under 5 years of age. After a variable prodrome of malaise, about 75% of cases present with an initial lesion called a ''herald patch.'' This is a 2–5 cm annular, erythematous, scaly plaque with a raised border and central clearing, seen anywhere on the body. The generalized eruption that follows 4–10 days later characteristically consists of small, ovoid papules with a fine scaly border. The long axis of these lesions follows the cleavage lines on the back and trunk in a so-called ''Christmas tree'' pattern. Generally the rash spares the distal extremities, face, and scalp, although this is not always true in younger children. Also, papules, vesicles or pustules occur in younger patients. Lesions continue to occur for up to 2 weeks, with clearing in 6–8 weeks. Postinflammatory hypo- or hyperpigmentation can result.

DIAGNOSIS

The history of the herald patch and the characteristic nature of the lesions of the generalized eruption usually suffice to confirm the diagnosis of pityriasis rosea. However, the herald patch may resemble a *tinea corporis* infection, although these grow slowly and are not followed by a generalized eruption. Several other diseases are characterized by diffuse erythema and scaling, including *guttate psoriasis, nummular eczema, drug reactions,* and *seborrheic dermatitis,* but the face and distal extremities are often involved and there is no "Christmas tree" pattern. The eruption of *secondary syphilis* can look very similar, but may involve the palms and soles. Obtain a VDRL if the patient is sexually active or if the rash involves the palms or soles.

ER MANAGEMENT

For most patients no treatment is necessary. Antihistamines (hydroxyzine 2 mg/kg/day or diphenhydramine 5 mg/kg/day) alleviate the pruritis. Topical corticosteroids may be useful in very inflammatory cases, but generally do not shorten the course of the disease. Refer patients with lesions persisting for more than 12 weeks to a dermatologist.

REFERENCE

1. Cavanaugh RM Jr: Clin Pediatr 22:200–203, 1983

Scabies

INTRODUCTION

Scabies is caused by infection with the itch mite. It is acquired by close personal contact, although spread via fomites (clothing, linens, and towels) is possible as the organism can survive for about 2 days away from humans. Pruritis is most likely due to an acquired sensititivity to the mite's feces, since the average person is infected with less than 10 to 15 organisms.

CLINICAL PRESENTATION

The usual complaint is generalized pruritus, especially at night. The most common sites are the interdigital webs, the flexor aspects of the wrists, the nipples, the axillae, the extensor surfaces of the elbows, and the abdomen. However, the head, neck, palms, and soles are frequently involved in infants and young children. The characteristic lesion is the burrow, a short serpiginous ridge that ends with a vesicle. Erythematous, excoriated papules and vesicles are common findings with secondary crusts, eczematization, and bacterial infection. The lesions will vary, based on the duration of infection and degree of sensitization of the individual.

DIAGNOSIS

Scabies is a "great imitator" of other pruritic eruptions; however, a history of contact, intense pruritis, and the variable lesions suggest the diagnosis. *Atopic dermatitis* most commonly occurs on the flexor surfaces and not in the interdigital webs. The lesions of *pityriasis rosea* are well circumscribed and not on the distal extremities. *Folliculitis* can be identified by the hair shaft in each lesion. Since the lesions of scabies can become impetiginized, differentiation may be very difficult, although pruritus is not intense in *impetigo*.

To confirm the diagnosis of scabies, place a drop of mineral oil on a nonexcoriated papule, then gently scrape with a no. 15 scalpel blade until the top is removed. Place the scrapings on a microscope slide, cover with a coverslip, and then examine at 10x magnification. Identification of eggs, the mites, or oval brown feces is diagnostic.

ER MANAGEMENT

Present modes of treatment are effective against the mites but less so against the eggs. The age of the patient must be considered when choosing a medication as some (eg, lindane) are more toxic in infants. The issue of treating asymptomatic household contacts has not been resolved, although sexual contacts and bedmates are particularly at risk. Bed clothes and linens should either be washed or stored for several days after treatment is given.

Lindane 1.0% (gamma benzene hexachloride; Kwell, Scabene). Apply 8–12 hours, after bathing, to the entire body from the neck down.

Approximately 30 cc are needed to cover the average child. Repeat the application 5–7 days later to kill any newly hatched mites. Uncommonly, acute central nervous system toxicity manifested by nausea, vomiting, headache, dizziness, and convulsions occurs. The risk of these toxic effects in infants and small children may be greater because of their relatively greater surface area.

Treat children less than 2 years of age and pregnant females with the alternative medications listed below:

Crotamiton 10% (Eurax). This is a safe alternative to lindane for young infants and pregnant women. No systemic side effects are reported, although the rate of cure may be somewhat lower. Apply after bathing, and reapply 24 hours later. Forty-eight hours after the second treatment take a cleansing bath.

Precipitated Sulfur 6–10% in Petrolatum. This is recommended for infants and small children, although it must be specially formulated by a pharmacist. Apply nightly after bathing for 3 consecutive nights. Its major problems are odor, messiness, and staining of clothing and linens.

REFERENCE

1. Orkin M, Malbach HI: N Engl J Med 298:496–498, 1978

Seborrheic Dermatitis

INTRODUCTION

Seborrheic dermatitis is a scaling eruption of unknown etiology generally limited to the areas of the body with the greatest number of sebaceous glands. The disease usually presents between 2 and 8 weeks of age and resolves by 1 year. It may then reappear during adolescence.

CLINICAL PRESENTATION

In the infant, the disease presents as a nonpruritic, dry, erythematous scaling of the scalp (''cradle cap''), often accompanied by retroauricular scaling and occipital lymphadenopathy. The eruption may progress to involve the forehead and face, with the development of characteristic salmon-colored greasy scales on a well-demarcated erythematous base. In the diaper area, the eruption has a similar appearance with involvement of intertriginous areas. Secondary candidal infection can occur.

Seborrhea in adolescents typically appears as excessive scaling of the scalp (dandruff), eyebrows, eyelids, and moustache and beard.

DIAGNOSIS

The typical picture of cradle cap and retroauricular scaling usually presents no diagnostic difficulty. Infants with *atopic dermatitis* are unhappy, with severe pruritis. Often there is a positive family history of eczema, hayfever, asthma, or allergies. In the diaper area, *irritant dermatitis* does not involve the intertriginous areas, while *Candida,* which can complicate seborrhea, causes scaling borders with satellite papules and vesicles. When the diagnosis is in doubt, microscopic examination of some scale after mixing with 10–20% potassium hydroxide and gently heating reveals budding yeasts and pseudohyphe in candidal infections.

Tinea capitis can cause a dandruff-like picture. However, alopecia and hairs broken off at the scalp level ("black dots") are features of tinea infection. *Psoriasis* is rare in infants, but in older patients there may be lesions on the elbows, knees, and sacral area.

ER MANAGEMENT

Usually treating the infant's scalp also clears the remainder of the eruption. For mild cases, apply mineral oil to the scalp and leave it on for 15 minutes. Afterwards, brush the scalp vigorously or comb with a fine-toothed comb, then shampoo. For more severe cases, an antiseborrheic shampoo, such as Zetar or Sebulex, is effective when used twice each week. Facial eruptions respond to applications of 1% hydrocortisone cream tid. Treat secondary *Candida* infections with nystatin cream tid.

REFERENCE

1. Jacobs AH: Pediatr Clin North Am 25:209–224, 1978

Tinea

INTRODUCTION

Superficial dermatophytoses are called tinea, although tinea versicolor is caused by pityrosporum orbiculare (not a dermatophyte). The name of the particular infection is based on the clinical location.

CLINICAL PRESENTATION

Tinea Capitis. Tinea capitis is caused by infection of the hair shaft. Patchy alopecia with scaling, erythema, and infected hairs that are broken off at scalp level (''black dots'') may be seen. A hypersensitivity reaction with a boggy, inflammatory mass (kerion) associated with fever, leukocytosis, and lymphadenopathy can develop acutely.

Tinea Corporis. Tinea corporis or ringworm, is an infection of the glabrous (nonhairy) skin commonly associated with contact with puppies and kittens. The lesions are well-circumscribed annular patches or plaques, with central clearing, and a raised, scaly, papular or vesicular border.

Tinea Cruris. Tinea cruris or ''jock itch'' is an infection of the groin and upper thighs rarely seen before puberty. More frequent in hot, humid environments and in obese or very athletic people, tinea cruris is exacerbated by tight-fitting and chafing clothing. Sharply demarcated, bilaterally symmetrical, scaly, erythematous plaques that spare the scrotum and labia are typically seen. Secondary candidal infection can occur.

Tinea Pedis. Tinea pedis, or ''athlete's foot,'' is a pruritic eruption that is exceedingly unusual in prepubertal children. The findings range from mild scaling to marked erythema, maceration, fissuring, and vesiculation involving the toes and interdigital webs. The infection may spread to the soles and sides of the feet, but the dorsal aspects of the toes are usually spared. An allergic response to the fungus (id reaction) occasionally causes an erythematous vesicular eruption on the trunk and upper extremities.

Tinea Unguium. Tinea unguium (onychomycosis) is a fungal infection of the nail plate that usually occurs in association with dematophytosis elsewhere (hands, feet). The infection begins in the tip of the nail, which becomes discolored, lusterless, and friable with subungal hyperkeratosis and separation of the distal nail from the nail bed (onycholysis).

Tinea Versicolor. Tinea versicolor (pityriasis versicolor) is an infection of the upper trunk and back, proximal arms, and neck that is particularly common in warm climates. Hypo- or hyperpigmented, well-demarcated, scaling, oval macules without erythema or pruritus are seen. It is diagnosed more commonly in the summertime as the involved areas will not tan while the surrounding uninfected skin does.

DIAGNOSIS

Differentiating fungal infections from other conditions is facilitated by scraping the lesions, mixing the scale with 10–20% potassium hydroxide, heating gently, then examining microscopically. Hyphae or spores are seen in these fungal infections, while tinea versicolor has a characteristic "spaghetti and meatballs" appearance. In addition, if the diagnosis is in doubt, culture the fungus on Sabouraud agar or DTM. Finally, a minority of tinea capitis and all tinea versicolor infections fluoresce under Wood lamp examination.

Tinea capitis is the only common etiology of childhood alopecia that causes scalp inflammation; the eruption may fluoresce under a Wood light and black dots may be seen. The scalp is normal in *alopecia areata, traction alopecia,* and *trichotillomania. Seborrheic dermatitis* causes scaling without hair loss.

Tinea corporis can resemble *contact dermatitis,* the herald patch of *pityriasis rosea,* and *nummular eczema.* The characteristic central clearing and raised, well-demarcated scaly border usually suggests the diagnosis.

Tinea cruris can be confused with *contact dermatitis, intertrigo,* and *erythrasma,* a *Corynebacterium* infection that fluoresces coral-red under Wood lamp examination. In addition, secondary candidal infection can occur and distort the picture, although therapy is not altered.

Before the diagnosis of tinea pedis is made in a prepubertal patient, consider *dishydrotic eczema* and *contact dermatitis* which can involve the dorsum of the foot.

Tinea unguium must be confirmed with a positive culture, as

psoriasis, eczema, trauma, and *congenital ectodermal syndromes* can all give a similar appearance.

Tinea versicolor resembles *pityriasis alba, postinflammatory hypopigmentation, vitiligo, seborrheic dermatitis,* and *secondary syphilis.* However, none of these conditions fluoresce under Wood's lamp examination.

ER MANAGEMENT

Tinea capitis cannot be treated topically. Obtain a culture (p. 61) and give the patient oral griseofulvin (10 mg/kg/day microsize; 5 mg/kg/day ultramicrosize) for 6 to 8 weeks. Although not very common, neutropenia and hepatotoxicity can occur. Discontinue the drug if the absolute neutrophil count drops below 1000/mm^3 or the liver transaminases exceed two and one-half times normal. Topical antifungals (clotrimazole, miconazole, tolnaftate) and selenium shampoos (Selsun) may decrease the period of infectivity. Also treat *tinea unguium* with oral griseofulvin, although a much longer course (6–18 months) is necessary.

Treat *tinea corporis, tinea cruris,* and *tinea pedis* with the topical antifungal medications mentioned above two or three times a day for 2–3 weeks. In addition, soak inflammatory lesions with normal saline or 5% Burow's solution compresses. Keep affected areas dry—this is particularly important for tinea pedis and cruris, where antifungal powders are indicated. Instruct the patient to wear cotton (instead of synthetic) underwear and socks to help dissipate moisture.

Tinea versicolor responds to the application of 2.5% selenium sulfide shampoo, which can be left on for 30 minutes three times a week, or daily for 5 minutes in the shower. Although the pruritus and scaling respond rapidly, continue therapy for 3–4 weeks, at which time the lesions no longer fluoresce under Wood light and normal pigmentation returns. Topical antifungals are also effective but more expensive.

REFERENCE

1. Esterly NB: PIR 3:41–49, 1981

Toxic Epidermal Necrolysis

INTRODUCTION

Toxic epidermal necrolysis (TEN) encompasses two entities. Most cases occur in infants and young children and are caused by toxin-producing coagulase-positive staphylococcci (staphylococcal-scalded skin syndrome [SSSS]). In patients over 10 years old, TEN is usually a drug reaction (sulfonamides, penicillins, and other antibiotics; barbiturates and phenytoin; allopurinol).

CLINICAL PRESENTATION

SSSS begins with a generalized macular erythema after a period of fever and irritability. The eruption becomes scarlatiniform (sandpapery) and tender, with wrinkling, bullae, sheet-like exfoliation, and a positive Nikolsky sign (peeling of skin with light pressure). Crusting radiating out from the orifices (mouth, nose, eyes) is typical, but mucous membrane involvement is rare. Despite the marked skin tenderness and irritability, these patients are not terribly ill. If hydration is maintained, recovery occurs in 1–2 weeks.

Drug-induced TEN has a similar appearance, although it tends to be more severe, with more widespread skin involvement, a longer course (2–3 weeks), and a higher mortality (10–50%). The reaction can occur weeks or months after the patient has started taking the offending drug. Nikolsky sign is positive only on lesions, not on clinically normal skin, as in SSSS. Mucous membrane involvement and fluid and electrolyte imbalances are more common.

DIAGNOSIS

Differential diagnosis may be difficult in the first day or two, as the eruption may resemble *scarlet fever* (nontender skin, pharyngitis and strawberry tongue, negative Nikolsky), *Kawasaki disease* (conjunctival, lip, oral mucosa, and tongue involvement with negative Nikolsky), and *Stevens-Johnson syndrome* (target lesions, mucous membrane involvement, but positive Nikolsky). TEN is suggested by the characteristic perioral crusting without mucous membrane involvement, sheet-like peeling, and positive Nikolsky sign.

The diagnosis of SSSS is confirmed by isolation of staphylococci from body orifices, or, rarely, the blood. However, often the differentiation between SSSS and drug-induced TEN can be made by skin biopsy only. Suspect a drug reaction in an older child who is taking one of the offending agents.

ER MANAGEMENT

If SSSS is suspected, obtain cultures from *all* body orifices (including conjunctiva) and the blood. Admit the patient and treat with IV anti-staphylococcal antibiotics (oxacillin 100 mg/kg/day or clindamycin 40 mg/kg/day). If a drug reaction is likely, stop the presumptive agent and give systemic corticosteroids (prednisone 2 mg/kg/day, or the equivalent). When the differentiation is not clear, use both treatment modalities until a dermatologist can perform a skin biopsy.

Pay meticulous attention to fluid and electrolyte status, as if the patient has a second-degree burn. Topical antibiotics are not indicated.

INDICATION FOR ADMISSION

- All cases of TEN (including SSSS)

REFERENCE

1. Amon RB: Dimond RL: Arch Dermatol 111:1433–1437, 1975

Urticaria

INTRODUCTION

Urticaria, or hives, represents a cutaneous allergic reaction secondary to the release of the chemical mediators of immediate hypersensitivity, especially histamine. Angioedema is a similar process occurring in the deep dermis or subcutaneous tissues. The most common causes are listed in Table 4-1, although in 80% of cases no definite etiology is discovered.

TABLE 4-1. COMMON ETIOLOGIES OF URTICARIA

Foods	Infections
Eggs	Viral upper respiratory
Peanuts	Strep
Shellfish	Hepatitis B
Drugs	Mycoplasma
Penicillins	Infectious mononucleosis
Aspirin	Physical Agents
Nonsteroidal antiinflammatories	Cold
Insect Bites	Heat
Intense Emotions	Exercise

Urticaria that persists longer than 6 weeks is arbitrarily called chronic urticaria, and is sometimes associated with systemic illnesses such as juvenile rheumatoid arthritis, systemic lupus erythematosus (SLE), acute rheumatic fever (ARF), viral hepatitis, and lymphomas. Therefore a thorough work-up is indicated to determine the etiology.

CLINICAL PRESENTATION

Hives are pruritic, poorly demarcated, erythematous elevations of the skin or mucous membranes. The centers are blanched and most lesions are evanescent; individual wheals rarely last longer than 12–24 hours. Hives are found anywhere on the body, varying in size from a pinpoint to 10 cm or more.

DIAGNOSIS

Obtain a complete history, seeking a possible offending agent. In general, no laboratory testing is required for patients with acute urticaria who are otherwise well. For children with chronic urticaria, on the other hand, perform a thorough physical examination looking for signs of a systemic disorder (fever, weight loss, arthralgias, or weakness). Initial screening tests for chronic urticaria include a CBC with differential, erythrocyte sedimentation rate (ESR), VDRL, heterophile antibody, FANA, rheumatoid factor, and liver function tests. If these results do not indicate the etiology, refer the patient to an allergist.

ER MANAGEMENT

Acute urticaria is best treated by removing or avoiding the offending agent, if it can be identified. Antihistamines of the H1 class are the drugs of choice. Among these, hydroxyzine (Atarax 2 mg/kg/day) is the most effective. Diphenhydramine (Benadryl 5 mg/kg/day) and cyproheptadine (Periactin 0.5 mg/kg/day) are acceptable alternatives. If the patient has particularly severe pruritis or angioedema, subcutaneous 1:1000 epinephrine (0.01 cc/kg up to 0.3 cc) or Susphrine (0.005 cc/kg up to 0.15 cc) often gives prompt relief.

The first step in the treatment of chronic urticaria is to remedy the underlying condition or, if possible, avoid the precipitant. Use hydroxyzine, diphenhydramine, or cyproheptadine as for acute urticaria. If unsuccessful, refer the patient to an allergist for further management.

REFERENCE

1. Twarog FJ: Pediatr Clin North Am 30:887–898, 1983

Verrucae

INTRODUCTION

Verrucae, or warts, occur in 5–10% of children between the ages of 10 and 16. They are benign tumors of the epidermis caused by a DNA (papilloma) virus that spread via autoinoculation and person-to-person contact. Local trauma seems necessary to promote infection with the virus, so that lesions are most common on the fingers, hands, elbows, and plantar surfaces. The incubation period is 1–6 months and, while the course is extremely variable, two-thirds of all lesions spontaneously resolve within 2 years. A patient can have anywhere between one and several hundred warts.

CLINICAL PRESENTATION

Common Warts. Common warts (verruca vulgaris) occur predominantly on the dorsal surfaces of the hands and the periungal regions. They usually begin as pinpoint, flesh-colored papules that grow larger

(1–10 mm), with roughened surfaces, grayish color, and sharply demarcated borders. Often these lesions are studded with black dots (thrombosed capillaries). Periungual warts most commonly occur in children who bite their nails.

Flat Warts. Flat warts (verruca plana) are tan to flesh-colored, soft, flat, small (2–6 mm) papules that occur primarily on the face, neck, arms, and hands. These are particularly common in shaved areas. Contiguous lesions can become confluent and plaque-like.

Plantar Warts. Plantar warts (verruca plantaris) usually occur in weight-bearing areas of the sole of the foot. They are flat with sharp margins, and black dots are seen within the lesions. Pressure forces them into the tissues of the foot and this leads to marked tenderness when walking. They often coalesce into a single large plaque called a mosaic wart.

Venereal Warts. Venereal warts (condylomata acuminata) are soft, reddish-pink filiform lesions that may coalesce into larger, cauliflower-like clusters. They are located primarily on the genitalia and around the anus. Proctoscopic examination may reveal involvement of the rectal mucosa as well. Condylomata acuminata are usually sexually transmitted, but in a third of cases may be associated with warts elsewhere on the body.

DIAGNOSIS

The diagnosis of common or flat warts can be confirmed by the presence of black dots (thrombosed dermal capillaries) beneath the surface. Gentle paring with a scalpel causes small bleeding points, and which represent intact capillaries.

Periungal warts can be confused with the periungal fibromas of *tuberous sclerosis*. However, other cutaneous manifestations of tuberous sclerosis usually are present (adenoma sebaceum, ash-leaf spots, shagreen patches).

Plantar warts can be confused with calluses, corns, and black heel (talon noir). *Calluses* do not have sharp, well-demarcated margins and no black dots are seen. *Corns* typically occur at the metatarsal-phalangeal joints. There are no black dots, but they have sharp margins and a characteristic translucent particle at the core. *Black heel* occurs in athletes who make frequent sudden stops, causing blackish pinpoint hemorrhages. The margin is not well demarcated and paring does not reveal bleeding points.

Condylomata acuminata must be differentiated from the *condylomata lata* of secondary syphilis. These lesions are 1–3 cm grayish-pink nodules occurring in the same regions. Dark field microscopy and serology (VDRL and FTA) are necessary to confirm the diagnosis.

ER MANAGEMENT

Adjust therapy for the type of wart, the location and duration of the lesion, and the age of the patient. The physician must consider the high rate of spontaneous resolution and the discomfort to the patient of the treatment. Often benign neglect is the best approach.

Keratolytic therapy may be instituted in the ER for a patient with a few lesions. The usual combination is salicylic acid (10–16%) with lactic acid (10–16%) in flexible collodion. This is applied daily after bathing, after which the lesion is covered for 24 hours with a waterproof adhesive bandage. The procedure is repeated after paring the wart with the side of a scalpel. Commercially available salicylic acid plaster is useful for plantar warts. Cut it to fit the lesion, tape it in place for 4–5 days, then pare the necrotic tissue and reapply the plaster, if necessary.

Refer patients with lesions on the face, multiple hand warts, periungual and subungual warts, large plantar warts, or venereal warts to a dermatologist. Other available therapies include liquid nitrogen, cantharidin, electrodessication and curettage, and podophyllin.

REFERENCE

1. Schmidt LM: Pediatr Ann 5:782–790, 1976

5

Ear, Nose, and Throat Emergencies

Acute Otitis Media

INTRODUCTION

Two-thirds of all children will have at least one episode of otitis media by 2 years of age. The incidence is much higher during the winter months, corresponding to the greater frequency of viral upper respiratory infections.

The most common etiologic organism is *Streptococcus pneumoniae,* followed by nontypable *Haemophilus influenzae.* Less frequently, *Branhamella catarrhalis, Streptococcus pyogenes,* and type B *Haemophilus* have been implicated. The gram-negative enteric organisms (*Escherichia coli, Klebsiella, Proteus, Pseudomonas*) and *Staphylococcus aureus* are responsible for about 15% of cases in the first few months of life, but are exceedingly rare afterwards. Currently, anaerobes, *Mycoplasma pneumoniae, Chlamydia trachomatis,* and viruses are not considered to be significant causes of acute otitis media. However, on routine bacterial culture, about one-third of middle ear cultures are found to be sterile.

CLINICAL PRESENTATION

Earache and tugging at the ears are the most frequent complaints. The older child may complain of dizziness or decreased hearing. Occasionally, there is a history of severe ear pain that resolved abruptly when a bloody or yellowish discharge began to drain from the external canal. In infants, there may be nonspecific symptoms such as vomiting, diarrhea, irritability, or decreased feeding. In many cases, however, the patient is asymptomatic or only has a fever or a persistent upper respiratory infection. Therefore, examine the ears of all such children, even if otoscopy in the last day or so did not reveal an otitis media.

DIAGNOSIS

Examine the tympanic membrane for shape (concave, retracted, bulging), color (pearly gray, injected, erythematous, yellow), the presence of landmarks (light reflex, malleus), and mobility. Redness alone is not sufficient to make the diagnosis since crying can cause erythema of the drum. The most sensitive of all these characteristics is the mobility of the tympanic membrane. A combination of erythema, bulging, loss of the usual landmarks, and decreased mobility is the characteristic picture of an acute otitis media. Tympanic membrane perforation with recent onset of bloody or purulent ear discharge is also diagnostic. The findings on pneumoscopy can be confirmed by tympanometry (flat tympanogram).

ER MANAGEMENT

The antibiotic treatment of patients over 8 weeks of age is summarized in Table 5-1. The usual duration of therapy is 10 days.

Antihistamine-decongestant combinations are not routinely indicated. Use them only when treatment of a specific symptom (rhinitis) is desired.

Afebrile, well-appearing infants under 8 weeks of age can be treated with amoxicillin. However, if there is fever (>100.6°F), toxicity, or a previous hospitalization with antibiotic treatment, admit the baby to the hospital. Perform a full sepsis evaluation, including a lumbar puncture, and give parenteral antibiotics (ampicillin 100 mg/kg/day and gentamicin 7.5 mg/kg/day or chloramphenicol 75 mg/kg/day, if over 4 weeks old) until culture results are available.

The ambulatory patient should be afebrile within 48–72 hours after beginning antibiotic therapy; persistence of fever suggests a treatment failure. Reexamine the child, looking for other sources of fever. If none is found, give an alternative antibiotic (see Table 5-1).

Reexamine the patient at the completion of therapy. A sterile effu-

TABLE 5-1. ANTIBIOTIC TREATMENT OF ACUTE OTITIS MEDIA (OVER 8 WEEKS OF AGE)

Antibiotic	Daily Dose	Frequency
First line agents:		
Amoxicillin	40 mg/kg	q 8h
Ampicillin[a]	100 mg/kg	q 6h
Erythromycin-sulfisoxazole	50 mg/kg of E	q 6h
Second line agents:		
Trimethoprim-sulfamethoxazole[b]	8 mg/kg of TMP	q 12h
Cefaclor[c]	20 mg/kg	q 8h
For vomiting or noncompliance:		
CR bicillin IM	50,000 units/kg	once
and		
Sulfisoxazole	150 mg/kg	q 8h

[a]Do not use if the patient has diarrhea.
[b]Does not adequately cover *S. pyogenes;* do not use if patient has pharyngitis.
[c]Expense does not justify use as a first-line agent.

sion commonly persists, but if the tympanic membrane continues to appear infected, either continue the same antibiotic or change to an alternative one. Reexamine the patient 1 week later.

Tympanocentesis is indicated for systemic toxicity, severe unremitting pain, unresponsiveness to conventional therapy, a suppurative complication (mastoiditis, meningitis, brain abscess), or immunocompromise.

INDICATIONS FOR ADMISSION

- Infants less than 8 weeks of age with a temperature over 100.6°F, toxicity, or previous inpatient antibiotic treatment
- Immunocompromised patients with fever over 101°F
- Suppurative complication (mastoiditis, meningitis, brain abscess)

REFERENCE

1. Paradise JL: Pediatr 65:917–943, 1980

Cervical Adenopathy

INTRODUCTION

Cervical adenopathy can be considered in three broad etiologic categories—reactive, infectious, or associated with systemic illness. The majority of cervical lymph nodes are reactive, found in conjunction with a viral or bacterial infection of the head or neck. Palpable cervical lymph nodes are present in approximately 80–90% of young, school-age children, especially if they have had a recent upper respiratory tract infection. These nodes are generally benign and no workup or specific treatment is necessary.

An adenitis is an infection of the lymph node itself, most commonly caused by *S. aureus* or group A strep, although other organisms such as anaerobes have been implicated. Tuberculous adenitis often occurs in conjunction with pulmonary disease. Atypical *Mycobacterium* and cat-scratch fever can result in a node with all the signs of acute infection.

Systemic diseases, especially infectious mononucleosis and mono-like syndromes (CMV, toxoplasmosis, leptospirosis, brucellosis, and tularemia) can cause cervical as well as generalized lymphadenopathy. The possibility of a malignancy (leukemia, Hodgkin's disease, non-Hodgkin's lymphoma) is always a concern.

CLINICAL PRESENTATION

Reactive nodes are usually multiple, discreet, firm, <1–2 cm in diameter, nontender, and mobile. The overlying skin is neither erythematous nor adherent. In general, reactive adenopathy subsides in 2–3 weeks, but it can persist. With an adenitis, the node becomes enlarged, tender, and fluctuant. The overlying skin is warm, erythematous, and occasionally adherent. An atypical *Mycobacterium* infection causes the node to suppurate.

Mono and mono-like illnesses can present with generalized tender lymphadenopathy, sometimes in association with a pharyngitis, macular rash, and hepatosplenomegaly. These nodes are firm and mobile.

A malignant node is fixed, hard, matted, and possibly supraclavicular in location. Weight loss, weakness, pallor, fever petechia, and ecchymoses are other possible findings.

DIAGNOSIS

Perform a thorough examination of the head and neck, to find a source of infection draining into the affected node(s). Enlargement of the parotid gland obscures the angle of the mandible. Infectious *parotitis* may cause unilateral or bilateral swelling with severe tenderness. Intraoral examination may reveal swelling, erythema, or a discharge from the opening of Stensen duct (opposite the second upper molar). Weakness, fever, rash, hepatosplenomegaly, and generalized lymphadenopathy are all indicative of a *systemic disease*. Weight loss, pallor, bleeding manifestations, and high fever are associated with *malignancies*.

There are seven features of the affected node(s) to consider:

Single or Multiple (Unilateral or Bilateral). Enlargement of a single node generally occurs in an adenitis, although tuberculous adenitis causes bilateral involvement. Reactive adenopathy and systemic diseases most often result in multiple, bilateral involvement, although a single, reactive node can be seen.

Location(s). The location of a reactive node can suggest the site of the primary infection (preauricular-conjunctiva; occipital-scalp; submental and submandibular-intraoral). Supraclavicular adenopathy is suspicious for a malignancy, while posterior cervical suggests a viral illness. Generalized lymphadenopathy most commonly occurs during mono or a mono-like infection, although leukemia is a possible etiology.

Size. Reactive nodes are typically small (<2 cm). Massive enlargement can occur with an atypical *Mycobacterium* infection.

Rate of Growth. Nodes that slowly enlarge suggest a malignancy, while rapid enlargement occurs in an infected or reactive node.

Mobility. In general, a freely movable node is benign. A node that is fixed to adjacent structures or matted to other nodes suggests a malignancy, mycobacterial infection, or cat-scratch fever.

Consistency. Soft or firm nodes are benign. Fluctuance occurs in adenitis, especially bacterial. A rubbery consistency is noted in sarcoid nodes and malignant nodes are usually rock hard.

Overlying Skin. Bacterial adenitis causes erythema and warmth of the overlying skin. However, adherence occurs in cat-scratch fever and atypical *Mycobacterium* infection. A reactive node does not affect the overlying skin.

ER MANAGEMENT

"Benign" reactive nodes found in conjunction with a head or neck infection require treatment of the primary illness, only. If the pharynx is erythematous, obtain a throat culture.

When adenitis is diagnosed, obtain a throat culture, place a 5TU PPD, and give an antibiotic with staphylococcal and streptococcal coverage (dicloxacillin 50 mg/kg/day or erythromycin 40 mg/kg/day, divided qid). Warm compresses, applied for 15–30 minutes every 3–4 hours, are also necessary. See the patient in 48–72 hours to evaluate the response to therapy and check the PPD. If there is clinical improvement or a positive throat culture, continue the antibiotics for a total of 10 days. If the node has not responded to antibiotics and warm compresses, change to clindamycin (25 mg/kg/day, divided qid). If the node becomes fluctuant, incision and drainage are both diagnostic and therapeutic.

Admit patients with nodes unresponsive to oral antibiotic therapy for parenteral treatment (oxacillin 100 mg/kg/day or clindamycin 40 mg/kg/day). Obtain complete blood count (CBC) with differential, heterophile antibody, and a blood culture prior to starting intravenous therapy.

If the PPD is positive, consider *Mycobacterium* as the cause of the infection. Obtain a chest x-ray and admit the patient for surgical consultation, collection of culture specimens, and institution of antituberculous therapy.

When a mononucleosis syndrome is suspected, obtain a heterophile antibody or mono-spot test. Treatment is supportive (p 302). If a malignancy is suspected, consult a hematologist-oncologist (pp 265–267). Initial evaluation usually includes a chest x-ray and CBC with differential, platelet, and reticulocyte counts prior to admission.

Treat parotitis with analgesia (acetaminophen, asprin) and warm compresses.

INDICATIONS FOR ADMISSION

- Cervical adenitis unresponsive to oral therapy
- Evaluation of a suspected malignancy
- Institution of antituberculous therapy

REFERENCES

1. Barton LL, Feigin RD: J Pediatr 84:846–852, 1974
2. Marcy SM: Pediatr Infect Dis 2:397–405, 1983

Epistaxis

INTRODUCTION

Epistaxis usually involves a site on the anterior nasal septum. Trauma (nose picking, punch, fall), upper respiratory infections, excessive use of decongestants, overly dry environments, and foreign bodies are the major etiologic factors. Rarely, structural abnormalities (hemangioma, telangiectasia), a bleeding diathesis (usually thrombocytopenia), or hypertension are involved. While children are often rushed into the ER because of "massive" blood loss, clinically significant bleeding is unusual.

CLINICAL PRESENTATION

Usually an anterior septal source is evident. It is rare for the bleeding to be bilateral, but blood crossing behind the nasal septum can mimic a bilateral bleed. Sometimes, if the site is posterior or the child is sleeping, the blood may be swallowed and then present as hematemesis.

DIAGNOSIS

Examine the nasal cavity with the child sitting on the parent's lap, using a bright light (otoscope). If a bleeding source is found, the examination may be terminated, as multiple sites are unusual (except in the case of a fractured nasal septum). Occasionally, a mucosal hemangioma or telangiectasia is seen. If no cause is found, but blood is noted trickling down the throat, assume that there is a posterior source.

Examine the skin for hemangiomata or telangiectasias which may also be present in the nasal cavity. Jaundice, petechiae, purpura, lymphadenopathy, and hepatosplenomegaly may suggest a bleeding diathesis (p 256) and anemia (significant blood loss) may be reflected by pallor, tachycardia, gallop rhythm, or orthostatic vital sign changes.

In general, no work-up is required for a nosebleed in an otherwise well child with an anterior septal source. Obtain a spun hematocrit if anemia is suspected. Evaluate for a bleeding diathesis (PT, PTT, platelet count, and bleeding time) if the patient has any of the physical findings enumerated above, a long history of recurrent nosebleeds, or a family history of excessive bleeding.

ER MANAGEMENT

Most anterior bleeds respond to pressure. Pinch the nares together for a full 5 minutes with the child sitting upright (to prevent swallowing of blood). If this is unsuccessful, soak a cotton ball with 1:1000 aqueous epinephrine or ¼% phenylephrine and place it in the nasal cavity. Alternatively, pack the nose with vaseline gauze or Gelfoam. After hemostasis is obtained, the site can be cauterized for 3 seconds with a silver nitrate stick, although this is usually reserved for patients with recurrent bleeds. Treat hemangiomata or telangiectasias in the same way, but do not use cautery if a bleeding diathesis is suspected (possible tissue slough).

If routine measures are ineffective or the source is posterior, place a posterior pack. Anesthetize the nose with 4% lidocaine or benzocaine, pass an uninflated Foley catheter through the nose into the pharnyx, inflate the balloon, then pull the catheter back until it fits snugly posteriorly in the nose. Fill the nose with vaseline gauze up to the balloon and place a clamp across the catheter where it exits the nose.

INDICATIONS FOR ADMISSION

- Posterior pack, for 48 hours, until removal
- Bleeding diathesis or significant blood loss

REFERENCE

1. Kirchner JA: N Engl J Med 307:1126–1128, 1982

Foreign Bodies

INTRODUCTION

Children will place small objects into any orifice. Unfortunately, the signs and symptoms of a foreign body may be very subtle, although the complications can be life threatening.

CLINICAL PRESENTATION AND DIAGNOSIS

Aural. Foreign bodies in the ear cause pain, tinnitus, and in the case of a live insect, extreme discomfort. Although usually a benign condition, inexpert attempts at removal can push the object further into the canal, perforate the ear drum, and cause bleeding and swelling of the canal.

Nasal. Nasal foreign bodies present with a unilateral foul-smelling discharge with unilateral obstruction. Usually the object can be seen anteriorly in the nose, but swelling of the mucosa may obscure it.

Esophageal. An esophageal foreign body is an unusual but potentially serious problem. Though most objects pass into the stomach, possible sites for lodging include the inferior margin of the cricoid cartilage, the level of the aortic arch, and just superior to the diaphragm. Clinically, pain, dysphagia, and dyspnea (secondary to laryngeal compression) occur. After the initial discomfort there may be a quiet period. Subsequent edema can cause esophageal obstruction (dysphagia and drooling), upper airway obstruction, and possible perforation, ultimately leading to mediastinitis. On x-ray, the foreign body is in a coronal orientation.

Laryngeal and Tracheal. Laryngeal and tracheal foreign bodies classically present with a brief episode of coughing, gagging, choking, or cyanosis. Patients may present with dyspnea, a croupy cough, and stridor, although wheezing occasionally occurs. A tracheal foreign body can cause an audible slap and palpable thud as air passes the object. Chest x-rays are usually normal, although pneumonia and air trapping are sometimes seen. Orientation of a radioopaque body in the saggital plane on x-ray confirms its location in the larynx or trachea, instead of in the esophagus.

Bronchial. Bronchial foreign bodies also initially cause coughing and gagging followed by a quiet period of variable duration (up to months or occasionally, years). These children then present with cough, dyspnea, fever, recurrent pneumonias, or severe asthma a variable amount of time later (days, weeks, or months). On auscultation, wheezing or decreased air entry may be heard. Since many foreign bodies are radiolucent, plain AP and lateral chest films may not be conclusive, although air trapping, pneumonia, or atelectasis may be seen. Instead, inspiratory/expiratory views may reveal expiratory air trapping and mediastinal shift away from the affected side. Decubitus films may show an unexpected increased lucency of the affected side when that lung is in a dependent position. Fluoroscopy may be required to appreciate subtle degrees of air trapping or mediastinal shifting.

ER MANAGEMENT

Usually, removal of a foreign body in the *external auditory canal* is easily performed with suction, a wire loop, curette, or forceps. Irrigation can be used for nonvegetable objects. Drown a live insect with mineral oil or 95% alcohol, prior to removal. Occasionally, admission is necessary to remove the object under general anesthesia.

Prior to attempting to remove a *nasal* foreign body, restrain the child with the head immobilized, anesthetize the nasal mucosa with 4% lidocaine spray, shrink the edema with ½% phenylephrine nose drops, and suction the discharge to enhance visualization of the object. Use of a curette or small alligator forceps is generally successful. Alternatively, if space can be seen between the foreign body and the nasal mucosa, pass an uninflated Foley or Fogarty catheter through the involved nostril beyond the object, inflate the balloon, then pull the catheter out. Antibiotics are not required after successful removal of the foreign body.

The treatment of an *esophageal* foreign body is removal during esophagoscopy. Consult a thoracic surgeon, otolaryngologist, or gastroenterologist immediately.

The management of foreign bodies in the *larynx* or *trachea* is controversial. It is incorrect to withhold treatment if the airway is not totally obstructed, as the patient's own efforts at expulsion can ultimately lead to complete occlusion. If the patient has any degree of respiratory distress, summon an anesthesiologist and otolaryngologist and attempt an abdominal thrust. While standing behind a sitting or upright child, wrap your arms around the lower chest with the fists firmly in the epigastrium. Then apply a forceful compression, causing positive intrathoracic pressure and expulsion of the object. If the patient is supine, compress the epigastrium while kneeling over the child. Alternative maneuvers, such as suspending the child by the ankles, back blows, inserting an uninflated Foley catheter, or blindly trying to clear the airway are contraindicated, as the object might be moved into a position of total airway occlusion. Some authorities recommend chest thrusts, which can lead to sternal and rib fractures with damage to underlying organs. If the abdominal thrust is unsuccessful or if the child is seen after a latent period, consult an otolaryngologist or thoracic surgeon for removal under direct visualization. On rare occasions complete obstruction necessitates an emergency cricothyroidotomy.

Admit all children with *bronchial* foreign bodies for immediate removal by bronchoscopy and always consider the possibility that multiple objects were aspirated.

INDICATIONS FOR ADMISSION

- Esophageal, tracheal or bronchial foreign body
- Foreign body in the external auditory canal, nose or larynx that cannot be removed in the ER

REFERENCES

1. Heimlich HJ: Pediatrics 70:120–125, 1982
2. Blazer B, Naveh Y, Friedman A: Am J Dis Child 134:68–71, 1980
3. Cotton E, Yasuda K: Pediatr Clin North Am 31:937–941, 1984

Mastoiditis

INTRODUCTION

Although increasingly uncommon in the antibiotic era, mastoiditis continues to occur in all age groups, including young infants. The most common etiologies are *Streptococcus* and *S. aureus*.

CLINICAL PRESENTATION

The physical findings include swelling and erythema over the mastoid process behind the ear, along with abnormalities of the ipsilateral tympanic membrane consistent with otitis media. Classic earlobe elevation occurs in patients over 1 year of age, but displacement of the pinna down and out is seen in younger children. Fever >101°F is common.

DIAGNOSIS AND ER MANAGEMENT

Mastoid x-rays confirm the diagnosis in a child with the typical physical findings. Clouding of the mastoid air cells and temporal bone destruction due to the osteomyelitic process are evident.

Tympanocentesis is indicated to obtain fluid for Gram stain and culture, but mastoid drainage is generally necessary only if the patient is severely ill or intracranial spread of the infection (meningitis, cerebellar abscess) is suspected. Admit all children with mastoiditis and treat with a penicillinase-resistant drug such as oxacillin (100 mg/kg/day, IV for 10 days).

INDICATION FOR ADMISSION

- Mastoiditis

REFERENCE

1. Ginsburg CM, Rudoy R, Nelson JD: Clin Ped 19:549–553, 1980

Neck Masses

INTRODUCTION

Although the majority of neck masses in children are benign enlarged lymph nodes, the possibility of a malignancy is often a concern. In general, neck masses can be considered in four categories—lymph nodes (see p 267), congenital masses, benign tumors, and malignancies.

CLINICAL PRESENTATION AND DIAGNOSIS

Congenital Masses

Branchial Cleft Cyst. A branchial cleft cyst is usually not diagnosed until late childhood or early adulthood (average age 13 years) when it becomes infected. At that time a discrete, erythematous, tender, fluctuant mass is noted in the lateral neck, typically anterior to the sternocleidomastoid muscle. On occasion, there is a fistula anterior to the muscle with an orifice that drains mucus and retracts with swallowing. If the acute infection is properly treated with antibiotics, the cyst shrinks, but may reexpand during subsequent upper respiratory infections (URI).

Thyroglossal Duct Cyst. A thyroglossal duct cyst usually presents as an asymptomatic midline neck mass below the level of the hyoid bone. The sexes are affected equally and 50% of cases present prior to age 10 years. These frequently become infected and respond to antibiotics, only to reemerge during the next URI. In between, the mass is cystic or solid, nontender, and mobile. The pathognomonic feature is elevation of the mass when the tongue is protruded. Occasionally, ectopic thyroid tissue is present.

Congenital Muscular Torticollis. Congenital muscular torticollis presents at 1–2 weeks of age as a hard, nontender mass within the body of the sternocleidomastoid. Characteristically, while the head is tilted to the affected side, the child faces away from the lesion. The family may report that the baby looks in one direction only.

Benign Tumors

Cystic Hygroma. A cystic hygroma usually presents as an irregular, soft, painless, compressible lateral neck mass that transilluminates and can increase in size during straining. Fifty percent are present at birth and 90% are noted during the first 2 years of life. Massive enlargement can cause obstruction of the airway or the esophagus. Typical locations are the submental, preauricular, and submandibular areas.

Hemangioma. Hemangiomas, on the other hand, are more frequently present at birth and all are seen during the first year of life. Unlike cystic hygromas, there is a 3:1 female preponderance. Most are of the cavernous type, usually located within the parotid gland in the preauricular area. Infection or hemorrhage can cause acute enlargement and the mass becomes bluish in color when the infant is crying or straining.

Dermoid Cyst. A dermoid cyst typically is an asymptomatic, cystic midline mass located in the submental region. A *teratoma* has a similar presentation, but calcifications or teeth are often seen on x-ray.

Malignant Tumors

About one-quarter of all the malignancies of childhood occur in the neck and more than half of these are either Hodgkin disease or lymphosarcoma (pp 265–267). *Hodgkin* disease primarily (80%) presents in the upper neck as a painless, hard or firm, fixed, slowly enlarging unilateral node. Most patients are over 5 years old. Forty percent of *lymphomas* present extranodally in the neck throughout the pediatric age range, and the disease is often (40%) bilateral. Once again, a slowly growing, hard or rubbery, fixed mass is seen. Weight loss and hepatosplenomegaly are features of both diseases.

A *rhabdomyosarcoma* can originate in the nasopharynx or ear; symptoms are determined by the site. A nasopharyngeal mass presents as chronic adenoidal hypertrophy, with adenoidal facies, snoring, mouth breathing, serous otitis, and a serosanguineous nasal discharge. A mass in the ear causes chronic otitis, ear discharge, and mastoiditis. Weight loss occurs with either. Other rare neck malignancies include fibrosarcoma (mandible most common site), thyroid cancer (history of neck irradiation) and both primary (causing Horner syndrome) or metastatic (located in orbit, nasopharynx) neuroblastoma.

ER MANAGEMENT

Congenital Masses. During an acute bacterial infection, treat a *branchial cleft cyst* or *thyroglossal duct cyst* with dicloxacillin (50 mg/kg/day) or erythromycin (40 mg/kg/day) and warm soaks every 2 hours. Since these lesions have a tendency to become reinfected, refer the patient to an otolaryngologist so that elective excision can be performed. A thyroid scan is a prerequisite for thyroglossal duct excision, as the cyst may contain all of the patient's thyroid tissue. Instruct the parents of a child with a *sternocleidomastoid tumor* and torticollis to perform daily stretching exercises.

Benign Tumors. Refer patients with massive enlargement of a *cystic hygroma* or *hemangioma* causing life-threatening symptoms (airway or esophageal obstruction) or extreme disfigurement to an otolaryngologist. On occasion, a dermatologist or plastic surgeon should see the child so that cosmetic reconstruction can be planned. *Dermoids* and *teratomas* require elective excision.

Malignant Tumors. Suspect a malignancy when the mass is hard, nontender, and slowly growing. There may be systemic signs and symptoms (fever of unknown origin, weight loss, generalized lymphadenopathy, hepatosplenomegaly), or a clinical picture consistent with a mass in the ear or nasopharynx. Obtain a CBC with differential, platelet, and reticulocyte counts, order a chest x-ray to rule out mediastinal or hilar node enlargement. Admit the patient, and consult an oncologist.

INDICATIONS FOR ADMISSION

- Airway or esophageal obstruction
- Suspected malignancy

REFERENCES

1. May M: Ear Nose Throat J 57:12, 1978
2. Pounds LA: Pediatr Clin North Am 28:841–844, 1981

Otitis Externa

INTRODUCTION

Otitis externa, also known as swimmer's ear, is primarily a disease of the summertime, when swimming leads to the trapping of excess moisture in the external auditory canal. This results in a mixed infection of fungi (*Aspergillus* and *Candida*) and bacteria (*Pseudomonas, Klebsiella,* and *Enterobacter*).

CLINICAL PRESENTATION AND DIAGNOSIS

Frequently a history of recent swimming is elicited. The patient is usually afebrile, but complaining of ear pain or itching with a thick white, yellow, or green discharge from the external canal. Extreme discomfort upon pulling on the pinna or tragus distinguishes the discharge of otitis externa from that caused by a perforated tympanic membrane. Otoscopy reveals an erythematous, swollen canal often obscuring the tympanic membrane.

ER MANAGEMENT

Treatment consists of frequent use of antibiotic drops with a broad gram-negative spectrum. Some preparations also include a steroid to treat the inflammation (Corticosporin) or a topical anesthetic (Lidosporin). If a perforation of the tympanic membrane cannot be ruled out, use a medication that is less caustic to the middle ear structures (Corticosporin suspension rather than the solution). Instill the drops either directly into the canal or onto a cotton earwick which insures the delivery of the drug throughout the external canal. In addition, keep the canal dry; further swimming is not permitted unless the child wears earplugs. Complete resolution takes 5 to 7 days.

REFERENCE

1. Farmer HS: Am Fam Physician 21:96, 1980

Periorbital and Orbital Cellulitis

INTRODUCTION

The orbital septum, a fibrous membrane running from the periosteum of the orbital bones to the tarsal plates, separates the skin and subcutaneous tissues from intraorbital structures. Although the clinical pictures are similar, differentiation of periorbital (preseptal) cellulitis from orbital (postseptal) cellulitis is critical.

Periorbital cellulitis can be divided into two types. Most frequently, the infection is preceded by a break in the skin (insect bite, laceration, impetigo) and the causative organism is *S. aureus* or *Streptococcus*. Less commonly, the source of infection is hematogenously spread *H. influenzae* type B, with no loss of the normal skin barrier. The former infection can occur in any age patient, while the latter is more likely in patients 6 months to 5 years old. Orbital cellulitis is uncommon before 7 years of age and is associated with ethmoid and frontal sinusitis.

CLINICAL PRESENTATION

Both periorbital and orbital cellulitis present with warm, tender, erythematous lid swelling. Mild to moderate conjunctival swelling and hyperemia with a mucoid to purulent discharge may be present. Fever and regional adenopathy are seen, as well. However, there are a number of clinical features that differentiate these two diseases. With an orbital cellulitis, there may be proptosis, limitation of extraocular movement, a change in visual acuity, ocular pain, and chemosis. These do not occur with a periorbital infection. Also, the patient with an orbital cellulitis may have symptoms of a sinusitis, including cough, supra- or retrorbital headache, and nasal discharge.

With the common (nonbacteremic) type of periorbital cellulitis there is often a history of some break in the skin, or the entry point is noted on examination. These patients rarely have the toxic appearance, lethargy, or high fever seen in children with a bacteremic *Haemophilus* infection. These latter children are at risk for other foci of infection (meningitis, septic arthritis, pneumonia, etc).

DIAGNOSIS

Lid erythema and swelling may be caused by *conjunctivitis* (viral or bacterial), in which marked palpebral conjunctival injection is seen or an *insect bite* in which a punctum may be identified. *Allergic reactions* and the *nephrotic syndrome* can cause lid swelling (generally bilateral) in the absence of erythema, tenderness, or fever. Proptosis can be secondary to an *orbital tumor* although the signs of infection are usually absent, while hyperthyroid *exophthalmos* can be confused with proptosis.

If the distinction between periorbital and orbital infection is not clear on clinical grounds, sinus films may document the ethmoid or frontal involvement of an orbital cellulitis. However, there is a high incidence of false-positive sinus radiographs in periorbital cellulitis (probably secondary to the overlying cutaneous edema). If the diagnosis remains in doubt, a CAT scan of the orbit can confirm the presence of a postseptal infection.

ER MANAGEMENT

As mentioned above, when the distinction is not clear, radiologic studies can be helpful. However, since an orbital cellulitis can be a life-threatening illness, errors in diagnosis should be on the side of overdiagnosis of postseptal infection.

Periorbital cellulitis can be treated on an outpatient basis in an afebrile older patient who has clearly had a loss of skin integrity, is not at risk for *Haemophilus* bacteremia and does not appear toxic. Antistaphylococcal antibiotics (dicloxacillin 50 mg/kg/day; erythromycin 40 mg/kg/day; or cephradine 25 mg/kg/day all divided qid) for 10 days and warm compresses are effective. However, the patient must be instructed to return immediately if the infection is spreading or any of the signs or symptoms of an orbital cellulitis develop. Otherwise, follow-up is in 24 hours.

The treatment of *H. influenzae* type B periorbital cellulitis is intravenous ampicillin (100 mg/kg/day) and chloramphenicol (75 mg/kg/day), both divided q 6h. Obtain a CBC and blood culture, and if the child is lethargic or has meningeal signs, perform a lumbar puncture prior to initiating therapy.

Treat an orbital cellulitis with the same doses of intravenous ampicillin and chloramphenicol. Abscess drainage is indicated if there is extreme toxicity, evidence of intracranial spread (focal neurologic findings), or no response to 24 hours of antibiotics.

INDICATIONS FOR ADMISSION

- Periorbital cellutitis associated with fever or toxicity, or unresponsive to 24 hours of oral antibiotics
- Suspected *H. influenzae* periorbital cellulitis
- Orbital cellulitis

REFERENCE

1. Gellady AM, Shulman ST, Ayoub EM: Pediatr 61:272–277, 1978

Pharyngitis, Peritonsillar Abscess, and Retropharyngeal Abscess

INTRODUCTION

Pharyngitis is most often caused by viral infections (adenovirus, parainfluenza, rhinovirus, coronavirus, CMV, Ebstein-Barr virus, Coxsackie A virus). Approximately 20–30% of cases are caused by group A beta hemolytic streptococci ("strep throat"). Other rare etiologies include mycoplasma, toxoplasmosis, tularemia, and diphtheria (very rare).

Occasionally, a bacterial pharyngitis can evolve over several days into a *peritonsillar abscess* (quinsy). This usually occurs in an adolescent who has not been treated with antibiotics; however adequate antimicrobial coverage does not always prevent this complication. Virtually all cases of peritonsillar abscess are caused by group A beta hemolytic strep, although uncommonly *S. aureus* and anaerobes are implicated.

CLINICAL PRESENTATION AND DIAGNOSIS

The older child usually complains of pain on swallowing or difficulty swallowing, while the toddler may be noted to refuse food or fluids or to be more cranky than usual. Other findings may include drooling or difficulty handling secretions, fever, and tender anterior cervical lymphadenopathy. Infection of the pharynx causes erythema of the tonsils and tonsillar pillars with or without tonsillar enlargement.

Viral Infections. Low-grade fever (<101°F) associated with conjunctivitis, rhinitis or cough suggests a *viral* etiology. Tonsillar exudate, toxicity, and severe difficulty swallowing are unusual findings in the common viral infections. However, adenovirus can cause a severe pharyngitis with exudate and ulceration. Thick, gray mucus covering the tonsils can be seen in infectious mononucleosis and mono-like syndromes (CMV, toxoplasmosis, tularemia). Generalized lymphadenopathy, hepatosplenomegaly, an erythematous maculopapular rash, fever (>101°F), periorbital edema, urticaria, upper airway obstruction secondary to lymphoid hyperplasia, and severe, prolonged lethargy are other manifestations of infectious mononucleosis, especially in the adolescent.

Streptococcal Infection. Streptococcal infection is suggested by whitish-yellow exudate on the tonsillar surface, palatal petechiae, a red uvula, tender anterior cervical lymphadenopathy, and fever >101°F. On occasion, associated severe abdominal pain and vomiting can mimic acute appendicitis. Marked dysphagia, with drooling and difficulty breathing, occurs less frequently. Streptococcal scarlet fever causes an erythematous sandpaper-like rash (scarlatiniform) with perioral pallor. Other findings are a "strawberry" tongue, accentuation of the rash in the flexion creases (Pastia lines), and, late in the course, periungual desquamation.

Peritonsillar Abscess. A peritonsillar abscess causes extreme discomfort and toxicity, with difficulty opening the mouth (trismus), drooling, a "hot potato" muffled voice and swelling of the uvula with deviation to the unaffected side. The tonsil is markedly erythematous and covered with a whitish exudate. Anterior and superior to the tonsil there is swelling of the soft palate which is sometimes fluctuant. The head may be tilted to the unaffected side and tender cervical adenopathy is usually prominent on the same side as the abscess.

Retropharyngeal Abscess. A retropharyngeal abscess, now rare, is a complication of streptococcal pharyngitis, trauma, or an extension of a vertebral osteomyelitis (most often caused by *S. aureus*). The child presents with drooling, respiratory distress, and hyperextension of the neck. On examination the posterior pharyngeal wall can be seen bulging anteriorly.

ER MANAGEMENT

Swab the tonsils and pharynx, and perform a slide latex particle agglutination test (Culturette Brand). If the slide test is positive, swab the tonsils again and plate the secretions on 5% sheep blood agar. Also obtain a throat culture if the slide test is not readily available.

Treat pharyngitis symptomatically, with gargles, lozenges, and aspirin or acetaminophen. If the slide test or throat culture is positive for *strep,* treat with antibiotics to prevent rheumatic fever as well as to shorten the course of acute pharyngitis. Therapy consists of either one dose of intramuscular benzathine penicillin G mixed with procaine penicillin (600,000 units <60 pounds; 1,200,000 units >60 pounds) or oral penicillin VK (250 mg qid for 10 days). Oral erythromycin (40 mg/kg/day), in four divided doses for 10 days, can be given to the penicillin-allergic patient. At least 20% of *S. pyogenes* are resistant to tetracycline, while sulfonamides (including trimethoprim-sulfamethoxazole) do not reliably eradicate acute group A streptococcal infections and therefore should not be used. If a patient with a positive slide test proves to have a negative throat culture, discontinue the antibiotics.

Treat a *peritonsillar abscess* with intravenous penicillin G (50,000–100,000 units/kg/day) and, if fluctuant, incision and drainage by an otolaryngologist. A tonsillectomy is indicated 4–8 weeks after discharge to prevent recurrences. Treat a *retropharyngeal abscess* with intravenous nafcillin (100 mg/kg/day) and drainage in the operating room under general anesthesia. If these patients are allergic to penicillin, use clindamycin (25–40 mg/kg/day).

When the clinical picture is suggestive of *infectious mononucleosis* or if the child has been suffering an unusually prolonged or severe sore throat, an evaluation for mononucleosis is necessary. Obtain a white blood cell count with differential to look for atypical lymphocytosis and a mono spot test or heterophile antibody. If there is upper airway obstruction, insert a nasopharyngeal tube and give prednisone (2 mg/kg/day). The diagnosis and management of mono and mono-like illnesses is discussed on p 302.

INDICATIONS FOR ADMISSION

- Severe dysphagia preventing oral intake
- Peritonsillar or retropharyngeal abscess

REFERENCE

1. Pantell RH: PIR 3:35–39, 1984

Serous Otitis Media

INTRODUCTION

Serous otitis media is the presence of sterile, nonsuppurative fluid in the middle ear.

CLINICAL PRESENTATION AND DIAGNOSIS

Despite adequate treatment, serous otitis frequently follows an episode of acute otitis media. Usually, there are no complaints, although the patient may note decreased hearing or a subjective change in hearing quality.

On pneumoscopy, the tympanic membrane appears darkened and retracted. There may be an air–fluid level with bubbles visible behind the drum. Mobility is limited, as can be confirmed by impedance testing (retracted tympanic membrane with negative middle ear pressure).

ER MANAGEMENT

The management of serous otitis is both controversial and unsatisfactory. The empirical use of antihistamine-decongestant combinations (chlorpheniramine or brompheniramine with phenylephrine or pseudoephedrine) has been advocated by the manufacturers, although there has been no consistent documentation of any advantage of their use over a placebo.

Refer these patients to a primary care provider for a hearing evaluation, as well as assessment of the frequency of acute infections and the need for antibiotic prophylaxis.

REFERENCE

1. Cantekin EI, Mandel EM, Bluestone CD, et al: N Engl J Med 308:297–301, 1983

Sinusitis

INTRODUCTION

The paranasal sinuses develop as outpouchings of the nasal chamber. They enlarge as the child grows, so that the importance of a particular sinus varies with the age of the patient. The ethmoid cells are present at birth, while the maxillary sinuses are not clinically significant until 18–24 months and the frontals not until 6–8 years.

The organisms responsible for most cases of acute sinusitis are *Pneumococcus* and nontypable *H. influenzae*. Other etiologies include *B. catarrhalis* and *S. aureus*. Chronic sinusitis, on the other hand, is predominantly caused by anaerobes, *S. aureus*, alpha strep, and nontypable *H. influenzae*.

CLINICAL PRESENTATION

The most common signs and symptoms of acute sinusitis are cough, mucopurulent nasal discharge, and fever. The cough typically occurs at night or during naps. Children over 5 years of age may complain of a headache that is accentuated by leaning forward. Younger patients (<5 years) may have malodorous breath without any pharyngeal or dental infection. Facial pain and swelling are not as common as in adults.

DIAGNOSIS

If sinusitis is suspected, obtain radiographs (AP, lateral, and occipitomental). Complete opacification and air-fluid levels correlate well with acute sinusitis, while chronic disease is manifested by mucosal thickening (>5 mm). Transillumination is of limited value.

Various combinations of headache, cough, fever, and nasal discharge can occur with *viral URI, influenza,* or *pneumonia*. Malodorous breath may be secondary to a *dental abscess, pharyngitis,* or a *nasal foreign body*.

ER MANAGEMENT

Treat acute maxillary, ethmoid, or sphenoid sinusitis with ampicillin (100 mg/kg/day divided qid), amoxicillin (40 mg/kg/day divided tid), or if the patient is allergic to penicillin, trimethoprim-sulfamethoxazole

(8 mg TMP/kg/day divided bid) or erythromycin-sulfisoxazole (40 mg erythro/kg/day divided qid). Cefaclor (40 mg/kg/day divided tid) is useful as a second-line drug. In addition, most otolargyngologists prescribe oral decongestants (pseudoephedrine 1 mg/kg q 6h) and topical vasoconstrictors (¼% Neo-Synephrine qid; Afrin bid) for 48 hours. Continue the antibiotics for at least 14 days, but reevaluate the patient in 48–72 hours. If there is improvement, finish the antibiotic course. Otherwise, change to an alternative medication or consider consulting an otolaryngologist for sinus drainage.

Admit patient with frontal sinusitis for IV antibiotics (oxacillin and ampicillin or chloramphenicol, 100 mg/kg/day) and the adjunctive measures listed above.

Aspiration of the nasal sinuses is indicated for patients who are immunocompromised, unresponsive to medical therapy, toxic, or suffering from one of the rare intracranial complications (brain abscess, subdural empyema, cavernous sinus thrombosis) or orbital cellulitis. Chronic sinusitis, on the other hand, is best managed by drainage. In either case, nasopharyngeal cultures are of no value.

INDICATIONS FOR ADMISSION

- Frontal sinusitis
- Systemic toxicity
- Unremitting headache or incapacitating symptoms
- Orbital cellulitis or intracranial complication

REFERENCE

1. Wald ER: Pediatr Infect Dis 2:61–68, 1983

Upper Airway Infections

INTRODUCTION

Upper airway obstruction may be caused by supraglottic or subglottic infections. Noninfectious diseases that may mimic these include spasmodic croup, foreign body aspiration, and angioneurotic edema. The exclusion or diagnosis of epiglottitis is always the first consideration since immediate treatment is life saving.

CLINICAL PRESENTATION AND DIAGNOSIS

All forms of acute upper airway obstruction present with some degree of inspiratory stridor, suprasternal retractions, tachypnea, and tachycardia.

Supraglottic Conditions

In supraglottic infections, there is usually a sudden onset of fever, dysphagia, and drooling. The patient also has a muffled voice, soft stridor, and prefers to sit up.

Epiglottitis. Epiglottitis is a bacterial infection of the epiglottis and argepiglottic folds. It is almost always caused by *H. influenzae* type B, although rare cases are caused by *S. pneumoniae, S. aureus,* and group C *Streptococcus.* The disease occurs year round, primarily in children 3–7 years old, but any age child or young adult can be affected. The onset is rapid, with the development of high fever, toxicity, sore throat, dysphagia, drooling, a muffled voice, and soft stridor. Hoarseness and a barking cough are notably absent. The patient prefers to sit up, with the neck extended (''sniffing dog'' position).

The clinical picture is usually so characteristic that the diagnosis is suspected immediately and treatment instituted at once. Do not disturb the child, since any provocation (especially the use of a tongue blade) can precipitate total airway obstruction.

If the presentation is unusual (a prolonged course or a low fever), such that epiglottitis is possible, but *unlikely,* obtain a lateral neck x-ray (Fig. 5-1). In epiglottitis, the epiglottis appears ''thumb''-shaped (instead of narrow), the normal cervical lordosis is lost, and the hypopharynx is distended with air. In viral croup, the supraglottic structures are normal, but there is an infraglottic haze. If epiglottitis cannot be absolutely ruled out in the ER, treat the patient as if he or she has it (see below).

Peritonsillar Abscess. Peritonsillar abscesses (p 117) most commonly occur in older children and adolescents. Clinical findings include fever, trismus, dysphagia, drooling, and a muffled (''hot potato'') voice. Swelling of the soft palate leads to uvular deviation, and the head is often tilted away from the side of the abscess.

Retropharyngeal Abscess. Retropharyngeal abscesses (p 117) are rare, occurring primarily in children under 5 years of age. Patients complain of sore throat, fever, and dysphagia. Drooling, neck hyper-

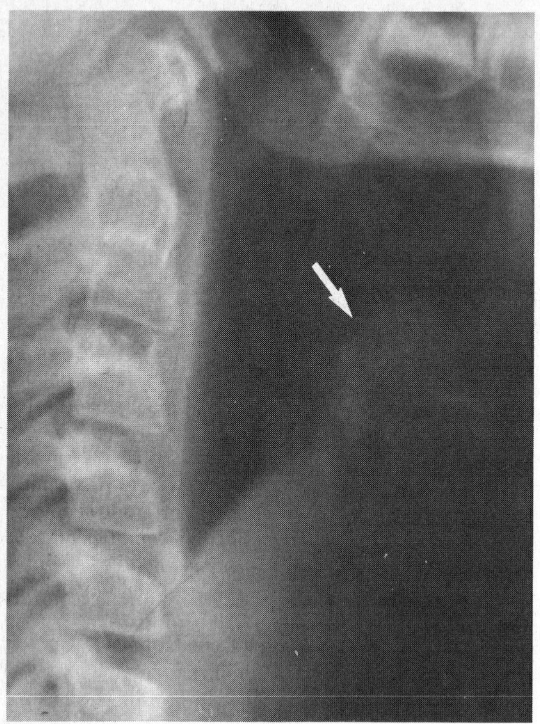

Figure 5-1. Lateral neck x-ray. **A.** Epiglottitis. (*Courtesy of Dr. H. Goldman.*)

extension, and occasionally, meningismus, occur. Bulging of the posterior pharyngeal wall can lead to airway obstruction.

Infectious Mononucleosis. Infectious mononucleosis (p 302) can present as upper airway obstruction secondary to lymphoid hyperplasia. Clinically, stridulous breathing in association with fever, exudative pharyngitis, cervical adenopathy, and fetid breath occur. An atypical lymphocytosis and a positive mono spot test suggest the diagnosis.

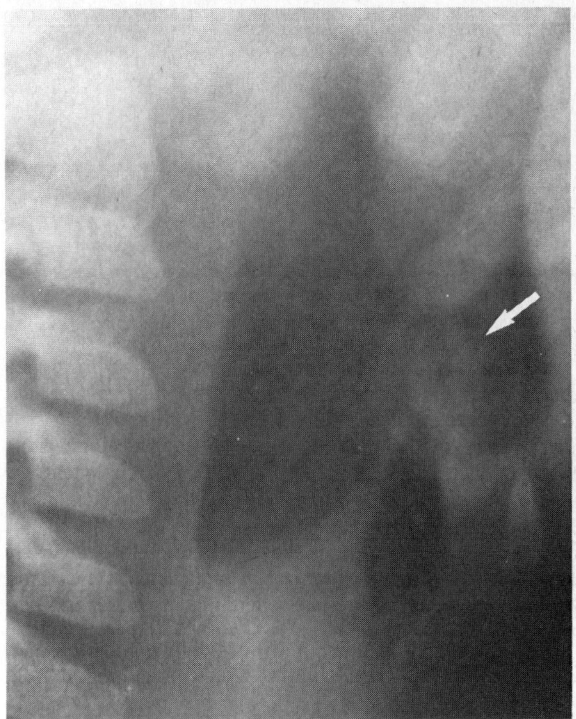

Figure 5-1. Lateral neck x-ray. **B.** Normal epiglottis. (*Courtesy of Dr. H. Goldman.*)

Angioneurotic Edema. Angioneurotic edema (see anaphylaxis, p 10) can cause acute upper airway obstruction immediately after exposure to an offending protein (bee sting, milk protein, antibiotics, contrast dye, etc). Wheezing, urticaria, and hypotension may be present.

Subglottic Conditions

Subglottic infections present more gradually, usually after a prodromal illness. There is more prominent inspiratory and expiratory stridor (secondary to tracheal edema), low-grade fever, hoarse voice (vocal cord edema), and a barking cough.

Viral Croup. Viral croup (acute laryngotracheitis) usually occurs in the fall and winter in children 3 months to 3 years of age. It is predominantly caused by parainfluenza 1 virus, although influenza A and B, RSV, and *Mycoplasma pneumoniae*, are other causative agents. Viral croup typically begins with a 12–48 hour URI prodrome of cough, coryza, and low-grade fever. The infection then spreads to the trachea and larynx, producing inspiratory and expiratory stridor, a hoarse voice, and a barking cough. The illness may last from 3 days to 2 weeks and tends to worsen at night. The diagnosis is made clinically, although in unusual cases (rapid onset with high fever) a lateral neck x-ray may be necessary to rule out epiglottitis.

Spasmodic Croup. Spasmodic croup is probably an allergic disease. It frequently occurs in patients with personal and/or family histories of asthma and allergies. A child with a mild URI awakens suddenly in the middle of the night with severe dyspnea, loud stridor, and a croupy cough. This tends to recur on successive nights. Dysphagia, drooling, high fever, and toxicity are notably absent.

Foreign Body. Consider an aspirated foreign body (p 107) in a toddler who suddenly develops respiratory distress, especially in the absence of a preceding URI. Coughing, gagging, and cyanosis may occur. Confirmation of the diagnosis may require decubitus or inspiratory–expiratory chest x-rays or chest fluoroscopy.

Bacterial Tracheitis. Bacterial tracheitis is a rare disease, probably caused by bacterial superinfection in a child with viral croup. Sudden onset of high fever, toxicity, and severe respiratory distress occur in a patient who has had croup for several days.

ER MANAGEMENT

The priority is the expedient diagnosis and treatment of epiglottitis and airway obstruction.

Epiglottitis. If epiglottitis is suspected, summon the most experienced anesthesiologist and otolaryngologist available, to meet the child in the ER. Then, with the ER physician in attendance, proceed to the operating room. Delay blood drawing and establishing an IV until anesthesia is achieved (halothane and O_2). The procedure of choice is nasotracheal intubation, although an endotracheal tube is adequate. If the airway becomes obstructed before the patient reaches the OR, attempt bag and mask ventilation. If this is unsuccessful an immediate cricothyroid puncture is indicated. After the airway has been secured, obtain a complete blood count and blood culture, start an IV, and administer antibiotics (ampicillin, 100 mg/kg/day divided qid; chloramphenicol 75 mg/kg/day divided qid)..

If epiglottitis is unlikely but still possible, obtain a lateral neck x-ray. A physician, equipped with face mask and bag, must stay with the patient at all times. Keep the child *upright* while the radiograph is being obtained.

Peritonsillar Abscess. Treat with intravenous penicillin (100,000 units/kg/day) and if necessary, incision and drainage by an otolaryngologist (p 119).

Retropharyngeal Abscess. Surgical drainage, in addition to intravenous oxacillin (100 mg/kg/day), is required (p 119).

Infectious Mononucleosis. Treat with mist, steroids (prednisone 2 mg/kg/day, divided qid), and a nasopharyngeal airway (p 304) if obstruction occurs.

Angioneurotic Edema. Treat for anaphylaxis (p 10), with subcutaneous epinephrine (0.01 cc/kg up to 0.3 cc), aminophylline, hydrocortisone, and diphenhydramine.

Viral Croup. The mainstay of therapy is humidification of inspired air, with a vaporizer, fog generator, or hot shower.

If the patient remains stridulous at rest despite humidification, arrange for admission and give racemic epinephrine (Vaponephrine) delivered via mask and nebulizer over 15–20 minutes (add 0.5 cc to 3.5 cc of normal saline). The Vaponephrine acts as a local vasoconstrictor to shrink swelling; since rebound edema can occur, hospitalization is mandatory. Obtain a CBC with differential and arterial blood gas. Intubate (preferably nasotracheally) patients with severe respiratory distress, hypoxia, or CO_2 retention. Use a tube one size smaller than usual to prevent pressure necrosis of the airway lumen.

Spasmodic Croup. Usually, only mist is required. Often, the child improves remarkably while en route to the hospital. Caution the parents that the disease may recur the following night.

Bacterial Tracheitis. Treat in an intensive care setting with intravenous antibiotics (oxacillin 100 mg/kg/day) and intubation and mechanical ventilation.

Foreign Body Aspiration. Arrange for immediate removal by an otolaryngologist or thoracic surgeon (p 107).

INDICATIONS FOR ADMISSION

- Epiglottitis, peritonsillar abscess, retropharyngeal abscess, bacterial tracheitis, and foreign body aspiration
- Viral croup with persistent stridor at rest or severe respiratory distress
- Infectious mononucleosis with upper airway obstruction

REFERENCES

1. Maze A, Bloch E: Anesthesiol 50:132–145, 1979
2. Levison H, Tabachnik E, Newth CJ: Curr Prob Pediatr 12(3):38–65, 1982
3. Davis HW, Gartner JC, Galvis AG, et al: Pediatr Clin North Am 28:859–880, 1981

Upper Respiratory Infections

INTRODUCTION

Upper respiratory infections (URI), caused by numerous organisms, are responsible for countless ER visits. In some cases, however, a URI is the initial presentation of a more serious illness (otitis, pneumonia, sepsis, meningitis, etc).

CLINICAL PRESENTATION

Most often, the patient is afebrile, or has a low-grade temperature, with watery or mucoid rhinorrhea. Sneezing, coughing, and conjunctival injection are other features. Infants may have decreased appetite or noisy breathing.

DIAGNOSIS

Inquire about fever, cough, appetite, vomiting, treatments given at home, diarrhea, and whether anyone else at home is ill. Perform a complete examination, looking for evidence of bacterial infection such as purulent nasal discharge, *otitis media,* nuchal rigidity, and decreased breath sounds or rales (*pneumonia*). Also, ascultate for wheezing suggestive of an *asthma* attack or *bronchiolitis.*

A patient with high fever (>103°F) or a toxic appearance does not have an uncomplicated URI.

ER MANAGEMENT

Although there are myriad over-the-counter cold remedies, there are little data proving efficacy. The recommendations of bedrest, fluids, and aspirin or acetaminophen are valid. For infants, give normal saline nose drops (2 drops in one nostril at a time), followed by aspiration with a bulb syringe. A vaporizer may be helpful for all age groups.

An antihistamine-decongestant combination (½ tsp qid <4 yr; 1 tsp qid >4 yr) may be used in children older than 1 year.

REFERENCES

1. Lampert RP, Robinson DS, Soyka LF: Pediatrics 55:550, 1975
2. Walson PD: Pediatrics 74(Suppl):937–941, 1984

6

Endocrine Emergencies

Acute Adrenal (Addisonian) Crisis

INTRODUCTION

Acute adrenal crisis (Addisonian crisis) is a life-threatening emergency secondary to a relative or absolute deficiency of cortisol and aldosterone. The most common cause of an inadequate adrenal response to stress is congenital adrenal hyperplasia (inherited defect in steroid biosynthesis). Other etiologies include autoimmune adrenalitis (Addison's disease), iatrogenic insufficiency (following supraphysiologic glucocorticoid administration), fulminant infections, tuberculosis, and pituitary (adrenocorticotrophic hormone [ACTH]) deficiency. The precipitant of a crisis may be a bacterial or viral infection, fever, or a dental or surgical procedure. Immediate treatment is essential.

CLINICAL PRESENTATION

The presentation of acute adrenal crisis is nonspecific, so that the key to making the diagnosis is to suspect it. Weakness and lethargy are followed by gastrointestinal symptoms of anorexia, nausea, epigastric abdominal pain, and vomiting. Dehydration with decreased skin turgor and tachycardia ensue. Finally, the patient becomes hypotensive with postural (orthostatic) vital sign changes: a fall of the systolic pressure by 20 mm Hg or more or a pulse increase of at least 20 beats/min (see pp 12–13). Less common findings are petechiae and purpura (overwhelming sepsis) and hypoglycemic seizures. A subtle, but valuable, clinical finding is increased skin pigmentation in areas of friction (knees, elbows, knuckles) and sunlight exposure (face, neck), the skin creases, oral mucosa, and conjunctiva. This is indicative of ACTH hypersecretion, and suggests primary adrenal insufficiency. The course of adrenal crisis can be fulminant and sudden death can occur.

The prominent gastrointestinal symptoms of adrenal crisis can resemble *gastroenteritis* (diarrhea is frequent), an *acute abdomen* (involuntary guarding and rebound tenderness), or *intestinal obstruction* (bilious vomiting).

If acute adrenal crisis is suspected, do not delay treatment while awaiting the results of confirmatory laboratory tests. Prior to starting therapy, however, obtain blood for a cortisol level, complete blood count (CBC) with differential, and electrolytes. A serum cortisol sample at this time is of crucial importance for later confirming the diagnosis. In shock from any other etiology, the cortisol level is high, as compared to low or normal during Addisonian crisis. Acute adrenal insufficiency causes hyponatremia and hyperkalemia with a decreased Na/K ratio (usually less than 30).

ER MANAGEMENT

Once the diagnosis is suspected, institute treatment without delay. Adrenal function can be assessed when the acute emergency has passed.

Acute Crisis

1. Fluid: Clinical assessment tends to underestimate the severity of the hypovolemia. Consider the patient to be at least 10% dehydrated and give 20 cc/kg of normal saline intravenously over 30 minutes. Repeat the bolus until the patient becomes normotensive. Once the blood pressure is normal, continue with D5 normal saline for patients with salt-losing adrenal insufficiency. Change non-salt losers to D5 ½ to ⅔ normal saline. Total fluid requirements are in the range of 2000–3000 cc/M^2/day. Add potassium once the patient voids; cortisol administration will rapidly induce kaliuresis and a fall in the serum potassium.
2. Hydrocortisone: Give Solucortef 3 mg/kg (or 100 mg/M^2) intravenously (IV) at once, followed by 1 mg/kg IV every 6 hours.
3. If shock persists, a plasma expander such as plasmanate or a vasopressor such as dopamine may be needed. Vascular response to pressors requires that adequate cortisol replacement be given first.

4. Mineralocorticoid replacement is not necessary in the ER, provided that normal saline is used as the intravenous fluid, since high-dose glucocorticoids have sodium-retaining action. For a salt loser, once the vital signs are stabilized, desoxycorticosterone acetate (DOCA), 1–2 mg intramuscularly (IM), diminishes the salt requirement and permits use of ½ to ¾ normal saline. Do NOT give Florinef (9-alpha-fluorocortisol).
5. Identify and treat the underlying cause, if any.
6. Monitor the patient carefully for the complications of therapy, including fluid retention, hypernatremia, hypokalemia, hypertension, pulmonary edema, and congestive heart failure.

Minor Illness

Stressed patient receiving *maintenance* cortisol: double or triple the usual oral dose of hydrocortisone.

Patient taking *pharmacologic* amounts of steroids to treat an illness (asthma, nephrotic syndrome, idiopathic thrombocytopenia purpura [ITP], leukemia, collagen vascular disease): Double the dose if the stress is *trauma* or *surgery*. If the stress is a *serious infection,* lower the steroid dose to a level that prevents adrenal crisis, but does not suppress defense mechanisms (50 mg/M^2/day).

The patient has *recently completed a* 10-day or longer *course* of steroids: Give 2–3 mg/kg/day of hydrocortisone.

If any of the above at-risk patients are nauseated, but without vomiting or orthostatic vital sign changes, give 1 mg/kg of hydrocortisone IM. Do not send the patient home unless the vital signs are normal and oral intake is adequate without vomiting.

INDICATIONS FOR ADMISSION

- Addisonian crisis
- Vomiting, inadequate oral intake, or postural vital sign changes in a patient known to be at risk for adrenal insufficiency
- Family is unable to reliably give stress doses of steroids

REFERENCES

1. Kaplan SA: Pediatr Clin North Am 26: 77–89, 1979
2. Fass B: Pediatr Clin North Am 26: 251–256, 1979

Diabetes Insipidus

INTRODUCTION

Deficiency of antidiuretic hormone (ADH, vasopressin) causes central diabetes insipidus (DI), a syndrome characterized by an inability to concentrate urine. A variety of acquired hypothalamic lesions can cause DI, including tumors, basilar skull fractures, neurosurgical complications, granulomatous diseases, vascular lesions, meningitis, and encephalitis. In approximately 50% of cases, however, no obvious primary lesion can be found (idiopathic, congenital defect).

Nephrogenic DI is caused by renal unresponsiveness to ADH. The defect may be congenital or secondary to hypercalcemia or hypokalemia.

CLINICAL PRESENTATION

DI causes renal loss of water, which leads to enormous urine output and acute thirst. If water intake is not increased, the patient rapidly develops hypernatremic dehydration. Infants are usually irritable but eager to suck, often exhibiting a distinct preference for water over milk. Constipation, unexplained fever, and failure to thrive are other presentations.

Older children usually present with abrupt onset of polyuria and polydipsia and later develop nocturia, enuresis, vomiting, and constipation. These patients may compensate for water loss by increasing intake, but this is not possible in infants and unconscious patients. In awake patients, dehydration is unusual unless the thirst center is involved. Central nervous system (CNS) manifestations such as irritability, altered consciousness, increased muscle tone, convulsions, and coma are secondary to hypernatremia and correlate with both the degree and rapidity of rise in the sodium level.

DIAGNOSIS

The cardinal diagnostic features are a high rate of dilute urine flow in the presence of clinical signs of dehydration, urine osmolality that is distinctly less than the serum, and a mild to marked degree of serum hypernatremia and hyperosmolality. Urine-specific gravity is usually 1.001 to 1.010 in the presence of an increased serum osmolality. However, if there is severe dehydration or a low glomerular filration rate (GFR), urine output decreases and osmolality increases to a level above serum osmolality. This may temporarily disguise the diagnosis.

DI must be differentiated from other causes of polyuria such as *compulsive water drinking* (hypothalamic lesion involving thirst center, psychogenic), osmotic diuresis (*diabetes mellitus, chronic renal insufficiency*) and *urinary tract infection*. A large urinary volume can lead to bladder distension which can mimic *obstructive uropathy*.

ER MANAGEMENT

If DI is suspected, obtain urine for specific gravity, dipstick and microscopic analysis, sodium and potassium, and culture. Obtain blood for electrolytes, calcium, blood urea nitrogen (BUN) and creatinine, and osmolality. The diagnosis is confirmed if hypernatremia and hyperosmolality, with or without dehydration, are found in association with large volumes of dilute urine (specific gravity $\leq$1.010 and urine osmolality $\leq$ serum). Admit patients who are conscious and not dehydrated for further diagnostic testing and management, including a complete neurologic examination with visual fields evaluation and CT scan.

If the patient is dehydrated, hyperpyrexic, or has a depressed level of consciousness, treatment may be necessary in the ER. Give intravenous vasopressin, either 1–2 U/M^2 or a constant infusion of 0.5 mU/kg/min. Infuse maintenance fluids, along with one-half of the excess urine output as solute-free water (D5W).

INDICATION FOR ADMISSION

- New onset or symptomatic

REFERENCES

1. Robinson AG: New Engl J. Med 294:507–511, 1976
2. Czernichow P, Pomarede R, Basmaciogullari A., Bravner R. Rappaport R J Pediatr 106:41–44, 1985

Diabetic Ketoacidosis

INTRODUCTION

Diabetic ketoacidosis (DKA) may be the initial presentation of a new diabetic or a complication in a previously diagnosed patient. Infection is the most common precipitating factor, but trauma, pregnancy, emotional stress, and poor diabetic control are other causes. An absolute or relative insulin deficiency is present, along with increased levels of counterregulatory hormones (glucagon, cortisol, growth hormone, and catecholamines) leading to deranged metabolism, hyperglycemia, osmotic diuresis, hypertonic dehydration, and ketoacidosis.

CLINICAL PRESENTATION

The patient usually presents with abdominal pain, nausea, vomiting, dehydration, and tachypnea. The history often reveals polydipsia, polyuria, nocturia, enuresis, and, with new onset diabetes, recent weight loss. Characteristic Kussmaul breathing (deep sighing breathing) can be present, but respirations may be depressed if the patient is severely acidotic (pH <6.9).

DIAGNOSIS

In the known diabetic, consider DKA when the patient complains of abdominal pain, vomiting, or malaise. In patients presenting for the first time, the diagnosis may be more difficult to make (Table 6-1).

In addition to metabolic acidosis and ketonemia, significant hyperglycemia (>500 mg%) is common, although DKA can be associated with a glucose of 200–300 mg%.

Although sodium stores are depleted, the serum concentration of sodium may be low, normal, or high, depending on water balance. The measured sodium is lower than the true value because of both the shift of water to the extracellular space (Na^+ decreases 1.6 mEq/L per 100 mg% rise in glucose) and the increased lipid and protein in the serum (pseudohyponatremia). In addition, the low sodium level may reflect water retention secondary to increased secretion of antiduiretic hormone.

TABLE 6-1. DIFFERENTIAL DIAGNOSIS OF DKA

Metabolic acidosis
- Severe gastroenteritis with hypovolemia
- Salicylate poisoning
- Other ingestions
  - Ethanol
  - Methanol
  - Ethylene glycol
  - Phenformin
  - Isoniazid
  - Iron

Coma
- Hypoglycemia
- Sedative hypnotic or narcotic overdose
- Lactic acidosis
- Nonketotic hyperosmolar coma
- CNS trauma, infection, bleeding

Polyuria, nocturia, abdominal pain
- UTI

Hyperglycemia
- Salicylate poisoning (hyperglycemia is moderate, <300 mg%)
- Hypernatremia
- Stress
- Sepsis

Ketonuria
- Fasting states
- Gastroenteritis with vomiting
- Anorexia of any etiology
- Salicylate poisoning

In spite of a total body potassium deficit, the initial serum potassium concentration is usually normal or elevated. The causes are hemoconcentration and a shift of potassium to the extracellular space secondary to the acidosis and insulin deficiency. The measured potassium rises 0.6 mEq/L for every 0.1 drop in the pH, so that a low initial potassium level (<3.5 mEq/L is an unusual and ominous finding.

Finally, in the absence of infection, the total white count may be elevated to 18,000–20,000/mm^3 in patients with DKA, secondary to the increase in catecholamines.

ER MANAGEMENT

Initial blood tests include electrolytes, serum glucose, CBC, venous pH and osmolality. Blood cultures are necessary in patients with fever, and an SMA 12 and aspirin level may be indicated when the diagnosis is not evident. In 20–60% of patients in DKA, the amylase, CPK, and transaminases (serum glutamic-oxaloacetic transaminase [SGOT], serum glutamic-pyruvic transaminase [SGPT]) are transiently elevated. Obtain a rhythm strip to assess the degree of hyperkalemia (symmetrical, narrow based, peaked T-waves), and continuously monitor the electrocardiogram (ECG).

The initial objective is to restore circulatory volume and improve perfusion. Consider the patient to be 10% dehydrated and give 20 cc/kg of normal saline (no glucose or potassium) over 30 minutes. The initial fluid bolus may lead to considerable improvement in serum glucose, osmolality, and pH, so repeat these tests and obtain an ECG before changing the intravenous therapy. If the patient remains hypotensive, repeat the saline bolus. Otherwise, if the patient is normotensive and not tachycardic, and the serum osmolality and sodium have started to correct, change the solution to half-normal saline (replace the fluid deficit over 24–48 hours).

Continue the normal saline for patients with high osmolality (>310 mosm/kg) and low serum sodium (<130 mEq/L). Severe hyperosmolality (>340) may cause stupor. However, consider other causes, particularly *sepsis*, if the patient is stuporous without hyperosmolality. If the osmolality cannot be directly measured, it can be estimated by the equation:

$$\text{Osmolality} = 2(\text{Na}^+ + \text{K}^+) + \text{glucose}/18 + \text{BUN}/2.8$$

Hypokalemia with subsequent cardiac arrest are complications of improper bicarbonate use and delay in potassium administration. Following the initial saline bolus, if the patient has voided and the T-waves on the ECG are not peaked, add 40 mEq of potassium (one-half as K^+ acetate and one-half as K^+ phosphate) to each liter of hydrating solution. However, patients with severe hypokalemia ($K^+ < 3.5$ mEq/L) may need as much as 80 mEq/L.

Consider giving bicarbonate only if the pH is less than 7.1. Even then it is rarely needed since the initial saline bolus usually has a marked effect on restoring a normal pH. Because bicarbonate diffuses slowly into the CSF while CO_2 enters readily, a paradoxical cerebral acidosis can develop as a result of excessive use of bicarbonate. However, if after the fluid bolus the pH remains below 7.1, 1–2 mEq/kg of $NaHCO_3$ may be added to 500 cc of IV fluid and infused at twice the maintenance rate. Once the pH is above 7.1, no further alkali is required.

Restoring euglycemia too rapidly may increase the risk of acute cerebral edema. Therefore, treat DKA with a continuous insulin infusion if the serum glucose is greater than 600 mg% or the patient is acidotic (pH <7.25). Make the insulin solution by adding 1 cc of U100 regular insulin (100 units) to 500 cc of normal saline. Fill and flush the tubing with 50 cc of this solution before it is connected to the patient's IV line in order to saturate all the insulin-binding sites in the tubing. The solution contains 0.2 U/cc; infuse it at a rate of 0.1 U/kg/hr (0.5 cc/kg/hr). The blood glucose should fall at a linear rate of 75–100 mg%/hr. When the serum glucose approaches 250 mg% and the pH is >7.25, change the IV solution so that the patient receives about 1 unit of insulin for every 5 grams of glucose (0.05 U/kg/hr of insulin; D5 ½ normal saline with 40 mEq K^+ at 1½ maintenance). This will maintain the glucose level at a steady state.

The insulin infusion is indicated until the acidosis is corrected (pH 7.25–7.3). If the patient is acidotic (pH <7.25) but not hyperglycemic, add more glucose (D7.5) to the IV solution or increase the rate (twice maintenance) rather than slowing the insulin infusion. While the patient is in the ER check the pH, glucose, and osmolality every hour, and the blood pressure, heart and respiratory rates, urine output, and mental status more frequently. A flow sheet helps to organize these data.

INDICATIONS FOR ADMISSION

- Newly diagnosed diabetes
- pH <7.25, serum glucose >600 mg%, or altered level of consciousness
- Persistent vomiting

REFERENCES

1. Kreisberg RA: Ann Int Med 88: 681–695, 1978
2. Sperling MA: Pediatr Clin North Am 31: 591–610, 1984

Hypercalcemia

INTRODUCTION

Hypercalcemia is defined as a serum calcium greater than 11 mg/dl. Etiologies include increased bone resorption (primary hyperparathyroidism, parathyroid hormone [PTH], secreting tumors, skeletal metastases, immobilization, thyrotoxicosis), increased GI absorption (vitamin D intoxication, milk-alkali syndrome, idiopathic hypercalcemia of infancy), and decreased renal calcium clearance (thiazide use). Traumatic vaginal delivery of large infants can cause subcutaneous fat necrosis, with resultant transient hypercalcemia.

CLINICAL PRESENTATION AND DIAGNOSIS

Patients with hypercalcemia usually have a nonspecific presentation with weakness, listlessness, irritability, gastrointestinal complaints (nausea, vomiting, constipation, abdominal pain), and neurologic symptoms (confusion, depressed consciousness). Hypotonia is a striking finding in the newborn, while older children may have failure to thrive. Hypercalcemia can cause a renal concentrating defect, with resultant polyuria, polydipsia, and dehydration. Long-standing hypercalcemia may lead to band keratopathy, nephrocalcinosis, renal stones, and renal failure with hypertension. Idiopathic hypercalcemia of infancy is associated with elfin facies (upturned nose, long philthrum, hypotelorism, receding chin, and strabismus), supravalvular aortic stenosis, and mental retardation.

The diagnosis is confirmed by documenting an elevated serum calcium, usually in association with a decreased phosphorous, normal or increased alkaline phosphatase, and hyperchloremic acidosis. X-rays may reveal generalized bone demineralization, lytic skull lesions (''salt and pepper'' pattern), nephrocalcinosis, or renal stones.

ER MANAGEMENT

Treatment must be instituted at once, as CNS and renal damage can result from hypercalcemia. If the calcium is ≥ 11 mg/dl or the patient is symptomatic, give intravenous isotonic saline at 2–3 times the maintenance rate along with furosemide (1 mg/kg q 6h) to induce calciuresis and natriuresis. Corticosteroids (prednisone 2 mg/kg/day or hydrocortisone 10 mg/kg/day) also help decrease the serum calcium, although the effect may take 4–5 days and rebound hypercalcemia can occur if steroids are discontinued abruptly. Consult an endocrinologist prior to instituting other therapies (calcitonin, mithramycin, dialysis).

INDICATION FOR ADMISSION

- All patients requiring treatment for hypercalcemia

REFERENCE

1. Tsang RC, Noguchi A, Steichen JJ: Pediatr Clin North Am 26: 223–249, 1979

Hyperthyroidism

INTRODUCTION

Hyperthyroidism primarily affects children over 6 years of age. Etiologies include diffuse toxic goiter (Grave's disease), thyroiditis with hyperthyroidism, thyroid adenoma, and exogenous overdosage. Thyroid storm, or thyroid crisis, is a life-threatening complication rarely seen in children.

CLINICAL PRESENTATION

The onset of hyperthyroidism is usually gradual, with complaints of palpitations, sweating, heat intolerance, weight loss, tremor, nervousness, increased frequency of bowel movements, and emotional lability. Short attention span, inability to concentrate, and deteriorating school performance may occur. Other complaints are attacks of dyspnea and, in the postmenarcheal female, oligomennorrhea and irregular menses.

On examination, virtually all patients (except in the case of exogenous overdose) have a goiter, and a characteristic bruit may be heard over the thyroid. The skin is warm and moist, and tachycardia (particularly increased resting pulse), increased systolic blood pressure, and widened pulse pressure are common. Eye signs include lid retraction, staring, lid lag, and exophthalmos. Deep tendon reflexes are often brisk, and fine tremors of the eyelids, fingers, or tongue may be noted.

There is usually an abrupt onset of thyroid storm and in 50% of cases there is an identifiable precipitating factor (stress, infection, surgery, childbirth). The clinical picture includes high fever (up to 106°F), cardiovascular symptoms (tachycardia, arrhythmia, heart failure, shock), neurologic findings (agitation, tremor, psychosis, stupor, coma), and gastrointestinal complaints (abdominal pain, vomiting, diarrhea, hepatomegaly, jaundice).

DIAGNOSIS AND ER MANAGEMENT

In most cases the diagnosis is confirmed by radioimmunoassay of T_3 and free T_4; treatment can be deferred until these values are known. If thyroid storm is suspected, immediate treatment is indicated after blood is obtained for thyroid function tests (T_3, FT_4, thyroid stimulating hormone [TSH], T_3 resin uptake, antithyroid antibodies). To decrease thyroid hormone levels, give propylthiouracil (PTU, an initial loading dose of 600–1200 mg/day divided q 8h) followed 1 hour later by iodide (Lugol solution, 10 gtts tid PO). In addition, give propranolol (0.1 mg/kg/day IV divided q 6h or 4 mg/kg/day PO divided q 6h) to inhibit the peripheral hormone effects.

Treat thyrotoxicosis not in crisis with PTU (5–10 mg/kg/day divided q 8h) and propranolol (1–2 mg/kg/day divided q 6 to 8h).

INDICATION FOR ADMISSION

- Thyroid storm

REFERENCE

1. Howard CP, Hayles AB: Clin Endocrinol Metabol 7: 137, 1978

Hypocalcemia

INTRODUCTION

Hypocalcemia is defined as a total serum calcium <7 mg/dl or an ionized calcium < 2.5 mg/dl. Most cases are secondary to hyperventilation-induced alkalosis. Other less common causes include hypoparathyroid conditions (idiopathic, pseudo-, transient neonatal, post-thyroid surgery, hemochromatosis), renal failure, massive transfusion, hypomagnesemia, hyperphosphatemia, and vitamin D deficiency or defective metabolism.

CLINICAL PRESENTATION

Clinical manifestations of hypocalcemia primarily involve the nervous system. Mild hypocalcemia may cause nonspecific hyperreflexia, but more serious decreases lead to muscle cramps and paresthesias of the hands, feet, and perioral region. Hypocalcemic tetany causes flexion at the wrists and metacarpophalangeal joints, extension at the interphalangeal joints, and adduction of the thumb into the palm (carpopedal spasm). In the extreme situation, seizures and life-threatening laryngospasm can occur.

Other nonspecific symptoms include lethargy, emotional lability, irritability, imparied cognition, vomiting, and diarrhea. The newborn may present with poor feeding, vomiting, lethargy, and cyanosis.

Characteristic physical findings include the Chvostek sign, facial muscle twitching elicited by tapping the facial nerve just anterior to the ear, and Trousseau sign, wrist and finger flexor contraction elicited by maintaining a blood pressure cuff at just above systolic pressure for 2–3 minutes.

Typically, the hyperventilating patient is an adolescent who presents with anxiety, tachypnea, and labored breathing in addition to the signs of hypocalcemia. There may be a history of recent emotional upset or past psychiatric disorders.

Findings in patients with long-standing hypocalcemia may include cataracts, metastatic calcifications, dry and brittle hair and nails, and dry, coarse skin.

DIAGNOSIS

Hyperventilation. Suspect hyperventilation-induced hypocalcemia in an older child or adolescent who presents with tachypnea, anxiety, and carpopedal spasm. Obtain an arterial or venous blood gas. An increased pH, decreased pCO_2, and normal O_2 (arterial) confirm the diagnosis and rules out other causes of hyperventilation, such as *hypoxia* or a *metabolic acidosis*.

Other Etiologies. Immediately obtain an ECG for corrected QT (QTc) interval. This is calculated by dividing the actual QT interval by the square root of the R-R interval. The QTc should not exceed 0.425.

In addition, obtain blood for total or ionized calcium, electrolytes, phosphorous, magnesium, and alkaline phosphatase. There must be a low serum total calcium (<7 mg/dl) or ionized calcium (<2.5 mg/dl) to confirm the diagnosis of hypocalcemia.

Phosphorous is elevated (> 6 mg/dl in young child; >5 mg/dl in older child) in *hypoparathyroidism,* but low in vitamin D deficiency. Alkaline phosphatase is generally normal in hypoparathyroidism, but elevated in *vitamin D deficiency*.

Moniliasis or increased skin pigmentation suggests *autoimmune hypoparathyroidism,* while a round face, stocky build, mental retardation, and short fourth and fifth metacarpals and metatarsals suggest *pseudohypoparathyroidism*.

ER MANAGEMENT

Hyperventilation. Instruct the patient to breath in and out slowly into a paper bag. This causes rebreathing of CO_2 leading to a decreased serum pH and thus, an increased ionized calcium. Occasionally, sedation with hydroxyzine (0.5 mg/kg/dose) or diphenhydramine (1–2 mg/kg/dose) is required.

Once the hyperventilation has stopped, try to discover the precipitating cause. Reassure the patient and family as to the benign nature of the episode and arrange for primary care follow-up within 1 week.

Other Etiologies. Give symptomatic patients (seizures, laryngospasm, tetany) 10% calcium gluconate (1–2 cc/kg) slowly intravenously, while continuously monitoring the ECG. Cessation of the symptoms, along with shortening of the QTc interval, are the endpoints of ER therapy. A continuous intravenous infusion or repeated bolus infusions may be required in an intensive care setting.

Treat nonsymptomatic patients with oral calcium (75 mg/kg/day of elemental calcium, divided q 6h).

INDICATIONS FOR ADMISSION

- Symptomatic patients (except hypoventilating patients)
- Asymptomatic patients with a first episode of hypocalcemia

REFERENCES

1. Tsang RC, Steichen JJ, Chan GM: Crit Care Med 5: 56, 1977
2. Missri JC, Alexander S: JAMA 240: 209, 1978

Hypoglycemia

INTRODUCTION

Hypoglycemia is an abnormally low blood glucose concentration. For children and infants over 72 hours old, the lower limits of normal glucose values are 40 mg/dl in capillary or whole blood and 45 mg/dl in plasma or serum.

Although there are many etiologies of hypoglycemia (Table 6-2), it is most commonly secondary to insulin overdose in a diabetic or fasting in a nondiabetic under 8 years of age.

CLINICAL PRESENTATION

Neonates present with jitteriness, apnea, cyanosis, irregular respirations or tachypnea, hypotonia, seizures and an abnormal cry. Infants and older children can have gastrointestinal symptoms (hunger, nausea, abdominal pain) or neurologic complaints (headache, speech and vision disturbances, weakness, anxiety, behavior changes, short attention span, ataxia, seizures, coma). These symptoms may occur with or without sweating, pallor, or tachycardia (catecholamine excess).

TABLE 6-2. ETIOLOGIES OF HYPOGLYCEMIA

Decreased Glucose Intake	Ingestions
Fasting	Alcohol
Malnutrition	Salicylates
Malabsorption	Oral hypoglycemic agents
Hormone Deficiencies	Propranolol
Growth hormone	Other Etiologies
Cortisol	Sepsis
Glucagon	Ketotic hypoglycemia
Thyroid hormone	Islet cell adenoma
Liver Disease	
Fulminant hepatitis	
Reye syndrome	
Glycogenoses (type I, III)	
Galactosemia	
Fructosemia	

DIAGNOSIS

If hypoglycemia is suspected or the patient has an altered mental status or seizures, estimate the blood sugar with a dextrostix or chemstrip BG. Confirm the hypoglycemia with a laboratory determination (preferably in a grey-top tube).

If the patient is not a known *diabetic*, obtain blood for cortisol, growth hormone, and insulin prior to any treatment. Also, obtain blood for liver function tests, alanine (decreased in *ketotic hypoglycemia*), lactate (increase suggests *inborn error of metabolism*), serum electrolytes, ketone bodies (negative in *hyperinsulinism,* positive in ketotic hypoglycemia), venous pH, and thyroid function tests. Test the urine for ketone bodies and reducing substances.

If the symptoms followed a meal, determine whether *fructose* or *galactose* was the sole sugar consumed. Ask about possible *alcohol or oral hypoglycemic agent ingestion*. The family history may reveal other infants with hypoglycemia or metabolic acidosis. Vomiting suggests *acidosis, gastroenteritis, food poisoning,* or *acute liver disease*.

Short stature, microphallus, and midline defects (cleft palate, single maxillary central incisor) suggest *hypopituitarism*. Increased skin pigmentation may indicate compensatory ACTH release (*primary adrenal insufficiency*). Hepatomegaly occurs in *glycogen storage diseases,* inborn errors of carbohydrate metabolism, and *liver disease,* but not in ketotic hypoglycemia.

ER MANAGEMENT

Regardless of etiology, the treatment of hypoglycemia is glucose. Give the older child 1–2 cc/kg of 50% glucose (0.5–1 g/kg) intravenously. The dose for small children is 2–4 cc/kg of D25; give neonates a smaller bolus (1–2 cc/kg of D25). Follow bolus therapy with a continuous infusion of 10% glucose, with maintenance electrolytes, at a maintenance rate. If the blood glucose falls below 40 mg/dl, change to 15 or 20% glucose.

If the hypoglycemia persists, give glucagon (30–50 μg/kg, up to 1 mg IV, IM, or subcutaneously) and hydrocortisone (Solu-cortef, 100 mg/m^2 for infants, 3 mg/kg for children IV). However, glycemic response to these hormones requires adequate amounts of substrates.

INDICATIONS FOR ADMISSION

- Hypoglycemic episode in a nondiabetic
- Hypoglycemia in a diabetic if the cause is unclear or self-destructive behavior is likely

REFERENCE

1. Pagliara AS, Karl IE, Haymond M, Kipnis DM: J Pediatr 82: 365–374, 558–577, 1973

7

Environmental Emergencies

Burns

INTRODUCTION

The evaluation of a burn injury includes an estimation of the percent of body surface area involved, the thickness or depth of skin burned, and the presence or absence of associated injuries such as smoke inhalation, fractures, and head injury.

First-Degree Burns

CLINICAL PRESENTATION AND DIAGNOSIS

Evidence that a burn is first degree (eg, sunburn) includes the lack of blister formation, intact light touch and two-point discrimination, an inability to peel the skin, and blanching when the skin is depressed.

ER MANAGEMENT

Treatment includes aspirin (10 mg/kg q 4h) for pain relief and topical application of over-the-counter sunburn remedies or soothing lotions. Hydrocortisone cream (1%) may help reduce the pain and swelling of severe sunburn, especially if the eyelids and face are involved. Cool showers and baths are also helpful. The severe itching that occurs after a few days can be treated with diphenhydramine (5 mg/kg/day, divided qid).

Second-Degree Burns

CLINICAL PRESENTATION AND DIAGNOSIS

Second-degree burns can be divided into superficial partial-thickness burns that heal spontaneously in less than 2 weeks and deep partial-thickness burns that should be considered for skin grafting. Distinguishing them may be difficult, as both are likely to have blisters. The deeper burns, however, have less erythema, may not have as much fluid transudation across the injured dermis, and may contain areas of extremely pale or white, blanched dermis. All second-degree burns are extremely painful, and the skin appendages (hair follicles, sweat glands, sebaceous glands) remain intact.

ER MANAGEMENT

Immediate treatment involves the application of cold water or ice compresses which relieve the pain and stop the burning process. Give aspirin (10 mg/kg q 4h) by mouth or rectum as well as parenteral analgesia such as IV Demerol (2 mg/kg) and Phenergan (1 mg/kg) or intravenous (IV) morphine sulfate (0.05–0.1 mg/kg), if needed. Gently clean the burned surface with saline-soaked gauze. Trim broken blisters, but unbroken blisters must be left intact. After cleaning and debriding, cover small superficial partial thickness burns with a medicated gauze dressing such as Xeroform, secured in place with a gauze wrap. For deeper injuries, treat with an antibiotic cream such as Silvadene, wrap with gauze, and evaluate daily until the healing process is progressing nicely. If Silvadene is used, it must be completely removed and reapplied at each dressing change. Encourage the patient to bathe daily at home.

Third-Degree Burns

CLINICAL PRESENTATION AND DIAGNOSIS

Full-thickness injuries are generally caused by fire (clothing burned) or prolonged contact with boiling water or hot grease. There is little edema and no pain. Unless very small (<2% of the body surface area), these wounds must be treated with surgical excision of the dead tissue and skin grafting.

ER MANAGEMENT

Emergency management includes cooling the burned surface, cleaning the wound with saline and gauze, removing loose or hanging skin, and applying Silvadene.

GENERAL APPROACH TO THE BURNED CHILD

1. Stop the burning process by removing burned clothing and copiously lavaging all chemical burns. Apply cold soaks to reverse the thermal gradient and relieve pain (second-degree burns), but avoid hypothermia.
2. Assess and maintain ventilation and check for inhalation injury (singed naries or vibrissae; carbonaceous material in the hypopharynx or sputum; edema or inflammation of the pharynx, glottis, or larynx). Obtain an arterial blood gas (ABG), and if there are any of the above findings, immediately perform laryngoscopy to rule out involvement of the epiglottis or vocal cords. Obtain a carboxyhemoglobin level in all closed-space fire victims using 0.5 cc heparinized venous or arterial blood.
3. Initiate intravenous fluid therapy. Immediately place a large bore intravenous catheter in all children with second-degree burns in excess of 15% body surface area (BSA) or third-degree burns in excess of 5% BSA. Calculate the 24-hour fluid requirement for the first day after injury as 4 cc of normal saline or lactated Ringer per percent BSA burn per kilogram body weight. Adjust this figure to obtain a urine output of 1 cc/kg/hr in children under 30 kg. Give half the estimated fluid requirement in the first 8 hours and the other half over the subsequent 16 hours. Make these calculations after the IV has been started and urine output has been established and documented. Insert an indwelling urinary catheter using aseptic technique into any burn victim needing IV fluids in order to strictly monitor output (see p 14). Discard any urine obtained when the catheter is inserted as this may have been in the bladder before the burn injury. Check the urine (with dipstix) for hemoglobin or myoglobin.
4. Take a careful history. Inquire about the cause of the burn, the presence or absence of preexisting illnesses, chronic medications, and allergies. Ascertain the tetanus immunization status; give 0.5 cc of tetanus toxoid booster if the last immunization was

more than 5 years ago. If there has been no previous immunization, give 0.5 cc of tetanus immune globulin.

5. Estimate the extent and depth of burn using the "rule of 9s" in patients > 10 years of age. According to the "rule of 9's," the body surface is divided as follows:

head	=	9%
arm	=	9%
anterior trunk	=	18%
posterior trunk	=	18%
leg	=	18%
genitals	=	1%

For younger patients, subtract 0.5% from each leg for every year less than 10 and add the same percentage to the head.

6. Perform a careful physical examination. Check for corneal injury using fluoroscein stain. Ophthalmologic consultation is required if the lids are burned, the eyelashes have been singed, or any eye damage is suspected. Evaluate the patient for associated injuries, especially fractures and head trauma.
7. Insert a nasogastric tube and attach it to suction if the burn exceeds 20% of the total BSA or if there is nausea, vomiting, or abdominal distention.
8. Give pain medication as needed (IV morphine sulfate, 0.05–0.1 mg/kg every 30–60 minutes).
9. Obtain a throat culture to rule out streptococcal infection, although prophylactic antibiotics are not indicated.
10. Perform the initial burn wound care as described above.
11. Examine the patient for circumferential injuries. Remove all rings, bracelets, and restrictive clothing. Look carefully for signs of impaired circulation including cyanosis, impaired capillary refill, changes in sensation, deep tissue pain, or paresthesias. If present, call a burn surgeon or a plastic surgeon as an escharotomy may be necessary.

INDICATIONS FOR ADMISSION

- First-degree burns: Total body involvement or if the patient is at risk for dehydration

- Second-degree burns: More than 5% BSA in infants, 10% BSA in children, or 15% BSA in adolescents; or when the burns involve critical areas such as the face, hands, feet, or genitalia.
- Third-degree burns: More than 2% of the BSA; or involvement of the face, hands, feet, or perineum.
- Transfer the patient to a special burn treatment facility if the total burn is >20%, or if there are third-degree burns covering >10% of the BSA
- Patients with any size burn whose family seems unable or unwilling to cope with recommendations for care and follow-up, or if the circumstances surrounding the injury seem suspicious

REFERENCE
1. Moncrief SA: JAMA 242: 72–74, 179–182, 1979

Electrical Injuries

INTRODUCTION

Electrical injuries are worse with high voltage, alternating current, and wet skin. Most preadolescent electrical injuries involve low voltage (110 volts) household current, while high voltage injuries occur predominantly in adolescents. Electrical burns are painless, bloodless, necrotizing lesions that can extend a variable distance. They occur at the sites of entrance and exit of the current, and tissue damage is more widespread than the initial presentation suggests.

CLINICAL PRESENTATION AND DIAGNOSIS

Low Voltage. Small children, especially toddlers, frequently sustain low voltage electrical injuries when they insert objects (pins or keys) into household sockets or chew electrical cords. A localized burn injury to the corner of the mouth and tongue or to the fingers and hand results, unless the child is able to conduct electricity, in which case low voltage current might be fatal. Fortunately, conduction is rare so these are usually limited injuries.

High Voltage. These occur most commonly in adolescents who have contacted power lines or live third rails. Extensive tissue coagulation at the entrance or exit wound sites, flash burns, and contact surface arc burns of the axilla, antecubital fossa, popliteal fossa, and groin may be seen. These injuries are associated with hemolysis, rhabdomyolysis, fractures, ruptured viscera, direct burns of the lung or viscera, cardiac arrhythmias, neurologic injuries, and renal failure.

ER MANAGEMENT

Low Voltage. Perform a careful physical examination looking for evidence of both an entrance and an exit wound and obtain an electrocardiogram (ECG). For the common electrical burn of the mouth, local wound management includes oral hygiene and direct wound care with topical bacitracin. When significant portions of the lips, especially the oral commissures are involved, consult a plastic surgeon or oral surgeon. If localized tissue charring is present and there is any suggestion of injury to underlying structures, immediate surgical consultation is necessary. The parents are to be warned that between 5 and 14 days after the injury, as the burned tissue begins to separate, bleeding from the labial artery may occur. This bleeding can be controlled by local pressure but occasionally requires a trip to the ER for suture ligation.

High Voltage. As soon as the patient arrives in the ER, make a quick assessment of the adequacy of ventilation, obtain an ECG, and secure an IV. If the patient is in cardiopulmonary arrest, intubate and begin cardiopulmonary resuscitation (CPR, pp 1–9). Initial blood tests include an arterial blood gas (ABG), complete blood cell count (CBC), blood type, electrolytes, and cardiac enzymes. Use lactated Ringer as the initial IV fluid, infused rapidly enough to maintain a brisk urine output of 3–6 cc/kg/hr. Do not add potassium for the first 24 hours. If transportation to a specialized facility is necessary, the intravenous lines should be well secured and the urine output established prior to transfer.

The initial management also includes placement of a nasogastric tube and a Foley catheter and performing a urine dipstix. The presence of hemoglobin or myoglobin on urine dipstix is an indication of significant deep tissue injury and predicts renal failure unless a brisk urine output is quickly established. To prevent precipitation of pigment in the renal tubules, keep the urine pH alkaline (> 7) by infusing sodium bicarbonate (1 mEq/kg) over 30 minutes. Use mannitol (0.5 g/kg) only if urine output remains inadequate after large volumes of IV fluid have been given.

The emergency surgical management of high voltage electrical injuries includes debridement of all obviously devitalized skin, muscle and bone; fasciotomy of all involved muscle compartments; and reduction and stabilization of all long-bone fractures.

INDICATIONS FOR ADMISSION

- The presence of both an entrance and an exit wound (confirms conduction of the current through the body)
- Any neurologic dysfunction, including a history of loss of consciousness, or any abnormalities on initial ECG (overnight observation)
- Children with mouth burns, unwilling or unable to take adequate fluids by mouth
- All high voltage electrical injuries

REFERENCES

1. Gifford GH Jr, Marty AT, MacCallum DW: Pediatrics 47: 113–119, 1971
2. Burke J, Quinby W, Bondoc C, et al: Am J Surg 133: 492–497, 1977

Frostbite

INTRODUCTION

Frostbite is a cold injury in which there is actual freezing of the tissues. The ambient temperature must be less than 22°F; wind, moisture, and local pressure are predisposing factors.

CLINICAL PRESENTATION

Frostbite is most common in the lower extremities, although the hands, ears, and nose may be involved. Incipient frostbite presents as blanching of the skin. This is followed by superficial frostbite, in which the involved area becomes numb, waxy white, and firm. Upon warming there is erythema, swelling, and pain. Deeply frostbitten skin appears bluish-white and hard, and becomes mottled-blue, swollen, and extremely painful upon warming. Vesicles and bullae form within 6–24 hours.

DIAGNOSIS

The clinical presentation along with a history of cold exposure makes the diagnosis obvious. However, early in the course, superficial and deep frostbite may appear very similar. Good prognostic signs after rewarming include intact pinprick sensation, warmth, clear vesicles that extend to the tips of the digits, and the absence of cyanosis. Cyanosis, the absence of edema, and hemorrhagic blebs that do not extend to the digit tips are poor prognostic signs.

ER MANAGEMENT

Rapidly warm the affected areas by immersion into a tepid bath (105–110°F) for 20–40 minutes. Since the water cools rapidly, monitor with a thermometer and repeatedly add hot water, taking care to avoid contact between the hotter water and the involved skin. Afterwards, apply sterile gauze wraps without rupturing any blebs, obtain plastic surgery consultation, and admit the patient for at least 48 hours of observation. Prophylactic antibiotics are not indicated.

INDICATION FOR ADMISSION

- All cases of frostbite

REFERENCE

1. The Medical Letter 22: 112–114, 1980

Heat Excess Syndromes

INTRODUCTION

Heat cramps, heat exhaustion, and heat stroke are seen primarily in hot weather. Heat cramps occur most commonly in inadequately conditioned athletes who tend to have higher sweat sodium than well-conditioned individuals.

Heat exhaustion occurs after prolonged standing or exercise in hot weather. Volume-depleted patients (diarrhea, diuretic use) are at particular risk, as vasodilation accentuates the intravascular hypovolemia.

Heat stroke can result from excess heat production (exertional heat stroke), secondary to extreme activity compounded by poor conditioning, nonbreathing sweat suits, and amphetamines. Alternatively, there may be impaired heat dissipation (classic heat stroke), as seen in epidemics during prolonged stretches of hot, humid, windless weather. In this type, the patient cannot dissipate heat to a surrounding environment that is warmer than body temperature, while high humidity and windlessness impair the effectivess of sweating. Classic heat stroke is most common in patients who are sedentary, chronically ill, taking sweat inhibiting anticholinergics (phenothiazines, tricyclics), or have no access to air conditioning.

CLINICAL PRESENTATION

Leg and occasionally abdominal *heat cramps* are seen after intense exercise in hot weather. Although the cramps may be severe, they are not dangerous.

Heat exhaustion victims complain of nausea, vomiting, headache, piloerection, and dizziness; fainting may ensue. A low-grade fever may be present.

Heat stroke presents with hyperthermia (>105°F) and neurological abnormalities (headache, ataxia, confusion, seizures, coma). Exertional victims may be dry or soaked with sweat. They may suffer from disseminated intravascular coagulation, rhabdomyolysis, renal failure, and lactic acidosis. Classic heat stroke victims have dry skin. Either form may show cardiovascular collapse from volume depletion and/or vasodilation.

DIAGNOSIS

Suspect the heat excess syndromes during hot weather. The diagnosis of heat cramps is usually made by the history (cramping during exertion), while heat exhaustion may resemble a *syncopal episode* or severe *gastroenteritis*. However, the history of standing or activity in hot weather usually suggests the diagnosis.

Similarly, the diagnosis of exertional heat stroke is evident from the history of extreme hot weather activity in a diaphoretic patient. Suspect classic heat stroke during a prolonged heat wave in a patient with some predisposing factor. Heat stroke may resemble overwhelming *sepsis* and *meningitis*. Evaluate every hyperthermic patient for signs of a serious infection (meningeal signs, petechial or purpuric rash), especially if there is no response to the treatment outlined below.

ER MANAGEMENT

Heat cramps: Treat with rest, muscle stretching, and saline solution (NS 10 cc/kg IV, Pedialyte or Gatorade PO).

Heat exhaustion: Intravenous saline (10–20 cc/kg) and resting in a cool place is usually all that is required.

Heat stroke: The treatment is cooling as *rapidly* as possible. Use ice, ice baths, cold water, alcohol, or fans, but discontinue the effort when the temperature has dropped to 102°F. Heat stroke victims (both forms) require intravenous rehydration with normal saline. Adolescents may require as much as 5 liters over the first 24 hours..

Obtain a CBC, electrolytes, blood urea nitrogen (BUN) and creatinine, urinalysis (for pigment), and ECG. Use lidocaine (1 mg/kg) for ventricular arrhythmias and phenytoin (10–15 mg/kg slow IV) for seizures.

INDICATION FOR ADMISSION

- Heat stroke

REFERENCE

1. Clowers GHA, O'Donnell TF Jr: N Engl J Med 291: 564–567, 1974

Hypothermia

INTRODUCTION

Hypothermia, a core temperature of 35°C (95°F) or less, is usually caused by accidental exposure. Infants are at particular risk, because of their large BSA, lack of fat insulation, inadequate shivering and inability to avoid the cold. Prolonged out of hospital resuscitation and cold water immersion are common causes of hypothermia, and drug and alcohol ingestion are predisposing factors in adolescence.

Although most cases of accidental exposure are seen in winter, hypothermia may occur during wet, windy, spring or fall weather. Hypothermia may develop within minutes in a cold water immersion victim, or require days in a neonate in a poorly heated home.

CLINICAL PRESENTATION

The initial response is vasoconstriction with shivering, teeth chattering, and clumsiness. Below 90°F shivering ceases, the patient is apathetic and disoriented, the pulse and blood pressure fall, and there may be a variety of arrhythmias (atrial fibrillation and sinus bradycardia are most common). Lethargy and a depressed gag reflex, combined with cold induced bronchorrhea and capillary damage, predispose to aspiration pneumonia. Below 86°F coma ensues, along with unreactive pupils, absent doll's eyes, areflexia, and imperceptible vital signs.

DIAGNOSIS

Consider a patient with cold skin, altered mental status, and bradycardia to be hypothermic until proven otherwise. Since the diagnosis of hypothermia rests on measuring the core temperature, insert a thermocouple probe 3–5 cm into the rectum.

Many authorities consider the J- or Osborne wave on ECG to be pathognomic for hypothermia. This is a "camel hump" appearing immediately after the QRS complex.

When a hypothermic patient arrives in the ER, investigate for precipitating and complicating factors such as *alcohol* or *drug intoxica-*

tion (barbiturates, phenothiazines), *near drowning, head trauma, sepsis,* or *hypoglycemia*. Consider other causes of hypothermia, such as *hypothyroidism*, and *Addison disease*, when a patient fails to respond to rewarming measures with a rise in core temperature of at least 1°C per hour.

ER MANAGEMENT

Because of the difficulty in distinguishing between hypothermia and death, the hypothermic patient should not be considered dead until "warm (>32°C) and dead."

Therapy consists of supportive measures and rewarming. Resuscitate cold water immersion victims unless there is dependent lividity, and continue the effort until the patient shows no response after warming. Since the cooled heart has a lowered fibrillation threshold, handle and move these patients cautiously and do not introduce a central line into the heart.

Treat mild hypothermia (>32°C), in a patient with otherwise stable vital signs who is able to generate heat by shivering, by passive external rewarming with blankets. Use intravenous fluids and humidified O_2 warmed to 45°C. Avoid active external rewarming (hot water bottles, electric blankets) since it causes cutaneous vasodilation. This in turn allows cold peripheral blood to return to the core, leading to a paradoxical drop in the core temperature (afterdrop).

For the seriously hypothermic patient (<32°C) with unstable or absent vital signs, the treatment of choice is active core rewarming. One method is peritoneal dialysis with a commercial dialysate or normal saline, initially potassium free, at 45°C, using two catheters to speed the exchange. Other modalities are colonic, gastric, and bladder lavage with warmed fluids and cardiopulmonary bypass.

Naloxone (5 ampules) and D50 (1 cc/kg) are indicated for all patients with an altered mental status. Do not overuse the usual resuscitation drugs; their effectiveness may be limited by the patient's temperature. Ventricular fibrillation may not respond to countershock or bretylium. Rewarm the patient as rapidly as possible and repeat the countershock when the core temperature has risen 2–4°C. Remember that arterial blood gases are distorted by hypothermia (for each degree centrigrade below 37°C: the pH decreases by 0.015, the pCO_2 increases by 4.4 torr, and the pO_2 increases by 7.2 torr).

INDICATION FOR ADMISSION

• Hypothermia

REFERENCE

1. Ferguson J, Epstein F, van de Leuv J: Emerg Clin North Am 1:619–633, 1983

Inhalation Injury

INTRODUCTION AND CLINICAL PRESENTATION

Smoke inhalation causes injury by two mechanisms. The first is carbon monoxide poisoning, which is the most common cause of death in victims of house fires. Carbon monoxide poisoning results in suffocation by blocking oxygen transport (shifting the oxyhemoglobin curve to the left). The second is by direct respiratory tract damage from toxic gases such as hydrochloric acid, nitrates, sulfur dioxide, and aldehydes. These substances are released when plastics and artificial fabrics are burned and are more common in fires in industrial sites, motor vehicles, airplanes, and public places such as theaters. In addition, some burning synthetics also release cyanide, phosgene, and other substances that are immediately fatal.

Despite the intense heat generated by some fires, thermal injury to the respiratory tract is unusual because of the effective heat-dissipating capacity of the airways. Thermal injury below the vocal cords occurs only in the rare case of steam inhalation.

Acute (first 24 hours) respiratory distress is caused by upper airway edema. Clinically, hoarseness and stridor are noted. Delayed acute pulmonary insufficiency occurs secondary to either blocking of surfactant production or poisoning of the ciliated mucosal cells, impeding clearance of the lung. Particulate matter in the smoke may cause foreign body reactions in the mucosa leading to tracheobronchitis, with bronchospasm and secondary pneumonia.

DIAGNOSIS AND ER MANAGEMENT

Assessment of the cardiorespiratory status takes precedence. Institute CPR in patients requiring life support (see pp 1–9). Regardless of the presence of symptoms, give all patients at risk for carbon monoxide poisoning 100% oxygen to breath (via nonrebreathing mask) and continuously monitor the ECG. As soon as a CBC, ABG, and carboxyhemoglobin level are obtained (0.5 cc of heparinized venous or arterial blood), a careful history and more thorough physical examination can be performed.

The likelihood of significant inhalation injury is increased if the fire occurred in a closed space or the patient was trapped inside a building or exposed to steam or burning synthetics (particularly plastics). Loss of consciousness or change in mental status at the scene of the fire may occur with carbon monoxide or other toxic inhalation. The presence of chest pain, especially on inspiration, may indicate a developing pneumonitis.

On physical examination, look for facial burns, singed nares or nasal hair, soot in the hypopharynx, carbonaceous sputum, respiratory distress, stridor, hoarseness, wheezing, decreased breath sounds, or tachypnea. If any of these signs or symptoms are noted, direct laryngoscopy must be performed immediately. If erythema of the glottis or vocal cords is noted or the patient is unconscious, intubate at once (preferably nasotracheally).

Arterial blood gases may initially be normal but the presence of decreased pO_2 or increased pH (hyperventilation) suggest inhalation injury. In the presence of any of the above-mentioned physical findings, a normal chest x-ray and normal blood gases do not exclude the possibility of lung damage that may not be clinicially evident for 12–24 hours.

A carboxyhemoglobin level >10% indicates significant inhalation injury regardless of partial pressure of oxygen. The treatment of a COHb >20% is hyperbaric O_2. If a chamber is unavailable, continue 100% 0_2 until the COHb level is ≤5%. Also treat patients with levels below 20% if they have specific neurologic symptoms (including depressed level of consciousness) or cognitive defects, were found unconscious at the scene of the fire, or are pregnant.

If it is clear that an inhalation injury has occurred, immediate bronchoscopy is indicated to evaluate the lower airway as well as to facilitate lavage and removal of foreign bodies and toxic chemicals from the tracheobronchial tree. For severe inhalation injury, give a bronchodilator (IV aminophylline 6 mg/kg loading bolus, then 0.9–1.3 mg/kg/hr), mucolytic agents (Mucomyst) and ventilatory support (3–5 mm of positive end expiratory pressure [PEEP]) as rapidly as possible. The use of steroids and antibiotics are contraindicated as primary treatments for inhalation injury in the ER.

INDICATIONS FOR ADMISSION

- Evidence of smoke inhalation injury (productive cough, wheezing, carbonaceous sputum) or a high probability of having sustained such injury
- Patients who meet the criteria for therapy with hyperbaric oxygen, for 24 hours of observation after the treatment is completed

REFERENCE

1. Stone HH: J Pediatr Surg 14: 48 1974

Insect Bites and Stings

INTRODUCTION

Insect bites and stings usually cause a local reaction. However, systemic reactions can occur, especially after Hymenoptera stings (honeybees, wasps, hornets, fire ants) in susceptible patients.

CLINICAL PRESENTATION

Reactions to insect bites and stings can be classified as immediate (within 2 hours) or delayed (after 2 hours). Immediate reactions may be local or systemic.

Immediate Reactions. These are most often local, with sharp pain, followed by erythema and swelling at the sting site. Local reactions usually last 24–48 hours and they can be extensive, although all involved skin is contiguous with the sting site. *Systemic* reactions occur at locations that are not contiguous with the sting site. These may be mild, with itching and urticaria, or severe, consisting of anaphylaxis with hypotension, wheezing, laryngeal edema, and shock. Severe systemic reactions usually occur within 1 hour of the bite or sting.

Delayed Reactions. These can occur after a 1-week interval. They present as large local reactions, serum sickness (fever, arthralgia, urticaria, lymphadenopathy), and, rarely, peripheral neuritis or vasculitis.

DIAGNOSIS

The diagnosis is usually made by history or by the typical appearance of a local reaction, particularly during the warm weather months. A *cellulitis* may look similar, but usually a bacterial infection does not abruptly appear over several hours. Also, a cellulitis may be associated with fever, lymphangitic streaking, local lymphadenopathy, leukocytosis, and an elevated erythrocyte sedimentation rate (ESR).

Consider other etiologies, such as *drugs* (penicillins, sulfonamides, contrast dyes) and *foods* (shellfish, eggs) in patients with systemic reactions. Try to ascertain whether the insect was a member of the Hymenoptera order and inquire about a history of allergies and any previous systemic reactions to insect stings.

ER MANAGEMENT

Local reactions: Remove the stinger (if still in place), cleanse the site, apply ice or cool compresses to the area, and give oral diphenhydramine (5 mg/kg/day divided qid). If the erythema has continued to spread during the 24 hours after the bite or sting, consider the wound to be infected; start an antistaphylococcal antibiotic (dicloxacillin 50 mg/kg/day or cephradine 25 mg/kg/day) and recommend warm compresses every 2 hours.

Systemic reaction: Treat mild reactions (itching, urticaria) with oral hydroxyzine (2 mg/kg/day divided qid). The management of severe systemic reactions is the same as for anaphylaxis (p 10). This includes intravenous and local epinephrine (each dose is 0.01 cc/kg of

1:1000), a tourniquet around the sting site, intubation (if necessary), intravenous fluids, intravenous aminophylline (6 mg/kg bolus), and intravenous hydrocortisone (10 mg/kg). Refer these patients to an allergist for evaluation and possible immunotherapy.

INDICATION FOR ADMISSION

- Anaphylactic reaction

REFERENCE

1. Fikar CR: Pediatrics 68: 744, 1981

Near Drowning

INTRODUCTION

Most childhood drowning results from either bathing accidents (infants, epileptics) or swimming accidents (young children). Trauma, alcohol or other drug use, and immersion hypothermia may endanger more experienced swimmers.

CLINICAL PRESENTATION

About 90% of drowning victims aspirate water, and aspiration of vomitus or particulate matter is commonplace. Hypertonic ocean water draws fluid from the plasma into the alveoli, whereas hypotonic fresh water rapidly enters the circulation and impairs surfactant function. Both types of fluid aspirations result in heavy lungs, distended alveoli, interstitial and alveolar hemorrhage, and pulmonary vascular congestion.

Despite the shifts in plasma volume, hypo- or hypervolemia is rarely significant in patients surviving to reach hospital. Central nervous system dysfunction is primarily secondary to hypoxemia, with resultant seizures or depression of sensorium. Pneumonia, lung abscess, and empyema may occur after the initial 24 hours.

DIAGNOSIS

For most submersion victims the diagnosis is obvious. However, unnoticed *head or cervical spine trauma* may dramatically alter the outcome. Therefore, assume that victims rescued from shallow water have a head or neck injury and immobilize the head until the cervical spine is cleared clinically and radiographically.

FIELD AND ER MANAGEMENT

Appropriate field management is most important in determining outcome. Perform a basic life support survey looking for responsiveness, spontaneous breathing, airway patency, and circulation. If no respirations are present, open the airway.

When cervical spine injury is suspected, the chin lift or jaw thrust (pp 1–9) are the preferred maneuvers. If mouth to mouth ventilation fails to inflate the lungs, sweep the oropharynx with your fingers. In older children or adolescents who still have airway obstruction, perform an abdominal thrust (p 108). After opening the airway, initiate artificial ventilation as well as closed chest massage, if no central pulse is felt. When supplemental oxygen is available, use the maximum concentration. Intubate patients who require closed chest massage, remain comatose, or threaten their airway with vomitus. Start an IV, and give 1 cc/kg of 50% dextrose and naloxone (5 ampules) to comatose patients after obtaining blood for a CBC, type and cross, and electrolytes. Monitor the patient electrocardiographically.

Once the patient has arrived in the ER, measure the vital signs and reasses the airway. Perform a careful neurologic examination and consider occult hemorrhage if hypotension persists after adequate oxygenation. Send an ABG and prepare to intubate patients who are hypoxemic, despite 100% oxygen by mask. Suction intubated patients to remove vomitus, secretions, particulate debris, and aspirated fluid. Obtain a chest x-ray, as well as a CBC, type and cross, glucose, BUN, and electrolytes, if these were not drawn in the field.

Aggressively treat victims of cold water submersion (<40°F), and warm patients with core temperatures below 90°F, using heated peritoneal dialysis (p 160) before discontinuing resuscitative efforts. Antibiotics and steroids are not routinely indicated for submersion victims. Fever and leukocytosis are common within the first 24 hours and do not imply a need for antibiotics, although all near-drowning victims must be watched for deterioration of gas exchange within 24 hours of submersion as well as for the development of pulmonary infection (purulent sputum, a fever spike after the initial resolution, a rising white count after the initial peak).

INDICATION FOR ADMISSION

- All submersion victims

REFERENCE

1. Kaizer KW: Emerg Clin North Am 1: 643–652, 1983

appendicitis DD–

- sickle cell crisis
- AGE
- Mesenteric Lymphad
- pyelo/stones
- Intussusepn
- Enteric dup
- HSP
- peritonitis
- basal pneumonia
- Ruptured ectopic
- mittleschmerz
- Endometriosis
- PID
- HUS
- IBD
- Leukemic ileocecal syn
- NEC
- Hirshsprung

Pelvic mass–

- Ectopic preg
- TOA
- Hydrometrocolpus
- ovary torsion/cyst

8

Gastrointestinal and Liver Disorders

Abdominal Pain

INTRODUCTION

Abdominal pain is an extremely common symptom, caused by a multitude of both abdominal and extraabdominal disorders. Although most cases are secondary to minor viral infections, care must be taken to rule out serious illnesses, such as appendicitis, intestinal obstruction or perforation, pelvic inflammatory disease (PID), ectopic pregnancy, sickle cell crisis, and urolithiasis.

CLINICAL PRESENTATION

Spasm or distention of an abdominal organ usually causes poorly localized and ill-defined visceral pain, often accompanied by nausea and vomiting. Upper gastrointestinal tract pathology commonly causes epigastric discomfort, proximal colonic disease is perceived as periumbilical pain, and distal colonic pain is referred to the hypogastrium. Stimulation of the parietal peritoneum is reflected as localized and defined somatic pain, often associated with reflex muscle spasm and aggravated by movement or cough.

Other clinical findings depend on the etiology, but may include fever, rash, pharyngitis, tachypnea and rales, jaundice, dysuria, and diarrhea.

DIAGNOSIS

Although there are many causes of acute abdominal pain, a careful history and physical examination will usually confirm an etiology, so that laboratory examinations often are not necessary.

Ascertain the character, duration, timing, severity, and localization of the pain, as well as factors that influence the discomfort (meals, posture). Intermittent, crampy pain is characteristic of *intestinal obstruction,* while a constant, aching pattern might be secondary to *vascular insufficiency* or *localized inflammatory processes.* Recurrent or chronic abdominal pain may be *functional* or caused by *constipation, lactose intolerance,* or *inflammatory bowel disease.* In general, the further the pain is from the umbilicus, the greater the likelihood of an underlying organic lesion. In addition, the severity of the pain is not always a reliable guide to the seriousness of the condition.

Other useful information includes the frequency and character of vomiting or bowel movements, if any. In *viral gastroenteritis,* vomiting and fever usually precede the abdominal pain and diarrhea. The presenting symptom of intestinal obstruction is usually abdominal pain, which is then followed by vomiting, possibly bilious. Bloody diarrhea suggests an infectious disease (*Salmonella, Shigella*) or a surgical abdomen (*intussusception, Meckel diverticulum*). Ask about fever, pharyngitis, respiratory symptoms, trauma, urinary symptoms, pica, history of sickle cell disease, travel out of the country, and emotional stress.

While the abdominal examination is of paramount importance, a careful and complete physical examination is necessary. Pharyngitis, pulmonary rales, jaundice, costovertebral angle tenderness all suggest specific etiologies for the abdominal pain.

First, observe the abdomen for evidence of prior surgery, trauma, petechiae or ecchymoses, rash, abdominal distention, or malnutrition. Auscultation may be significant for the high-pitched tinkling bowel sounds of mechanical obstruction or the absence of sounds of a paralytic ileus. Gently palpate for the presence or location of spasm, tenderness, organomegaly, or mass. Rebound tenderness, indicative of peritoneal irritation, may be elicited by gentle percussion or a simple request to cough. The severity of the pain may be reflected in the child's facial expression. A stool-filled colon can often be palpated in children with constipation. Variable tenderness, without signs of peritoneal irritation, can be elicited in children with *recurrent abdominal pain.* At the conclusion of the physical, a gentle rectal examination may be necessary to determine the presence of stool or pelvic tenderness or mass.

Rarely, sedation may be needed prior to performing a proper abdominal examination. Use Seconal 1–2 mg/kg IV; phenobarbital 5 mg/kg or Valium 0.1–0.2 mg/kg IM; or chloral hydrate 40 mg/kg rectally.

A pelvic examination is indicated if there is lower abdominal or pelvic pain associated with a vaginal discharge, bleeding, or history of sexual activity. Check for bleeding, a discharge, cervical motion tenderness, and adnexal mass (see pp 239–241).

ER MANAGEMENT

The priority is the expedient diagnosis and management of a surgical abdomen (appendicitis, intestinal obstruction, intussusception, Meckel diverticulum). Persistent right lower quadrant pain, a rigid abdomen, bilious or pernicious vomiting, currant jelly stools, massive bright red rectal bleeding, hypotension, or toxicity are indications for obtaining a complete blood count (CBC) with differential, spun hematocrit, electrolytes, glucose, blood urea nitrogen (BUN) and creatinine, urinalysis and culture, and a type and cross-match. Make the patient NPO and secure an IV, infusing 20 cc/kg of NS if the patient is dehydrated or has orthostatic vital sign changes. Unless an appendicitis is strongly suspected (p 172), obtain a KUB and upright abdominal films looking for air–fluid levels, obliteration of the psoas margins, free air, mass effects, or densities (fecalith, urolith). Immediate surgical consultation is necessary.

The management of nonsurgical cases of abdominal pain depends on the etiology (gastroenteritis p 186; hepatitis p 177; pharyngitis p 117; pneumonia p 458; sickle cell crisis p 273; lead poisoning p 361; pelvic inflammatory disease p 238; ectopic pregnancy pp 235–236; parasite infestation p 309). If the diagnosis is not clear, obtain a urinalysis and observe the patient for several hours. Persistent severe pain or an inability to tolerate PO fluids are indications for admission.

Refer patients with functional recurrent abdominal pain to a primary care provider who can provide close follow-up.

INDICATIONS FOR ADMISSION

- Surgical abdomen
- Dehydration or inability to take fluids
- Significant blood loss (tachycardia, orthostatic hypotension)

REFERENCES

1. Apley J: The Child with Abdominal Pain, 2nd ed. London; Blackwell, 1975
2. Farell MK: Pediatrics 74 (Suppl): 955–957, 1984

Acute Appendicitis

INTRODUCTION

Appendicitis is the most common illness requiring emergency surgery in childhood. The pathophysiology involves obstruction of the lumen, leading to necrosis and perforation of the appendiceal wall, with subsequent peritonitis. Early diagnosis is therefore of paramount importance.

CLINICAL PRESENTATION

In uncomplicated appendicitis there is a short history (usually <36 hours) of anorexia, nausea, and vomiting, with periumbilical pain that intensifies and shifts to the right lower quadrant. Low grade fever (<101°F) is common, and a change in stool pattern, either diarrhea or constipation, occurs in about 15% of patients. Tenderness will be greatest over McBurney point (one-third of the way along a line from the anterior superior iliac spine to the umbilicus) and there may be positive psoas and obturator signs (pain on passive hip hyperextension, pain on passive hip internal rotation respectively). Pain may also be elicited in the right lower quadrant while palpating the left side (Rovsing sign). Involuntary guarding (muscle spasm that persists when the abdomen is palpated with the hips flexed) and rebound tenderness (elicited by asking the patient to cough or jump) are frequently noted. Rectal examination may reveal right-sided tenderness. With retrocecal appendicitis, the pain may remain periumbilical, or maximal tenderness and rigidity may be found in the right flank.

In the patient with a ruptured appendix, the history is usually longer than 36 hours. There may be frequent vomiting, dyspnea secondary to elevation of the diaphragm, and a temperature above 101.3°F (38.5°C). A diffusely tender and rigid abdomen indicates peritonitis. Perforation occurs in 90% of infants with appendicitis. There is a short (few hours) history of anorexia, vomiting, and lethargy, and the physical examination reveals an ill infant with a distended and rigid abdomen.

DIAGNOSIS

Acute Gastroenteritis. In acute gastroenteritis, vomiting often appears simultaneously with the onset of abdominal pain, while in appendicitis periumbilical pain almost always precedes the vomiting. High volume diarrhea and the absence of signs of peritoneal irritation further distinguish this condition from appendicitis.

Pneumonia. Right lower lobe pneumonia may present with pain referred to the abdomen. Respiratory symptoms and signs and a positive chest radiograph confirm the diagnosis. In addition, pneumonia often causes a much higher temperature than appendicitis.

Urinary Tract Injection. A patient with a urinary tract infection can have fever, dysuria, and pyuria, in association with the abdominal pain.

Constipation. Constipation may cause right lower quadrant tenderness, although there should not be signs of peritoneal irritation or a history of migration of the pain. A rectal ampulla filled with stool and pain relief on defecation are characteristic.

Functional Abdominal Pain. Attacks of functional abdominal pain may be severe, but absence of clinical and laboratory signs of inflammation and improvement following a period of observation allow differentiation from acute appendicitis.

Other Considerations. Other considerations include *hepatitis, pancreatitis, lead poisoning, urolithiasis,* and *diabetes.* In the adolescent female, *PID, ectopic pregnancy, threatened abortion,* or a *twisted ovarian cyst* can mimic acute appendicitis, although the pain is usually lower in the abdomen and vaginal bleeding or a discharge may be present.

ER MANAGEMENT

When the diagnosis is evident from the history and physical examination, make the patient NPO and start intravenous hydration with D5 1/2 NS at a maintenance rate. Obtain blood for a CBC and type and cross-match, and notify a surgeon. If perforation is suspected, give the first doses of antibiotics (ampicillin, 100 mg/kg/day; clindamycin, 40 mg/kg/day; and gentamicin, 6 mg/kg/day).

When the diagnosis is unclear, a KUB may be useful since identification of a fecolith confirms the diagnosis of appendicitis. Patients with tachypnea, cough, or other pulmonary signs or symptoms or unexpectedly high fever, should have a chest x-ray as well. A CBC is not helpful in making the diagnosis of appendicitis, although a white blood count (WBC) >18,000/mm^3 suggests rupture or a bacterial process (gastroenteritis or pneumonia). A urinalysis is necessary to rule out diabetes (glycosuria) and a urinary tract infection, although leukocytes (usually 5–10/hpf) can be seen in the urine with appendicitis. Possible findings on pelvic examination in the postmenarchal female include vaginal bleeding (ectopic, threatened abortion) or discharge (PID), adnexal mass (PID, ovarian cyst, ectopic pregnancy), or cervical motion tenderness (PID).

When appendicitis cannot be excluded and alternative diagnosis cannot be confirmed, make the patient NPO and admit him for careful observation. However, if appendicitis seems unlikely, the patient may be sent home on a clear liquid diet (and no analgesics), to return for reexamination in *6–8 hours,* or *sooner* if symptoms increase.

INDICATION FOR ADMISSION

- Suspected appendicitis

REFERENCES

1. Ballantine TVM: Surg Clin North Am 6:117, 1981
2. Savrin RA, Clatsworthy HW: Pediatrics 63: 37–43, 1979

Acute Liver Failure

INTRODUCTION

Acute hepatic failure is an uncommon syndrome resulting from severe impairment of hepatic function. In infants, infections (TORCHS, hepatitis B virus) and inborn errors of metabolism (galactosemia, fructose intolerance, tyrosinemia) are the most common etiologies. During childhood and adolescence, the etiology is most often infectious (hepatitis A, hepatitis B, non-A non-B hepatitis, herpes, adenovirus), toxic (acetominophen overdose; isoniazid, methotrexate, valproic acid, oral contraceptive, phenothiazine, or halothane use; exposure to carbon tetrachloride or benzene), or metabolic (Reye syndrome).

CLINICAL PRESENTATION

Often there is a history of exposure to viral hepatitis or toxins, or an antecedent infection. Findings include persistent anorexia, nausea, vomiting (especially in Reye syndrome), lethargy, fever, right upper quadrant pain, and jaundice (except in Reye syndrome). Bleeding manifestations may be present (ecchymoses, prolonged bleeding after venipuncture, hematuria, hematochezia, melena). Progressive neurologic deterioration ensues and can be classified into four stages. In stage 1, mild confusion and sleep disorders are noted. This is followed by irritability, confusion, inappropriate behavior, hyperventilation, and somnolence during stage 2. Hyperreflexia, liver flap (asterixis), and slowing of the electroencephalogram (EEG) may also be present. Obtundation develops during stage 3, although the patient may be arousable. In stage 4, the coma is deep, with areflexia, seizures (focal or generalized), decerebrate rigidity, and apneic episodes.

DIAGNOSIS

Liver failure is usually manifested by transaminases (serum glutamic oxaloacetic transaminase [SGOT], serum glutamic pyruvic transaminase [SGPT]) greater than 3000 U/L, with hypoglycemia, hypoalbuminemia, prolongation of the prothrombin time, elevated blood ammonia, and hyperbilirubinemia (except in Reye syndrome).

For the infant, inquire about the neonatal course including birth weight (*TORCHS*-infected infants may be small for gestational age), hemolysis or anemia (TORCHS), feeding history (*galactosemia, fructose intolerance*), and maternal history of hepatitis (*congenital hepatitis, biliary atresia*), or genital *herpes*. In older patients, ask about possible *drug ingestion* (acetaminophen, isoniazid, phenothiazines, valproic acid, methotrexate oral contraceptives), *toxin exposure* (carbon tetrachloride, halothane, benzene derivatives), and exposure to *hepatitis*. Always consider *acetaminophen* overdose in the adolescent.

On examination, check for jaundice, scleral icterus, papilledema, hepatomegaly, and right upper quadrant tenderness. Perform a thorough neurologic examination, including assessment of the level of consciousness and orientation, pupillary response, extraocular movements, motor response, and reflexes.

ER MANAGEMENT

Obtain blood for CBC with differential, electrolytes, glucose, BUN and creatinine, liver function tests (SGOT, SGPT, creatine phosphokinase [CPK], lactic dehydrogenase [LDH], alkaline phosphatase, bilirubin, total protein and albumin), prothrombin time and partial thromboplastin time, and ammonia. Insert an IV and infuse a 10% dextrose solution at a maintenance rate. Monitor the glucose frequently and increase the dextrose concentration if the patient becomes hypoglycemic. Give fresh frozen plasma, (5 cc/kg IV) and vitamin K (5 mg IM) if there are any clotting study abnormalities or evidence of bleeding.

Admit the patient to an intensive care setting where measures to lower the ammonia level (enemas, oral neomycin, oral lactulose) can be instituted. Patients with Reye syndrome require intensive management of increased intracranial pressure (see p 397). This may include a cooling blanket, mannitol, dexamethasone, and hyperventilation, with continuous monitoring of central venous and intracranial pressures.

INDICATIONS FOR ADMISSION

- Hepatic failure (prothrombin time 5 seconds over control, bleeding, hypoglycemia)
- Hepatic encephalopathy
- Reye syndrome

REFERENCES

1. Rogers EL, Rogers MC: Pediatr Clin North Am 30:701, 1980
2. Hoyumpa AM, Dedmond AV, Avant GR: Gastroenterol 76:184, 1979

Acute Viral Hepatitis

INTRODUCTION

Viral hepatitis is most commonly caused by hepatitis A virus (HAV) and hepatitis B virus (HBV), whose clinical and epidemiologic characteristics are summarized in Table 8-1.

However, as much as 25% of sporadic hepatitis and 90% of post-transfusion hepatitis cannot be serologically related to either HAV or HBV and is attributed to the agents(s) designated as hepatitis non-A, non-B. In addition, other organisms cause acute infectious hepatitis, including Epstein-Barr virus, cytomegalovirus, toxoplasmosis, herpes simplex, leptospira, and yellow fever virus.

TABLE 8-1. CLINICAL AND EPIDEMIOLOGIC CHARACTERISTICS OF HAV AND HBV

Clinical Features	HAV	HBV
Peak pediatric incidence	1st decade	2nd decade/neonatal
Route	Fecal-oral	Parenteral/sexual/perinatal
Incubation	15–50 days	40–180 days
Onset	Acute	Subacute
Fever > 101°F	Common	Less common
Anorexia	Severe	Moderate
Nausea/vomiting	Common	Less common
Rash	Rare	Common
Arthralgia/arthritis	Rare	Common
Epidemiologic Features		
Common source epidemics (food, water)	Yes	No
Day care center contact	Yes	No
IV drug abuse	No	Yes
Blood, blood products	No	Yes
Homosexuality	?	Yes (males)
Asians, Eskimos	No	Yes
Dialysis patients	No	Yes
Institutionalized persons	?	Yes

CLINICAL PRESENTATION

Anicteric hepatitis is the most common form (over 90% of cases), and it may be completely asymptomatic. With icteric forms, there is usually a 1-week prodrome of fever, lethargy, anorexia, nausea, vomiting, and right upper quadrant abdominal pain. With HBV, urticaria, purpura, papular acrodermatitis (Gianotti-Crosti syndrome), arthralgias, or arthritis may also occur. These symptoms resolve rapidly with the onset of jaundice associated with an enlarged, tender liver, dark urine, and light colored stools. The icteric phase lasts 1–4 weeks, with complete recovery in most cases. A prolonged cholestatic form, lasting 2–6 months, is rare in children. In about 0.1–1% of all cases, a fulminant hepatitis results in hepatic coma and possibly death.

Although infection with HAV is not associated with long term sequelae, HBV hepatitis can progress to chronic liver disease and cirrhosis. There is also a carrier state for HBV, which can be asymptomatic or associated with chronic liver disease.

DIAGNOSIS

If hepatitis is suspected, obtain a CBC with differential, liver function tests, prothrombin time (PT) and partial thromboplastin time (PTT), serum electrolytes and glucose, hepatitis B surface antigen (HBsAg), heterophile antibody, and IgM anti-HAV (if available). In general, transaminase levels (SGOT, SGPT) increase during the prodromal period and return to normal after the appearance of jaundice. Conjugated hyperbilirubinemia predominates during the icteric stage, and bilirubin levels may be extremely high if there is associated renal disease or hemolysis. Alkaline phosphatase is elevated, but albumin is normal. Leukopenia with atypical lymphocytes may be seen during the prodrome. Abnormalities of clotting factors occur only in severe cases, and a prolonged PT (2 or more seconds over control) is a poor prognostic sign.

The presence of anti-HAV IgM confirms HAV infection within the previous 4 weeks, while anti-HAV IgG implies infection occurred more than 4 weeks prior to testing.

The most commonly used test for diagnosing HBV is the surface antigen, HBsAg, which appears in the blood 4–6 weeks after exposure, but 1 week to 2 months before any elevation of the transaminases. HBsAg usually disappears 1–13 weeks after the onset of clinical disease. Persistence beyond 6 months defines chronic carriage

TABLE 8-2. HEPATITIS B VIRUS SEROLOGY

Stage of Disease	HBsAg	Anti-HBs	Anti-HBc
Incubation	+	−	−
Illness	+	−	+
Early convalescence (serologic gap)	−	−	+
Late convalescence	−	+	+
Postrecovery	−	+	+
Chronic carrier	+	−	+

or chronic hepatitis. Antibody against HBsAg (anti-HBs) is protective, lasts indefinitely, and implies recovery from infection and absence of infectivity. It does not appear until after resolution of the clinical hepatitis and is usually not measurable until several weeks after the disappearance of the HBsAg. This means that there is a serologic "gap" when both HBsAg and anti-HBsAg are absent from the blood. This gap is filled by another (core) antibody, anti-HBc, which is not protective. HBV serology is summarized in Table 8-2.

During the prodromal phase, viral hepatitis may be confused with a *flu-like illness* or *gastroenteritis*. A tender enlarged liver, bilirubinuria, and increased transaminases suggest the correct diagnosis. During the icteric stage, consider other causes of jaundice such as *obstruction* (right upper quadrant colicky pain and mass), *toxins* (hydrocarbons, arsenic), and *drugs* (acetaminophen, chlorpromazine, isoniazid, valproic acid). *Carotenemia* is confirmed by the absence of scleral icterus and a normal serum bilirubin. In the neonate, intrauterine infections (*TORCHS*), *metabolic disease* (galactosemia), *biliary atresia,* and a *choledochal cyst* are the major differential diagnostic problems.

ER MANAGEMENT

There is no specific therapy for acute viral hepatitis. Neither dietary restrictions nor forced bedrest are necessary. Intravenous hydration may be necessary for patients with severe vomiting. Corticosteroids are contraindicated.

Effective prophylaxis is currently available only for infection caused by HAV and HBV. Give 0.02 cc/kg IM of immune globulin (IG) to all household and sexual contacts of patients with HAV. In day care center outbreaks give the same dose to all children, staff members, and household contacts of nontoilet-trained children attending the center. IG is not effective once there is clinical onset of the disease or if the time from exposure is more than 2 weeks. School contacts and health care personnel attending to a patient with HAV only require good handwashing and stool precautions, and not IG prophylaxis. When the index patient is known to be infected with HAV, serologic testing of contacts before IG administration is not necessary.

Postexposure HBV prophylaxis is summarized in Table 8-3. When there has clearly been an exposure (percutaneously or by mucous

TABLE 8-3. POSTEXPOSURE HBV PROPHYLAXIS

Exposure	Treatment
PERCUTANEOUS	
Blood known to be HBsAg (+)	HBIG 0.06 cc/kg IM immediately and begin HB vaccine series[a]
Blood from a known source but unknown HBsAg status	If the source is at high risk for having HBV (see Table 8-1) begin the HB vaccine series[a] and test the source for HBsAg: if (+) give HBIG 0.06 cc/kg IM in addition to the vaccine If the source is at low risk for having HBV begin HB vaccine series;[a] it is *not* necessary to test the source for HBsAg
Blood from an unknown source	Begin HB vaccine series[a]
PERINATAL	HBIG 0.5 cc IM and begin HB vaccine series,[a] both within 12 hours of birth if possible
SEXUAL	HBIG 0.06 cc/kg IM only if sexual contact within 14 days[b]. One dose only

[a]The HB vaccine series consists of the initial dose (0.5 cc IM $<$10 years, 1.0 cc IM $\geq$10 years), followed by repeat doses at 1 and 6 months

[b]For sexual contacts, give the vaccine in addition to HBIG to homosexual men and to any continuing sexual partner of an HBV carrier.

membrane contact) to blood that is positive for HBsAg, the treatment of choice is *both* hepatitis B immune globulin and HB vaccine. Give them as soon after the exposure as possible, at the same time but at different sites. Repeat the vaccine dose 1 month and 6 months later. In the event that vaccine is not available, give a second dose of HBIG in 1 month. If HBIG is not available, use IG (immune globulin, 0.06cc/kg). When there has been exposure to blood from a high-risk source (see Table 8-1) whose HBsAg status is not known, vaccinate the patient at once and send blood from the source for HBsAg testing: if the test is positive, give one dose of HBIG and then complete the vaccine series 1 month and 6 months later; if the test is negative, complete the vaccination series but HBIG is not necessary. In case the result of testing for HBsAg on the source blood will not be known for more than 7 days after the exposure, it may be advisable to give the exposed person a dose of IG pending the result. When there has been exposure to blood either from a low-risk source or from an unknown source, vaccinate the patient fully. HBIG is not necessary.

Treatment recommendations for perinatal and sexual exposures are also outlined in Table 8-3. Household, nonsexual contacts to persons with HBV infection do not routinely require prophylaxis unless there has been blood exposure (sharing razors, toothbrushes, etc.). Treat this type of exposure as a sexual exposure, with one dose of HBIG. If, however, the person with HBV infection becomes a chronic carrier, vaccinate all household contacts. An infant who has received intimate care from a person with HBV infection represents a special case because of the high risk for chronic carriage and morbidity in this age group. Although there is no official CDC recommendation for this situation, treatment of such an infant with one dose of HBIG and with HBV vaccine is advisable.

INDICATIONS FOR ADMISSION

- Fulminant hepatitis, with a prothrombin time more than 5 seconds over control or behavioral changes
- Inability to take adequately by mouth
- Neonates with jaundice

REFERENCES

1. Seto DSY: Pediatr Clin North Am 26: 305–314, 1979
2. MMWR 33:285–289, 1984
3. MMWR 34: 313–324, 329–335, 1985

Colic

INTRODUCTION

Colic (paroxysmal fussing of infancy) is a well-accepted entity whose etiology and pathogenesis are poorly understood.

CLINICAL PRESENTATION

Typically, at 2 or 3 weeks of age, an otherwise well baby begins to become fussy and cry after feedings. In mild cases, the fussiness occurs only in the evening, but in moderately severe cases, there are 2–3 episodes per day. With severe colic, the infant cries with each feeding and is often unable to finish the meal. The pain typically lasts 2–3 hours at a time, and the baby draws his legs up as if he has abdominal discomfort. He seems to feel better when rocked, moved back and forth, held close to the parent, or walked. When the particular activity is stopped, however, the crying resumes. Vomiting, diarrhea, and constipation are not features of colic and, in between episodes, the infant appears comfortable and alert. Weight gain as well as the physical and neurologic examinations are normal.

DIAGNOSIS

The key to making the diagnosis of colic is the parents' statement that the infant is perfectly fine between paroxysms. Perform a complete physical examination. If the baby cries during the examination, have him suck on a clean finger or nipple. If this does not stop his crying, lay the infant on his stomach or put him over your shoulder. When distracted, the colicky baby is alert and interested in his surroundings. He sucks vigorously on a nipple or pacifier. Upon gentle palpation, the abdomen is soft and nontender.

Systemic infections (sepsis, meningitis, urinary tract infection, septic arthritis, osteomyelitis, pneumonia), *supraventricular tachycardia, heart failure, congenital glaucoma, infantile spasms,* and *hypothyroidism* or other metabolic diseases can present with nothing more than fussiness. With these illnesses, however, the infant may be lethargic, feeding less vigorously, or have fever, vomiting, diarrhea, or constipation. The parents' description of a change in the baby's overall behavior is worrisome.

Diarrhea of any etiology may be associated with crampy abdominal pain, but diarrhea excludes the diagnosis of colic. Likewise, the constipated infant may have abdominal pain (mild to severe) that is related to feedings, with grunting, crying, and straining during bowel movements. Although some infants with colic may be constipated, it is necessary to alleviate the *constipation* before making the diagnosis of colic.

Volvulus or *intussusception* may initially present with crampy pain. However, vomiting quickly ensues, followed by signs of intestinal obstruction and rectal bleeding.

ER MANAGEMENT

The goal of the ER examination is to rule out other conditions that can present with colicky pain. Once the diagnosis is made, reassure the parents that the infant is not seriously ill, since this is usually their overriding concern. In general, formula changes or manipulation of the breast-feeding mother's diet are not successful in alleviating colic. However, discontinue any new foods or juices that were introduced just before the onset of the colic. If the mother smokes cigarettes, ask her to stop to see if the colic improves. Encourage the parents to burp the infant frequently during and after the feeding, if they are not doing so.

Simethicone drops (0.3–0.6 cc) just before or with each feeding may be helpful in some infants. Avoid antispasmodics since there is little evidence that they work, and they may be dangerous. Arrange for the patient to be seen again within a week, and refer the family to a primary care physician for close follow-up.

INDICATION FOR ADMISSION

- The family can no longer cope with the crying

REFERENCE

1. Carey WB: Pediatr Clin North Am 31:993–1005, 1984

Constipation

INTRODUCTION

Constipation is a condition in which the stools are infrequent, hard, and difficult to pass. Many parents complain that infants are experiencing infrequent stooling or apparent straining. However, in most cases the stools are soft and the baby is therefore not constipated. Infrequent (every 1–2 days), soft bowel movements are commonly seen with breast feeding and underfeeding. Functional constipation in infants being fed formula (especially iron fortified) or cow's milk is common, and an anal fissure can also cause constipation in infancy. Hirschsprung disease, hypothyroidism, diabetes mellitus, and cystic fibrosis are rare, but serious, etiologies.

After infancy, stool consistency is a function of intake and intervals of 1–2 days between bowel movements are common. Busy preschool and school-age children often "forget" to move their bowels (uncomplicated minor constipation). The major pathologic cause of constipation is functional stool retention, which occurs as a result of issues surrounding toilet training. Constipation can also be linked to serious emotional disturbances.

CLINICAL PRESENTATION

As mentioned above, constipation implies that the stools are hard, infrequent, and difficult to pass.

Parents may report infants straining during the passage of small, hard, "pebble-like" stools. In babies with *functional constipation of infancy,* there is often a positive family history of constipation in the first year of life and a diet of iron-fortified formula or cow's milk. With an *anal fissure,* there may be blood streaking on the stool or diaper, and the fissure or a sentinel tag of rectal mucosa may be seen.

After infancy, *uncomplicated minor constipation* occurs in active children who go 1–2 days between bowel movements. There is no encopresis, toilet-training difficulties, or serious emotional disorders.

Preschool children with *functional stool retention* often develop a constipation–obstipation cycle. This leads to abdominal distention and occasionally, encopresis secondary to an overflow of liquid stool leaking around a large mass of hard stool. *Emotionally disturbed* patients have soft stool in the ampulla, despite a similar history of constipation and encopresis.

Hirschsprung disease usually presents in males in the first 2 years of life with very infrequent (days to weeks), thin, ribbon-like stools associated with abdominal distention, failure to thrive, and possibly, signs of intestinal obstruction. On examination, the rectal ampulla is empty or has a markedly diminished amount of stool.

In general, constipation occurs in association with other, more specific findings in patients with *diabetes mellitus* and *hypothyroidism*.

DIAGNOSIS

No laboratory evaluation is necessary in the ER for constipated infants. Inquire about the bowel movements, especially the frequency, consistency, and presence of blood. Ask about the feedings, including type of formula or foods, frequency, and amount. Infrequent soft stools are normal in the breast-fed infant but suggest underfeeding in the formula-fed infant. *Functional constipation* is likely if there is a positive family history and the infant is being fed an iron-fortified formula or cow's milk.

After infancy, inquire about difficulties with toilet training, possible *emotional disturbances,* and encopresis. In the absence of any of these, *uncomplicated minor constipation* is likely. Otherwise, perform a rectal examination. An empty ampulla suggests *Hirschsprung disease,* soft stool is present with emotional disorders, and hard, impacted stools are noted in patients with *functional retention*.

ER MANAGEMENT

Constipation tends to be a chronic problem and, as such, the patient requires follow-up in a primary care setting. For the infant with *functional constipation,* either change the formula to one without iron, or instruct the parents to add 1 teaspoon of dark Karo syrup or malt extract (Malt Supex) to each 8 ounce bottle. Do not prescribe any stronger laxatives in the ER. If *underfeeding* is diagnosed, increase the volume to about 150 cc/kg/day.

Reassure the parents of a young child with *uncomplicated minor constipation* that he or she is normal. They may try avoiding constipating foods (bananas, rice cereal) and adding prune juice (15–30 cc/day) or bran to the diet.

Emotionally disturbed children and those with *functional constipation* cannot be adequately treated in the ER. Refer them to a primary care provider for ongoing care. If the patient is very uncomfortable, give a Fleets pediatric enema to empty the colon.

REFERENCES

1. Davidson M, Kugler MM, Bauer CH: J Pediatr 62:261, 1967
2. Fleisher DR: Pediatr Ann 5:700, 1976

Gastroenteritis And Dehydration

INTRODUCTION AND CLINICAL PRESENTATION

Most episodes of acute vomiting and diarrhea are caused by viral or bacterial infections or, in the case of food poisoning, by toxins elaborated by bacteria. A few cases are secondary to parasitic infection.

Rotavirus. Rotavirus, a wintertime infection in temperate climates, predominantly affects children from 6 months to 2 years of age. Vomiting is very common, especially early in the illness, followed by voluminous watery stools. The illness usually lasts from 5 to 8 days and is often followed by a secondary disaccharide intolerance.

Norwalk Virus Infection. Norwalk virus infection, which affects older school-age children and adolescents, lasts from 24 to 48 hours and consists of variable, host-specific symptoms of abdominal cramps, vomiting, diarrhea, malaise, myalgias, and low grade fever.

Shigella Diarrhea. *Shigella* diarrhea is characterized by the abrupt onset of bloody or yellow-green mucopurulent stools, often accompanied by high fever. Vomiting is uncommon, although seizures can accompany the illness, regardless of the severity of the diarrhea. Transmission is by the fecal-oral route, and ingestion of just a few organisms can cause the illness. Thus, *Shigella* gastroenteritis is easily transmitted from one family member to another.

Salmonella Gastroenteritis. Symptoms of *Salmonella* gastroenteritis are variable and include fever, vomiting, and malaise, in addition to diarrhea that may be watery, or dysentery-like. Bacteremia occurs in a third of cases associated with fever (>101°F) under 1 year of age. *Salmonella* gastroenteritis is a large inoculum disease; transmission is by contaminated food. It is rare, when normal hygiene is practiced, for the illness to spread through a family. More commonly, several family members become ill at the same time from a common source.

Escherichia Coli Diarrhea. Enterotoxigenic *E. coli* diarrhea is watery and persists when the patient is not being fed, while the enteropathogenic type produces a malabsorption-type diarrhea, and the enteroinvasive form causes a dysentery-like illness.

Campylobacter and Yersinia Infections. With *Campylobacter* and *Yersinia* infections, the stools are watery or mixed with pus and blood. Fever is common. *Campylobacter* is particularly common in infants and young children, and there sometimes is a history of a new puppy in the home.

Giardia Lamblia Diarrhea. *Giardia lamblia* causes a watery diarrhea which is often chronic (more than 3 weeks). Vomiting is rare, and fever is variably present. Although not a common cause of gastroenteritis in the United States, consider it in patients who attend day care centers.

Food Poisoning. Food poisoning presents with vomiting and diarrhea within a few hours of eating contaminated food. The diagnosis is evident when a number of people become ill at the same time. The temperature is usually normal. Some patients present with neurologic findings such as blurred vision and weakness suggesting *Clostridium botulinum. Infant botulism* (see p 292) which can progress to respiratory depression, presents with constipation and hypotonia. A history of eating honey may be obtained, since it is a source of botulinum spores.

DIAGNOSIS

With gastroenteritis of any etiology, patients can present with vomiting, diarrhea, or both; fever and abdominal pain are common. However, the abdomen should be soft and either nontender or diffusely

TABLE 8-4. STOOL EXAMINATION

1. Gross examination	Blood—bacterial Water margin—viral
2. Microscopic: Add 1–2 drops of methylene blue to dilute stool, cover with cover slip and examine under low power.	Sheets of white cells—bacterial
3. Test pH (use urine dipstick)	pH <6—viral (disaccharide intolerance)

Consult The Harriet Lane Handbook (10th ed), pp 44–45, for more specific test for sugar (reducing substances) in the stool.

tender with no guarding or rebound, and the vomitus should not be bilious.

Examination of the stool may help differentiate viral from bacterial etiologies (Table 8-4). Obtain a rectal swab for stool culture from patients with high fever (>103°F), toxicity, or mucus, blood, or pus in the stool. Culturing for *Shigella* and *Salmonella* is routine, but *Campylobacter* and *Yersinia* may have to be specifically requested.

The severity of the illness depends on the degree of dehydration (Table 8-5). Tachycardia out of proportion to the temperature elevation (>12 beats/min/°F) or orthostatic changes (a rise in heart rate of more than 20 beats/min or blood pressure fall of more than 20 mm Hg upon arising from the recumbent position) identify the hypovolemic patient.

Vomiting occurring in the absence of diarrhea and fever may not be secondary to a gastroenteritis (Table 8-6).

In infants, a *urinary tract infection* and *otitis media* are often associated with fever and diarrhea (''parenteral'' diarrhea). Infants who are *teething* may develop low grade fever and loose stools secondary to the swallowing of excessive amounts of saliva. In the older child and adolescent, consider *inflammatory bowel disease*, particularly if there is a history of weight loss or poor growth.

A urinalysis (including specific gravity) is indicated when there is any degree of dehydration, fever, weight loss, or diarrhea persisting despite proper management. Ketonuria (starvation) is a common finding but may indicate *diabetes mellitus* if associated with glycosuria

TABLE 8-5. ESTIMATION OF DEHYDRATION

	<5	5–7%	≥10%	15%
Heart rate	nl	mod ↑	Markedly ↑	Markedly ↑
Respiratory rate	nl	nl	Hyperpnea	Hyperpnea
Blood pressure	nl	Orthostatic drop	Narrowed pulse pressure	Hypotensive
Skin turgor	nl	nl-slightly ↓	Decreased	Decreased
Eyeballs	nl	nl	Sunken	Sunken
Mucous membranes	nl to dry	Dry	Dry	Dry
Fontanelle	nl	sl depressed	Sunken	Sunken
Mental status	nl	nl to irritable	Lethargic	Comatose
Urine output	nl to sl ↓	↓ to none	None	None
Urine SG	>1020	>1030	Maximal if urine obtained	

TABLE 8-6. DIFFERENTIAL DIAGNOSIS OF VOMITING

Process	Sign
Obstruction	Distended abdomen, bilious vomiting, crescendo vomiting, surgical scar on abdomen
Intracranial hypertension	Bulging fontanelle, altered mental status
Diabetes mellitus	Hyperpnea, polyuria, acetone breath
Adrenal insufficiency	Virilization, hyperkalemia, hyponatremia
Reye syndrome	Altered mental status
Pregnancy	Hypogastric mass, missed menstrual period
Toxic ingestion	Sudden onset, history of ingestion

and polyuria. Pyuria suggests a *urinary tract infection;* obtain a urine culture using sterile technique but avoid suprapubic aspiration in dehydrated patients.

ER MANAGEMENT

Determination of the state of hydration is the priority. Since the most accurate means of assessment of hydration is by comparison of the patient's present and premorbid weights, the patient must be weighed at every visit. In the absence of a previous value, rely on the other indicators of the state of hydration (see Table 8-5). If the patient is clinically dehydrated (>5%) or has serious associated symptoms (large bloody stools, hyperpnea), obtain serum electrolytes, pH, and a CBC. A blood culture is indicated if the patient appears toxic, is in shock, or is under 1 year of age with bloody diarrhea and fever (>101°F).

Patients who are less than 5% dehydrated can be treated symptomatically, but they may not be sent home from the ER unless they have stopped vomiting and it is clear that they can tolerate small feedings of clear liquids.

Treatment of Vomiting. Vomiting usually responds to small sips of clear liquids (soda, oral electrolyte solution, weak tea, fruit punch). A useful regimen is to wait at least 1 hour after the last vomiting episode and then give 5–10 cc every 20 minutes for an hour, followed by 15–20 cc every 20 minutes for a second hour, and then 30 cc (1 oz) every 20 minutes during the third hour. Fluid intake may be slowly liberalized after that time. If vomiting occurs, instruct the parents to wait an hour and then begin again. A second episode of vomiting requires a return visit to the ER. Once the infant or child is taking normal volumes of clear liquids, the diet may be advanced according to the patient's age:

1. Less than 2 months: return to breast feeding or half strength soy formula (advanced to full strength after 24 hours).
2. Over 2 months: either breast milk or half strength formula or cow's milk advanced as above.
3. Infants taking solid food: Give a bland diet (crackers, cereal, yellow vegetables, jello). Avoid milk and milk products for 24–48 hours.

Treatment of Diarrhea. Diarrhea responds best to large infrequent feedings. In breast-fed babies, diarrhea is less common and usually less severe, so there is generally no need to stop breast feeding. For formula-fed babies, temporarily discontinue the formula in favor of clear fluids. Oral electrolyte solutions with sodium concentrations between 30–60 mEq/L and 2–5 g% of glucose are adequate for mild dehydration. Never maintain a diet of clear fluids in young infants for more than 24 hours, since the calorie content of electrolyte solutions is low (100–200 cal/L). Older infants and children prefer soda, gelatin, broth, tea with sugar, or juice (do not use apple juice which may exacerbate diarrhea).

Once the diarrhea has improved, or after 24 hours of clear feeds, begin refeeding. If the diarrhea was not severe, give the formula the young infant was receiving as a half-strength solution. If diarrhea recurs or was severe, use a lactose-free soy formula. If this is not tolerated, change to an elemental formula. Gradually advance the formula to full strength. If lactose or sucrose intolerance was noted, wait 4 weeks to reintroduce the original formula.

In the older infant, follow the 24 hours of clear fluids with a BRAT diet (bananas, rice cereal, apple sauce, toast). Do not give milk or formula for several days.

Moderate dehydration (5–7%) requires careful evaluation and treatment. If the patient is not vomiting, oral rehydration can be attempted. Observe the child in the ER until it is established that he can drink without vomiting and that ongoing losses are not excessive. Be sure that the child is urinating and obtain a weight and urine specific gravity before sending him home. One day of a rehydrating solution with a higher sodium content such as Pedialyte RS (75 mEq/L of sodium) may be useful. Arrange for daily follow-up (including a weight) for all these patients.

Severe dehydration (10–15%) is a medical emergency. Greater than 15% dehydration may result in death. Rapid reexpansion of the intravascular volume is essential to establish adequate perfusion (see shock, p 11).

Do not use antiemetics and antidiarrheal medications since they may mask the signs and symptoms of ongoing losses in young children and, in bacterial infections, may promote the development of bacteremia.

Do not use antibiotics routinely in diarrheal illness but rather prescribe them only if cultures have documented a bacterial infection requiring antimicrobial therapy. Treat *Campylobacter* with erythromycin (40 mg/kg/day); use TMP/SMX (8 mg/kg/day of TMP) for *Yersinia* and *Shigella*.

The situation is less straightforward with *Salmonella* enteritis. Because of the high incidence (30%) of bacteremia in febrile infants (< 1 yr) with *Salmonella* enteritis, obtain a blood culture and CBC from all such patients, as well as from immunocompromised patients or patients who are toxic appearing.

Admit all febrile infants <6 months of age and toxic appearing or immunocompromised patients of any age. Well appearing infants >6 months old may be treated at home (TMP-SMX for 14 days) with daily follow up. If the blood culture is positive but the infant was sent home, reexamine him or her. Admit the infant if he or she remains febrile or is toxic appearing.

INDICATIONS FOR ADMISSION

- >7% dehydration, >5% (relative)
- Inability to take adequate fluids orally
- All infants <6 months and toxic-appearing infants 6–12 months of age with fever and a stool culture positive for *Salmonella*
- All patients with a blood culture positive for *Salmonella* unless afebrile > 48 hours

REFERENCES

1. Book LS: Pediatrics 74 (Suppl):950, 1984
2. Blacklow NR, Cukor, G: New Engl J Med 304:397, 1981
3. Finberg L, Harper PA, Harrison HE, et al: J Pediatr 101: 497, 1982
4. Diagnosis and Management of Acute Diarrhea. 13th Ross Roundtable Columbus, Ohio, Ross Laboratories, 1982
5. Cole CH (ed): The Harriet Lane Handbook (10th ed). Chicago: Yearbook Med Pub, 1984, pp 44–45

Hepatomegaly

INTRODUCTION

Palpation of the liver below the costal margin is a common finding in childhood. A liver edge 3 cm below the costal margin, in the midclavicular line, is normal during the first 6 months of life. Up to 2 cm

TABLE 8-7. NORMAL LIVER SPANS

	Males	Females
Age (Yr)	MEAN LIVER SPAN	MEAN LIVER SPAN
1	2.8	3.1
5	4.8	4.5
10	6.1	5.4
14	6.8	5.8
18	7.4	6.1

is normal until 4 years of age, and up to 1 cm throughout the rest of childhood.

Apparent liver enlargement may be caused by downward displacement secondary to intrathoracic conditions (hyperinflation, pneumothorax), subdiaphragmatic or retroperitoneal masses, and thoracic deformities. Normal liver spans, determined by percussion, are found in Table 8-7.

CLINICAL PRESENTATION AND DIAGNOSIS

The most likely cause of true hepatomegaly is *infectious mononucleosis* or a mono-like syndrome (CMV, toxoplasmosis). Malaise, weakness, fever, pharyngitis, generalized lymphadenopathy, and splenomegaly are associated findings. Other common causes include *viral hepatitis* (vomiting, jaundice, dark urine, acholic stools), *cirrhosis* and *chronic liver disease* (jaundice, spider angiomata, splenomegaly, ascites, hemorrhoids), *hemolytic anemias* such as thalassemia (peculiar facies, jaundice), and *congestive heart failure* (tachypnea, rales, cardiomegaly, edema). Serious, but less common, diseases include *leukemia* (pallor, bleeding, fever), *cystic fibrosis* (failure to thrive, recurrent pulmonary illnesses), and *Reye syndrome* (vomiting, neurologic dysfunction). Rare etiologies include *storage disorders* (Pompe disease, Tay-Sachs disease, tyrosinemia, von Gierke disease, galactosemia), *drugs* (acetaminophen overdose, carbon tetrachloride, methotrexate, chlorambucil), *Wilson disease, alpha-1-antitrypsin deficiency, hepatoma, liver hemangiomatosis, malaria,* and *liver abscess.* In the newborn, consider *congenital*

TORCHS infection, neonatal hepatitis, and *obstructive conditions* (biliary atresia, choledochal cyst).

ER MANAGEMENT

If true hepatomegaly is suspected and the patient does not appear seriously ill or jaundiced, work-up can be deferred, as a mono-like illness is most likely. The child should be reevaluated in 1–2 weeks. Alternatively, a CBC with differential, heterophile antibody, liver function tests and HBsAg can be obtained.

Jaundice, excessive vomiting, altered mentation, failure to thrive, and abnormal bleeding demand an immediate work-up. In addition to the above laboratory tests, a prothrombin time (PT) and partial thromboplastin time (PTT) should be obtained. Further evaluation is dictated by the clinical picture, but may include a bone marrow aspiration, CTT scan, liver–spleen scan, liver ultrasound, sweat chloride, alpha-1-antitrypsin assay, or liver biopsy.

INDICATIONS FOR ADMISSION

- Prothrombin time 5 seconds greater than control or partial thromboplastin time 20 seconds above control
- Altered mentation
- Severe vomiting that prevents adequate oral intake
- Suspicion of serious disease (leukemia, heart failure, cirrhosis, etc) for evaluation and management

REFERENCE

1. Walker WA, Mathis RK: Pediatr Clin North Am 22:929, 1975

Intussusception

INTRODUCTION

Intussusception is the most frequent cause of intestinal obstruction in infants beyond the immediate newborn period. It can occur at any age, although about 70% of cases are seen in the first year of life, especially between the ages of 4–10 months. The most common type is ileocolic, but intussusception may occur at any level of the GI tract.

Usually no etiology is found, although hypertrophy of Peyer's patches may play a role. In 5–10% of cases, especially in children over 6 years of age, there is a lead point such as a polyp, lymphoma, or a Meckel's diverticulum. Mesenteric venous engorgement, due to compression between the layers of the intussuscepted bowel, causes mucus secretion and blood seepage, and this accounts for the typical currant jelly stools. Later, necrosis, perforation, and peritonitis can occur.

CLINICAL PRESENTATION

Intussusception occurs primarily in healthy, well-nourished infants. Occasionally there is a history of a recent upper respiratory infection, diarrheal illness, or Henoch-Schönlein purpura. Characteristically, intermittent bouts of colicky pain occur more or less regularly, at 10- to 15-minute intervals. During these paroxysms the baby cries out, draws up his legs, and looks miserable. In between, the patient may initially appear well, but eventually becomes lethargic and apathetic. Vomiting follows the pain and may contain bile, suggesting intestinal obstruction. Classic currant jelly stools are present early in only 10% of cases, although they are eventually noted in 90% of infants and 65% of older children. Constipation, nonspecific diarrhea, and fever may also be seen. With recurrent intussusception and spontaneous reduction, symptoms may be subacute or chronic over a period of a few days to weeks.

Initially the abdomen is soft between episodes of pain, but later it becomes distended and tender. In 85% of cases, a sausage-like mass can be palpated in the right lower or upper abdomen. When the intussusception has progressed into the transverse colon, there may be absence of palpable viscera in the right lower quadrant (Dance sign). An abdominal mass may be appreciated on rectal examination, and blood on the examining finger is occasionally the first sign of the diagnosis. Bowel sounds are initially hyperactive, diminishing in time with circulatory compromise and bowel fatigue.

Occasionally, lethargy will be the most prominent sign. In these cases, the physician should inquire about a history of crampy abdominal pain and vomiting, and perform a careful physical examination for an abdominal mass and rectal bleeding. Consider the possibility of intussusception in any child with acute onset of encephalopathy, and especially when the working diagnosis is "r/o Reyes syndrome."

ER MANAGEMENT

If intussusception is suspected, immediately notify a pediatric surgeon, insert a nasogastric tube and an IV, obtain a CBC with differential, type and cross-match, serum electrolytes, and a venous blood gas, and order a KUB. A total white blood cell count of 10,000–18,000/mm^3 is common, while a higher leukocyte count suggests bowel necrosis. The abdominal film may show dilated small bowel loops, absence of air distal to the obstruction, and a soft tissue mass, usually in the transverse colon. Normal films, however, do not exclude the diagnosis. A barium enema is the diagnostic study of choice, showing the level of obstruction with a typical "coiled spring" appearance, caused by barium trickling around the intussusceptum.

Nonoperative hydrostatic reduction during the diagnostic barium enema is successful in 70–80% of cases. The child must be well sedated (IV morphine 0.1 mg/kg or Valium 0.3 mg/kg) or under general anesthesia. Barium is infused from a height not greater than 3 feet, abdominal manipulation is avoided during the reduction attempt, and the procedure is abandoned if reduction is not achieved after 10 minutes, although one repeat effort may be made after evacuation. The only criterion of complete reduction is free reflux of barium into the ileum. Because of increased risk of perforation, relative contraindications to nonoperative reduction include duration of symptoms over 36–48 hours, marked bleeding, and age less than 6 months. If there are clinical signs of perforation or shock, hydrostatic reduction is absolutely contraindicated. Give intravenous antibiotics: ampicillin (100 mg/kg/day divided q 6h) and gentamicin (2.5 mg/kg/dose divided q 8h) or clinidamycin (40 mg/kg/day divided q 6h) and arrange for surgery. Surgery is also indicated if hydrostatic reduction is unsuccessful.

INDICATION FOR ADMISSION

- Suspected intussusception

REFERENCES
1. Bergdahl S, Hugosson C, Söderlund S: J Pediat Surg 7:700, 1972
2. Gierup J, Jorulf H, Livaditis A: Pediatrics 50:535, 1972

Lower Gastrointestinal Bleeding

INTRODUCTION

Lower gastrointestinal (LGI) bleeding is common during childhood. It may appear as occult or gross rectal bleeding, or melena, either singly or in combination. The most common etiologies are summarized in Table 8-8.

CLINICAL PRESENTATION

Anal Fissure. With an anal fissure a small amount of blood is passed onto the diaper after the stool, or the stool is streaked with blood. The infant is alert, vigorous, and feeding well. There may be a history of recent diarrhea or constipation, but the stool may be normal by the time that the blood is first noticed. Usually at 12 or 6 o'clock there is either a tear in the rectal mucosa or a sentinel skin tag.

TABLE 8-8. ETIOLOGIES OF LOWER GASTROINTESTINAL BLEEDING

Under 1 Year Old	Over 1 Year Old
Anal fissure	Polyp
Bacterial colitis	Anal fissure
Volvulus (<4 months)	Bacterial colitis
Intussusception (>4 months)	Meckel's diverticulum
Milk protein allergy	Intussusception
	Inflammatory bowel disease
	Massive UGI bleeding

Polyps. Many cases of LGI bleeding in children over 1 year of age are due to polyps. The child, usually a male, presents with an episode of painless bright red rectal bleeding, occasionally accompanied by mild hypogastric tenderness. Most often the physical examination is unremarkable, although the polyp can sometimes be seen protruding from the rectum or palpated upon digital examination. Most cases involve a single polyp. There are several syndromes with multiple polyps and cutaneous findings, including Peutz-Jeghers (perioral pigmentation), Gardner (bony and soft tissue tumors), and Cronkhite-Canada (alopecia, dystrophic nails) syndromes.

Gastroenteritis. Gastroenteritis (p 186), especially bacterial, can cause bloody diarrhea with diffuse abdominal pain, fever, vomiting, and mucopurulent stools. Often other family members are affected.

Intussusception. Intussusception (p 194) causes the triad of colicky abdominal pain, LGI bleeding (currant jelly stools), and vomiting in patients 4 months to 4 years of age. Typically, a well child suddenly draws up his legs and cries out in pain. The discomfort subsides, only to have the cycle repeat. A tender sausage-shaped mass may be noted in the right upper quadrant (RUQ), while the right lower quadrant (RLQ) feels empty.

Volvulus. A volvulus causes bright red or maroon LGI bleeding in an infant or toddler. Bilious vomiting ensues, indicative of intestinal obstruction, and an abdominal mass may be noted.

Meckel Diverticulum. The most frequent cause of significant LGI bleeding in an otherwise healthy child is a Meckel diverticulum (p 201). There is painless massive bleeding, without hematemesis, and the physical examination is unremarkable. Anemia may be present in children over 3 years of age with repeated bleeding episodes.

Henoch-Schönlein Purpura. Henoch-Schönlein purpura may present with abdominal pain and mild LGI bleeding, with or without arthralgias and hematuria. The diagnosis is confirmed once the characteristic symmetric purpuric rash of the lower extremities appears.

Inflammatory Bowel Disease. LGI bleeding may accompany inflammatory bowel disease, but is rarely the presenting sign. There may be a history of watery diarrhea, weight loss, lower abdominal pain, and arthralgias.

Other Etiologies. Brisk upper gastrointestinal (UGI) bleeding (p 208) can lead to melena. *Gastroesophageal varices* cause massive UGI bleeding, usually in association with signs of chronic liver disease (splenomegaly, jaundice, caput medusa). *Peptic ulcers* cause coffee ground vomiting with epigastric pain that may be relieved by eating.

DIAGNOSIS

First, ascertain with a Hemoccult test that the red or black color in the stool is truly blood. Ingestion of beets, jello, Kool-aid, pyridium, ampicillin, and peaches may turn the stools red, while iron and licorice can cause "melena."

The nature of the bleeding suggests the most likely diagnoses. Bright red blood or streaking of blood on the stool surface suggests a low rectal lesion (*fissure*, polyp). Massive bleeding anywhere in the gastrointestinal tract can cause bright red LGI bleeding. Blood originating from the small bowel or upper colon (*polyp, gastroenteritis, intussusception, inflammatory bowel disease, HSP*) is darker, either mixed with the stool or unrelated to defecation. Melena, in association with UGI bleeding, is caused by lesions above the iliocecal valve (*varices, ulcers, polyps*). Occasionally, *genitourinary tract bleeding* can be confused with LGI bleeding, especially in patients wearing diapers. If the origin is not clear, perform a urinalysis.

Once the presence of blood is confirmed, inquire about a history of fever, vomiting, diarrhea, or constipation. Ask about aspirin or steroid usage (*ulcer*), previous bleeding episodes (*Meckel diverticulum, polyps*), weight loss or arthralgias (*inflammatory bowel disease*), and jaundice or liver disease (*varices*). On examination, look for signs of *liver disease* (jaundice, hepatosplenomegaly, caput medusa), purpura (*Henoch-Schönlein purpura*), perioral pigmentation (*Peutz-Jeghers* syndrome), an abdominal mass (*intussusception, volvulus*), and *anal fissure* or sentinel tag.

If the patient is having bloody diarrhea, a bacterial etiology is suggested by the presence of neutrophils in the stool. Smear a small amount of stool onto a slide, add 2 drops of methylene blue, cover with a coverslip. Wait several minutes, and examine for polymorphonuclear leukocytes (PMN) under low power.

If anemia is suspected (history of significant blood loss, pallor, tachycardia) obtain a spun hematocrit. Suspected inflammatory bowel disease (weight loss in association with abdominal pain or arthralgias) is an indication for an erythrocyte sedimentation rate (ESR).

ER MANAGEMENT

Stabilization of the vital signs is the priority. Check for signs of volume depletion (orthostatic vital sign changes, skin color and temperature, capillary filling, mental status). If volume depletion is present or bleeding is ongoing in the ER, insert a large bore IV and resuscitate with isotonic fluid (see shock, p 11). Obtain blood for CBC, spun hematocrit, platelet count, PT and PTT, type and crossmatch, electrolytes, glucose, and liver function tests.

If an *anal fissure* is noted, assume it to be the only source for the bleeding. Treat coexistent constipation (pp184–186), by adding a stool softener (malt extract, bran, prune juice) to the diet. If there is an associated *gastroenteritis,* treat with infrequent clear liquid feedings and examine a stool smear. If polys are seen, obtain a stool culture and, if the patient is febrile (>102°F) and under 1 year of age, a CBC and blood culture.

Patients with stable vital signs, who definitely had a *polyp* (past history, polyp seen or palpated), may be discharged with referrals to a primary care provider and pediatric gastroenterologist. If the diagnosis is not definite, consult a gastroenterologist for possible endoscopy.

If the patient has melena without hematemesis, insert a nasogastric tube and lavage the stomach, to determine whether the bleeding originates from the upper gastrointestinal tract. If blood or coffee grounds is found, lavage with iced saline until clear (see p 208).

The ER management of *intussusception* (p 194), *Meckel diverticulum* (p 201), and *volvulus* (intestinal obstruction, p 171) are detailed elsewhere.

INDICATIONS FOR ADMISSION

- Signs of intravascular volume depletion
- UGI bleeding or significant LGI bleeding
- Infants less than 6 months of age with fever and colitis (PMN in stool)
- Severe abdominal pain

REFERENCES
1. Berman WF, Holtzapple PE: Pediatr Clin North Am 23:885, 1975
2. Spencer R: Surgery 55:727, 1974

Meckel Diverticulum

INTRODUCTION

Meckel diverticulum is the most common intestinal malformation, occurring in 1–3% of the population. It is usually located within the terminal 100 cm of the ileum and may be connected by a fibrous cord to the abdominal wall. In about half of the cases there is ectopic mucosa, which is usually gastric (65–85% of cases), but pancreatic, small bowel, or colonic mucosa can also be present.

CLINICAL PRESENTATION

Most cases are asymptomatic, with the diverticulum an incidental surgical or postmortem finding. Signs or symptoms of hemorrhage, obstruction, or diverticulitis occur in 25–30% of the cases. Hemorrhage results from the ulceration of ileal mucosa that is adjacent to the ectopic gastric tissue. It is the most common presenting finding, seen in 40–60% of the symptomatic patients. Many children will have painless, massive, bright red bleeding, which can lead to shock. Alternatively, chronic blood loss, with normal or tarry stools, can occur.

Intestinal obstruction occurs in 20% of symptomatic patients. There can be intussusception with the diverticulum as a lead point, volvulus around the fixed tip of the diverticulum, internal herniation, or incarceration in an inguinal hernia. Half of the cases of intussusception occur in infancy, and the presentation is identical to idiopathic intussusception, although the risk of recurrences is higher.

Diverticulitis and perforation occasionally occur, possibly secondary to peptic ulceration. These are clinically indistinguishable from acute appendicitis, although the area of most intense pain is closer to the midline.

DIAGNOSIS AND ER MANAGEMENT

The ER management is dictated by the presenting symptom (see sections on abdominal pain, GI bleeding, intussusception, and appendicitis). A history of previous episodes of GI bleeding is important, as many patients with a bleeding Meckel diverticulum will have had a similar episode in the past. Once it has been established that the bleeding is coming from the LGI tract (see p 200), insert a large bore IV if there is active bleeding, orthostatic vital sign changes, or hypotension. A normal saline bolus (20 cc/kg) may be required. Obtain blood for a CBC, platelet count, type and cross-match, PT, and PTT.

Order a technetium 99m–sodium pertechnitate abdominal scan (Meckel scan) for patients with moderate to massive, relatively painless lower GI bleeding. It is a simple and noninvasive method for identifying a Meckel diverticulum with ectopic gastric mucosa, with an accuracy of 75–85%.

Treatment is operative after correction of anemia or fluid and electrolyte imbalances.

INDICATIONS FOR ADMISSION

- Positive Meckel scan
- LGI bleeding with profound anemia (Hgb <8mg/dL), orthostatic vital sign changes, hypotension, or other evidence of hypovelemia

REFERENCE

1. Schussheim A, Moskowitz GW, Levy LM: Am J Gastroenterol 68:25, 1977

Pyloric Stenosis

INTRODUCTION

Pyloric stenosis must always be considered in a young infant with vomiting, especially if there has been poor weight gain. It is four to eight times more common in boys than in girls, usually occurs in full term infants, and in about 5–7% of cases there is a positive family history in a parent or sibling.

CLINICAL PRESENTATION

The mean age of onset is 3 weeks, but symptoms may start at any time between birth and 5 months. The characteristic nonbilious, projectile vomiting is intermittent at first. Later, as more complete obstruction develops, it occurs after every meal. Peristaltic gastric waves, traveling from the left upper quadrant to the right lower quadrant, may be seen during feeding. When the course is prolonged, malnutrition and constipation may develop.

DIAGNOSIS

The diagnosis is confirmed by palpating the olive-sized pylorus. It is best felt after vomiting, usually slightly above and to the right of the umbilicus, but often under the liver edge. The olive is appreciated in 65–95% of the cases, but patience and experience are needed.

Because the obstruction is proximal to the ampulla of Vater, recurrent vomiting causes a hypokalemic, hypochloremic alkalosis. The ECG may reflect the hypokalemia (prolonged QT interval, and depression and broadening of the T-waves). Elevated hemoglobin and hematocrit levels are secondary to hemoconcentration. Indirect hyperbilirubinema may occur, possibly associated with decreased hepatic blood flow and glucuronyl transferase activity.

Radiologic studies are unnecessary when the pyloric tumor is palpated, but otherwise a barium swallow may show a dilated stomach with outlet obstruction and/or a narrowed, elongated pyloric channel that swings upwards (string sign). Recent experience suggests that an ultrasound may be equally accurate.

Antral web or *atresia* may cause gastric outlet obstruction, but symptoms occur earlier in life and the radiographic picture is diagnostic. The lack of bile rules out more distal lesions such as *duodenal stenosis* and *annular pancreas*. There is no gastric outlet obstruction in *gastroesophageal reflux*, but this condition may sometimes accompany pyloric stenosis. *Improper feeding practices* (large nipple hole, failure to burp the infant, etc.) and medical conditions, such as *sepsis, urinary tract infections, neurologic disorders,* and *congenital adrenal hyperplasia*, can present with recurrent vomiting but usually are easily differentiated from pyloric stenosis. None of these cause a hypochloremic, hypokalemic alkalosis.

ER MANAGEMENT

If an olive is palpated, make the patient NPO and insert a nasogastric tube. Obtain a CBC, electrolytes, and type and hold, perform a urinalysis with specific gravity determination, and start an IV. Initially, give 20 cc/kg of normal saline if the infant is volume depleted. Otherwise, D5 1/3 NS can be infused at maintenance rate. When the child is voiding well, add 20 mEq of KC1 to each liter. Surgery is performed when the fluid and electrolyte imbalances are corrected.

If an olive is not appreciated, observe the mother feeding the infant an electrolyte formula. If the infant does not vomit and is well hydrated, he may be sent home with a follow-up visit (including weight) scheduled for the next day. If the infant vomits the feed and/or appears dehydrated, admit him to the hospital for further evaluation after obtaining cultures of the blood and urine, and a venous pH, in addition to the laboratory tests outlined above.

INDICATION FOR ADMISSION

- Suspected pyloric stenosis

REFERENCES

1. Bell MJ: Surgery 64:983, 1968
2. Benson CD: Prog Pediatr Surg 1:63, 1970

Rectal Prolapse

INTRODUCTION

Rectal prolapse is usually a benign, self-limited condition that occurs predominantly in the first 2 years of life.

CLINICAL PRESENTATION AND DIAGNOSIS

Rectal prolapse appears as a sausage-shaped erythematous mass protruding a variable distance from the anus. Usually it occurs during stooling and recedes spontaneously. Etiologic factors include constipation, diarrhea, cystic fibrosis, parasites, and meningomyelocele.

ER MANAGEMENT

If the rectum does not reduce spontaneously, gentle finger pressure is usually effective. Appropriately treat any underlying constipation (p 185) or diarrhea (p 191), perform a careful physical and neurological examination (pay careful attention to the spine and lower extremities) and refer the patient for both a sweat chloride determination (cystic fibrosis) and serial stool collections (parasites).

Umbilical Lesions

INTRODUCTION

Most umbilical lesions are benign, although serious problems may be secondary to infection, abnormal intrauterine maturation of cord structures, and immune deficiency.

Generally, the umbilical cord begins to dry shortly after birth, then separates completely and falls off by the end of the second week. Delayed separation is defined as a cord that does not separate after 3 weeks. This may be associated with the application of triple dye antiseptic in the newborn nursery or, rarely, abnormal neutrophil function.

CLINICAL PRESENTATION

Umbilical Hernia. An umbilical hernia presents as a bulging out of the umbilicus that is noticed, and most marked, when the baby is crying or stooling. It is much more common in blacks, can be quite large, and usually closes within 2 or 3 years as the abdominal musculature grows. Infrequently, a piece of mesentery incarcerates, causing local pain and tenderness. Incarceration of bowel is exceedingly rare.

Persistent Omphalomesenteric Duct and Urachus. After the cord falls off, a persistent omphalomesenteric duct may present with fecal drainage, while a persistent urachus may allow the drainage of urine from the umbilicus. Either remnant may also persist as a blind sinus, with a purulent or egg-white-like discharge.

Granuloma. The most common of all umbilical lesions is persistence of the granulation tissue at the site of the cord separation. This presents with a small amount of a blood-tinged discharge and may enlarge into a granuloma, a reddish mass protruding from the umbilicus.

Omphalitis. Although a small rim of erythema around the base of the cord can be normal, omphalitis presents with erythematous streaking, particularly in the direction of the liver. The baby may be febrile, irritable, lethargic, and feeding poorly.

DIAGNOSIS

Immediately after separation, the surface of the umbilicus looks purulent. However, in the absence of erythema or tenderness of the surrounding skin, there is no infection. Normally there can be a small amount of blood-tinged, non-foul-smelling discharge. If the drainage smells like feces, consider a persistent omphalomesenteric duct. If there is a large amount of clear watery discharge, a persistent urachus is likely. Purulent drainage or material resembling egg whites suggests a persistent sinus secondary to one of the two preceding conditions.

Most often, when there is no umbilical hernia, folds of skin obscure the base of the umbilicus. It is not necessary to see a granuloma to make the diagnosis if the parents report some serosanguinous discharge.

ER MANAGEMENT

The treatment of an *umbilical hernia* is reassurance, since the vast majority resolve without intervention. Surgical repair is not indicated until at least 3 years of age. Instruct the parents to avoid using an abdominal binder, tape, or a large coin in a mistaken attempt to cure the hernia. These measures only lead to skin breakdown. Manually reduce incarcerated mesentery and arrange for surgical repair. Emergency surgical reduction is required if bowel incarcerates.

Omphalitis is potentially life threatening. Obtain a CBC and blood culture, and admit the baby for intravenous antibiotics (oxacillin 100 mg/kg/d and gentamicin 7.5 mg/kg/day).

If a *persistent omphalomesenteric duct* or *urachus* is suspected, consult with a pediatric surgeon to confirm the diagnosis and admit the patient.

The treatment of a *granuloma* is cautery with a silver nitrate stick. Moisten the stick with tap water, then roll it over the granuloma until the entire surface turns from red to grey. See the baby in 1 week and repeat the cautery, if necessary. If the granuloma cannot be visualized, blindly cauterize the base of the umbilicus by inserting the moistened silver nitrate stick. If the mass is particularly large when first seen, tie a ligature (3-0 nylon) around the base and see the baby again in 1 week. At that time, the granuloma can be severed at its base, which is then cauterized.

Obtain a CBC with differential if there is *delayed cord separation*. Instruct the parents to keep the cord dry and refer the baby to a primary care provider for follow-up within 1 week.

INDICATIONS FOR ADMISSION

- Omphalitis
- Incarcerated umbilical hernia
- Persistent omphalomesenteric duct, urachus, or sinus tract

REFERENCES

1. Bower TJ, et al: J Pediatr 101:932–940, 1982
2. Hayward AR, et al: Lancet 1: 1099–1101, 1979

Upper Gastrointestinal Bleeding

INTRODUCTION

UGI bleeding, from sites proximal to the ligament of Treitz, is uncommon in children. Most apparent cases are actually caused by the regurgitation of blood swallowed during episodes of epistaxis. Etiologies of true bleeding include gastritis and ulcers (use of aspirin, nonsteroidal anti-inflammatory agents, corticosteroids, or alcohol), esophagitis or Mallory-Weiss tear (forceful vomiting), and esophageal varices (portal hypertension).

CLINICAL PRESENTATION

The bleeding may appear bright or dark red if it is immediately vomited. Coffee grounds vomitus occurs if the blood was exposed to hydrochloric acid in the stomach. Occasionally melena is the only finding.

Patients with ulcers may report a history of epigastric pain relieved by eating and blood noted with the first emesis. In contrast, bleeding occurs after several episodes of vomiting in patients with gastritis, esophagitis, or Mallory-Weiss tears. Esophageal varices are usually associated with hepatosplenomegaly, hemorrhoids, caput medusa, and jaundice.

DIAGNOSIS

When the only evidence of bleeding is melena, the diagnosis of a UGI bleed must be confirmed by passing a nasogastric tube and aspirating the stomach contents (bright red blood or coffee grounds). Guiac the material, as red-colored foods or medicines may be mistaken for blood. Also, examine the nose for possible sites of *epistaxis*.

The priority is management. However, inquire about recent gastroenteritis, vomiting, nosebleeds, drug or alcohol use, chronic liver disease, and family history of *ulcers*. Perform a quick physical examination, looking for signs of *liver disease* (enumerated above) and evidence of shock.

ER MANAGEMENT

Insert a nasogastric tube and perform lavage with normal saline until the stomach aspirate is pinkish or clear. Infuse about 5 cc/kg, allow it to remain in the stomach for several minutes, and then aspirate via low suction. Use iced saline, except in young patients (<2 years) who may become hypothermic. While lavage is being accomplished, obtain blood for CBC, platelet count, type and cross-match, and if liver disease is suspected, liver function tests, PT and PTT. If necessary, transfuse 10 cc/kg of packed cells (pp 11–15) in the ER.

Admit these patients to an intensive care setting. Consult with a pediatric gastroenterologist, who may recommend immediate endoscopy. Cimetidine (10–30 mg/kg/day) and antacids (Maalox, 5–15 cc q 3–4h) are indicated for gastritis, ulcers, and esophagitis.

INDICATION FOR ADMISSION

- UGI bleeding

REFERENCE

1. Cox K, Ament ME: Pediatrics 63:408–413, 1979

9

Genitourinary Emergencies

Balanitis and Posthitis

INTRODUCTION

Balanitis is inflammation, with or without cellulitis, of the glans penis, while posthitis involves the foreskin. The etiology is poor penile hygiene, although in the circumcised boy balanitis is secondary to contact dermatitis from urine, laundry soaps, powders, and ointments.

CLINICAL PRESENTATION AND DIAGNOSIS

There is erythema, warmth, swelling, and tenderness of the glans and foreskin. There may be secondary meatitis with resultant dysuria and voluntary urinary retention.

Recurrent episodes of posthitis can result in phimosis and ultimately meatal stenosis, with dribbling of urine and a poor stream.

ER MANAGEMENT

The treatment is frequent warm water sitz baths, followed by thorough drying of the penis. If infection seems likely (purulent discharge, cellulitis), give either a topical (bacitracin ointment) or, for severe cases, an oral antibiotic (cephradine 25 mg/kg/day, dicloxacillin 50 mg/kg/day). If the cellulitis is widespread, recommend bedrest and a sheet cradle with the penis exposed.

Meatitis resulting in meatal stenosis requires an elective ventral meatotomy, while a predisposing phimosis is an indication for elective circumcision.

Meatal Stenosis

INTRODUCTION

Meatal stenosis is a narrowing of the urethral meatus, usually secondary to meatitis. Etiologies include ammoniacal diaper irritation (circumcised boys) and recurrent balanitis-posthitis (uncircumcised boys). Congenital meatal stenosis is very rare.

CLINICAL PRESENTATION

An abnormal urinary stream may be seen, with either spraying or upward deflection. Obstructive symptoms of hesitancy, straining, urgency, frequency, and postvoiding dribbling occasionally occur, although urinary retention is rare. If there is an associated meatitis, an erythematous, swollen meatus is noted, often with a purulent discharge or hematuria.

DIAGNOSIS

When the typical findings are present and the meatus is small, the diagnosis can be assumed to be meatal stenosis. However, observe the stream, since the subjective impression (on visual inspection) of a narrowed meatus does not constitute a valid diagnosis of meatal stenosis. Radiographic studies are seldom necessary to confirm the diagnosis, which is made on clinical grounds.

ER MANAGEMENT

Treat a purulent meatitis with sitz baths and 1% hydrocortisone cream tid. Refer all patients to a urologist for confirmation of the diagnosis and further evaluation.

For the rare occurrence of acute urinary retention, immediately consult a urologist for consideraton of catheterization.

INDICATION FOR ADMISSION

- Meatal stenosis causing urinary retention

REFERENCES

1. Allen JS, Summers JD, Wilkerson JE: J Urol 107:498, 1972
2. Comm. from the Urology Section: Pediatrics 61:778–780, 1978

Paraphimosis

INTRODUCTION

Paraphimosis results when a tight, phimotic foreskin is retracted proximal to the glans penis, without immediate reduction. This produces a tourniquet effect with resultant venous occlusion and glans edema.

CLINICAL PRESENTATION AND DIAGNOSIS

Glans edema is proportional to the duration of the paraphimosis. A swollen, blue, congested glans can progress to an ischemic white color, with eventual gangrene. Severe pain accompanies the edema, and marked vasoconstriction can cause urethral obstruction with difficulty in voiding and urinary retention.

ER MANAGEMENT

Place an icebag on the foreskin, then attempt manual reduction after sedating the patient (meperidine 2 mg/kg, promethazine 1 mg/kg, and chlorpromazine 1 mg/kg intramuscularly. Reduce the edema by squeezing the glans firmly for several minutes. Then, grasp the penile shaft with the index and third fingers of each hand, with the thumbs on the glans. Firm pressure on the glans against counterpressure on the shaft usually advances the foreskin back over the glans. Occasionally, there is tearing of the skin with bleeding which can be controlled by compression. Instruct the patient to avoid retracting his foreskin for several days.

If the paraphimosis cannot be reduced, consult a urologist for incision of the constricting tissue.

Arrange for an elective circumcision for all patients once the edema and inflammation have resolved.

INDICATION FOR ADMISSION

- Paraphimosis requiring incision

REFERENCE

1. Skoglund RW Jr, Chapman WH: J Urol 104:137, 1970

Phimosis

INTRODUCTION

Phimosis, an inability to retract the foreskin back over the glans penis, is considered normal until about 12 months of age. Afterwards, the accumulation of smegma under the foreskin can lead to infection, scarring, and subsequent secondary phimosis.

CLINICAL PRESENTATION AND DIAGNOSIS

Accumulated smegma may form aggregates that appear as whitish, globular masses under the nonretractile foreskin. Associated inflammatory conditions may coexist, including balanitis and posthitis (p 211) and meatitis (p 212).

With severe phimosis, the foreskin may balloon during voiding as the urine collects under it and dribbles out from the tight opening.

The adolescent may complain of pain on erection, secondary to tension on the foreskin from the glandular adhesions.

ER MANAGEMENT

Treat accumulated smegma without any associated infection with gentle retraction of the foreskin (as far as it can go) during bathing.

If there is no infection refer the patient to a urologist for elective circumcision. See p 212 for the treatment of accompanying posthitis or balanitis. Arrange for follow-up within 2 days.

If there is ballooning of the foreskin with a dribbling urinary stream, refer the patient to a urologist. Gentle dilation may be necessary, after which an elective circumcision is indicated.

REFERENCES

1. Boyce WT: PIR 5:26–30, 1983
2. Kaplan GW: Current Problems in Pediatrics 7(5), 1977.

Renal and Genitourinary Trauma

INTRODUCTION

Renal trauma occurs most frequently as a result of blunt injury (motor vehicle accidents, falls, athletic injuries); penetrating trauma (knife, gunshot) is less common. Because abnormal kidneys are more easily injured, in up to 20% of cases of traumatic hematuria an underlying congenital anomaly is found, including ureteropelvic junction obstruction, megaloureter, or ectopic or solitary kidneys. Although most renal trauma occurs as an isolated injury, in 25% of cases of blunt and 80% of penetrating abdominal trauma, other organs are injured, most commonly the liver.

Lower genitourinary tract trauma primarily involves the penis and scrotum. Penile skin is often caught in zippers and hairs encircling the penile shaft can lead to marked swelling. Penile and scrotal amputations are surgical emergencies. Bladder and urethral injuries usually occur secondary to blunt external trauma, often in association with pelvic fractures.

CLINICAL PRESENTATION AND DIAGNOSIS

Renal Injury. The cardinal signs are flank pain and tenderness and abdominal rigidity. Hematuria, either gross or microscopic, is nearly always present. A flank mass develops if there is extravasation of blood or urine into the perirenal tissues. Other findings include flank ecchymoses, fractured ribs, and pelvic fracture.

Bladder and Posterior Urethral Injuries. These most commonly occur in association with pelvic fractures, so that the signs of the bony trauma may obscure the urologic injury. A patient with a *ruptured bladder* presents with an inability to void, suprapubic and abdominal pain, and hematuria. Males with *posterior urethral injuries* have generally suffered severe blunt trauma and have significant associated injuries. Lower abdominal and pelvic swelling, tenderness, and ecchymosis are commonly seen, with hematuria and blood at the external meatus. Once again, the patient is unable to void.

Bulbar Urethral Trauma. Bulbar urethral trauma commonly accompanies a straddle injury. Perineal and scrotal hematomas may be noted along with bleeding from the meatus, and an inability to void.

On urinalysis, there are usually more than 10 RBC/hpf. However, there is no consistent relationship between the number of red cells and the degree of urinary tract injury, if any. In fact, the absence of blood does not exclude a major injury, as ureteral transection or occlusion of the renal artery may occur without hematuria.

ER MANAGEMENT

An intravenous pyelogram (IVP) is mandatory in all cases of suspected renal injury, whether the hematuria is microscopic or gross. Parenchymal swelling may interfere with the IVP interpretation unless it is performed within 6 hours of the injury. Therefore, obtain the IVP promptly (as soon as the blood pressure is stable). Nonvisualization of a kidney is most commonly secondary to an arterial injury. A renal scan (flow study) and an arteriogram must be performed if the kidney is not visualized. Cystoscopy and retrograde pyelography are rarely required in the ER setting.

Renal Injury. Four categories can be documented on the IVP. With a *contusion,* the renal outline is intact and there is no extravasation of dye. Bedrest and observation are all that are needed. A *laceration* disrupts the cortex and may extend into the collecting system, causing dye extravasation. Minor lacerations can be treated with bedrest, major lacerations may require surgical repair. A *collecting system injury* with dye extravasation is uncommon. Surgical repair and drainage are indicated. Finally, a *major vessel injury* is most commonly seen after acceleration–deceleration injuries. Nonvisualization on IVP demands an immediate arteriogram, or renal scan followed by surgical exploration.

External Genital Trauma. Treat *penile hair-tourniquet* with an ice-bag to ease the pain and shrink the swelling. Application of soapy water to the hairs facilitates their removal. Wrap any *penile amputation,* no matter what the size, in a saline gauze, put it in a plastic bag, and place it on ice with pressure and sterile dressings to the remaining shaft. Immediate reanastomosis surgery is frequently successful. Treat *amputation of scrotal skin* with sterile saline-soaked towels and immediate surgery. Treat a *urethral foreign body* with cystoscopy after percutaneous placement of a suprapubic catheter by a urologist. If gentle attempts to remove *penile skin caught in a zipper* are unsuccessful, inject 1% lidocaine (without epinephrine) into the foreskin. Then, the zipper can be closed, cut through at its base, and opened from the base, releasing the entrapped skin.

Bladder or Urethral Trauma. Inability to void, a distended bladder, and blood at the urethral meatus are warning signs. Call a urologist immediately. A rectal exam (boggy mass palpated in the area of urethral disruption) and retrograde urethrogram are indicated in the male and catheterization is necessary in the female (for a VCU). Urethral catheterization is *contraindicated* in the male.

INDICATIONS FOR ADMISSION

- Abnormal IVP (renal contusion, laceration, collecting system injury, major vessel injury)
- Penile or scrotal amputation
- Bladder or urethral contusion, laceration, or rupture
- Inability to void

REFERENCES

1. Guerriero WG: Surg Clin North Am 62:1047, 1982
2. Levitt SB in Edelman CM (ed): Pediatric Kidney Disease. Boston: Little, Brown and Co, pp 1145–1169, 1978
3. Mertz JHO, Widhard WN, Noorse MH, et al: JAMA 183:730, 1963

Scrotal Swellings

INTRODUCTION

Although a number of conditions can produce an acutely erythematous and tender hemiscrotum, expedient diagnosis of testicular torsion is always the first consideration when managing any case of scrotal swelling.

CLINICAL PRESENTATION

Testicular Torsion. Testicular torsion, the most common cause of acute scrotal swelling, is caused by twisting of the spermatic cord leading to venous, then arterial obstruction. Abrupt pain localized to the affected testis, groin, or lower abdomen occurs along with hemiscrotal swelling and erythema. The involved testis may lie higher in the scrotum, with a horizontal (rather than vertical) orientation. The hemiscrotal swelling does not transilluminate and elevation of the testicle is painful. Fever and dysuria are absent, and in about half of the cases there is a history of subacute bouts of scrotal pain (previous intermittent torsion).

Torsion of the Testicular Appendage. Torsion of the testicular appendage can mimic testicular torsion. On occasion, pain and tenderness are localized to the superior pole of the testis, and a bluish nodule can be seen through the thin scrotal skin at that site. The swelling does not transilluminate, although there may be an associated reactive hydrocele that does transilluminate. Elevation of the testis does not relieve the pain, and there is no fever or urinary symptoms. Previous subacute episodes are uncommon.

Epididymoorchitis. Epididymoorchitis may be confused with a testicular torsion, although it is uncommon in boys under 14 years of age. A recent history of mumps exposure or scrotal trauma facilitates the diagnosis of orchitis. Other etiologies include infectious mononucleosis, varicella, and Coxsackie virus. When epididymitis occurs in young boys, there is often a history of urinary tract anomaly (megaloureter, vesicoureteral reflux) or recent instrumentation, in association with a urinary infection. In postpubertal adolescents, the etiology of epididymitis is usually a sexually transmitted organism such as *Gonococcus, Ureaplasma,* or *Chlamydia* (p 241).

Testicular, and possibly abdominal, pain occurs in association with a nontransilluminating scrotal swelling, a thickened, tender epididymis, nausea, vomiting, fever, and dysuria. Manual scrotal elevation often relieves the pain in epididymoorchitis (Prehn sign), but not in testicular and appendiceal torsions.

Inguinal Hernia. Inguinal hernias are most common in the first year of life, especially if the infant was premature. Males are affected ten times more often than females, and hernias are more common on the right side. Typically, recurrent episodes of painless, nonerythematous scrotal and inguinal swelling occur, often when the baby is crying. Bowel sounds may be heard in the scrotum and transillumination is variable. Incarceration within the inguinal ring can ensue, with acute tenderness, erythema, and induration. With time, strangulation occurs, with bilious vomiting, decreased bowel sounds, abdominal distention, and fluid and electrolyte imbalances.

Hydrocele. Hydroceles are also most common in the first year of life, especially on the right side. Typically there are recurrent episodes of painless, nonerythematous scrotal swellings that vary in size. The mass transilluminates and the testicle is palpable posterior to the hydrocele. The swelling does not extend into the inguinal canal and intestinal obstruction does not occur.

Varicocele. Varicoceles are virtually always on the left side. They usually do not occur until puberty, at which time the patient complains of a sensation of weight in the scrotum. Examination in the upright position reveals a nontender, nonerythematous scrotum with a "bag of worms" inside.

Idiopathic Scrotal Edema Idiopathic scrotal edema is an inflammatory condition of unknown etiology causing a violaceous coloration and swelling of the scrotal wall with a normal underlying testis.

Hematocele. Hematoceles can occur after scrotal trauma or in association with a bleeding diathesis. A painful, bluish scrotal swelling is seen.

Testicular Tumor. Testicular tumors are rare, but most occur in patients under 3 years of age. There is diffuse or localized testicular enlargement that is firm or rock hard. There can be an associated reactive hydrocele that confuses the picture.

DIAGNOSIS

The diagnosis in patients with acute hemiscrotal pain and swelling is *testicular torsion* until proven otherwise. An appendicular torsion and epididymoorchitis may closely resemble a testicular torsion. If there is *any* suspicion of torsion, *immediately* obtain urological consultation.

With appendicular torsion, pain and swelling may be localized to the superior testicular pole and a blue dot may be seen through the thin scrotal skin. When there is any doubt, the diagnosis should be confirmed at surgery. However, there are useful laboratory tests that, if available within an hour of the patient's presentation, may help differentiate among the causes of an acute hemiscrotum. These include radioisotope scrotal scanning (cold in testicular torsion, normal or hot in appendicular torsion, hot with epididymoorchitis) and Doppler stethoscope (decreased blood flow in testicular torsion, increased with appendicular torsion and epididymoorchitis). Pyuria and dysuria may occur in epididymoorchitis, along with Prehn sign, fever, and an elevated white blood cell count.

Inguinal hernias, hydroceles, hematoceles, and varicoceles can usually be distinguished by the clinical findings. If a strangulated inguinal hernia cannot be ruled out, obtain a KUB test. Dilated intestinal loops with air-fluid levels may be seen along with a loop of bowel in the scrotum.

ER MANAGEMENT

Testicular Torsion. All suspected cases must be evaluated *immediately* by a urologist or general surgeon, as testicular survival depends on the duration of ischemia (100% survival at 4 hours, 0% at 24 hours). At surgery both testicles are sutured down. Duration of symptoms for more than 24 hours is not a reason to defer surgery, as the testis may tort and detort. The intermittent nature of the torsion increases the chance of survival in spite of the long duration.

In extreme circumstances, when a surgeon or operating room are unavailable, manual detorsion may be tried. Give morphine sedation (0.1 mg/kg intravenous [IV] repeated as needed), then rotate the testis

180–360 degrees clockwise, then counterclockwise until the torsion is relieved (as documented by pain relief or increased blood flow by Doppler). Surgery is still necessary, as retortion often occurs acutely.

Torsion of Appendage Testis. The only indications for surgery are when testicular torsion cannot be clinically excluded, or for chronic unremitting swelling or pain.

Epididymoorchitis. Treat the prepubertal male with antibiotics (trimethoprim/sulfamethoxazole, 8mg/kg/day of TMP or ampicillin 100 mg/kg/day) for 10 days, analgesics, bedrest, and scrotal support. The treatment of sexually transmitted epididymitis is detailed elsewhere (p 242).

Inguinal Hernia. An unincarcerated hernia requires no acute treatment. Refer the patient to a surgeon so that elective repair can be arranged. If the hernial sac contents cannot be easily pushed back into the abdomen, sedate the patient (meperidine 2 mg/kg, promethazine 1 mg/kg, and chlorpromazine 1 mg/kg) and place him in the Trendelenberg position, with an icebag on the hernia. After 30 minutes, attempt to push the hernia back into the abdomen. If this is not successful, admit the patient for correction of any fluid and electrolyte imbalances, prior to emergency herniorrhaphy.

Hydrocele. Almost all hydroceles spontaneously resolve prior to 24 months of age. Thereafter, refer the patient to a urologist.

Varicocele. Refer the patient to a urologist for ligation if the varicocele is on the right or persists when the patient is recumbant. The increased peritesticular temperature can lead to decreased fertility.

Idiopathic Scrotal Edema. No treatment is required, other than rest, analgesia, and antihistamines (diphenhydramine 5 mg/kg/day, divided qid).

Hematocele. Treat with rest and analgesia. If the patient has a bleeding diathesis, employ appropriate measures (see p 258) and consult with a urologist.

Testicular Tumor. If there is any suspicion of a testicular tumor, immediately refer the patient to a urologist for further evaluation and treatment.

INDICATIONS FOR ADMISSION

- Suspected testicular torsion
- Incarcerated inguinal hernia
- Testicular tumor

REFERENCES

1. Klauber GT, Sant GR in Kelalis PP, King LR, Belman AB (eds): Clinical Pediatric Urology. Phila: WB Saunders, 1985, 825–863
2. Kogan SJ in Whitehead ED, Leiter E (eds): Current Operative Urology. New York: Harper and Row, 1984, 1551–1553

Undescended Testes

INTRODUCTION

Spontaneous descent of an undescended testicle is unlikely after 1 year of age. Histologic deterioration begins during the second year of life, and this has been correlated with infertility, even in unilateral cases. Therefore, medical or surgical descent should be accomplished after the first birthday.

CLINICAL PRESENTATION AND DIAGNOSIS

Eighty percent of undescended testes are *palpable* in the groin, within the inguinal canal. Some of these testes are actually retractile and will reenter the scrotum during a warm bath. There may be an associated inguinal hernia.

Most *impalpable* testes are ultimately found within the inguinal canal or abdomen. In the remaining cases there is unilateral or bilateral testicular absence.

ER MANAGEMENT

No acute treatment is necessary. Refer infants under 1 year of age to a primary care provider and instruct the parent to examine the scrotum while the patient is in the bath. Refer patients at 1 year of age to a urologist. If an inguinal hernia is present, arrange for early surgical correction of the cryptorchidism and the hernia, regardless of the patient's age.

REFERENCE

1. Kogan SJ in Kelalis PP, King LR, Belman AB (eds): Clinical Pediatric Urology. Phila: WB Saunders, 1985, 864–887

Urethritis

INTRODUCTION

Urethritis is an inflammation of the urethral mucosa caused by irritation (bubble bath), anatomical lesions (urethral prolapse, polyp, diverticulum, valves), and foreign body insertion. Sexually transmitted infection is the most common etiology in sexually active adolescents, although infectious causes of urethritis are rare in prepubertal children.

CLINICAL PRESENTATION AND DIAGNOSIS

Irritation. Bubble bath causes a chemical irritation of the distal urethral and meatal mucosa in females. The patient presents with meatal pain, itching, and dysuria.

Anatomical Abnormalities. A prolapsed urethra most commonly occurs in young black females. The prolapsed mucosa is grossly visible and becomes irritated and congested, then hemorrhagic.

Other abnormalities, such as urethral diverticulum, urethral polyp, and valve of Guerin are uncommon. They usually present with gross hematuria, voiding pain at the dorsal glans penis, and blood spotting on the underpants.

Foreign Body. A urethral foreign body causes a bloody urethritis. There may be a clear history of insertion, the object may be palpable in the urethra, or it may be readily visible (radiopaque) on x-ray.

Posterior Urethritis. This is a nonspecific urethral inflammation in boys 5–15 years old. It presents with urethral discharge, urethral bleeding, or terminal hematuria. The physical examination is normal and routine cultures of the discharge and the urine are sterile.

Sexually Transmitted Urethritis. In males, gonorrhea, *Chlamydia,* or *Ureaplasma* cause dysuria, urethral discharge, and occasionally epididymitis or prostatitis. In females, *Chlamydia* commonly causes the acute urethral syndrome, with dysuria, urgency, suprapubic tenderness, and pyuria.

The diagnosis is discussed on pp 241–244. Obtain a urinalysis and routine urine culture (which should be negative), and perform a Gram stain (looking for gonococci) and culture (gonococci, *Chlamydia*) of the urethral discharge.

ER MANAGEMENT

Irritation. Discontinue the bubble baths, and if the symptoms are severe, give Pyridium (12 mg/kg/day to 300 mg divided tid).

Anatomical Abnormalities. Treat a prolapsed urethra with sitz baths, tid. If marked edema causes voiding difficulty, call a urologist for further evaluation.

Refer patients with gross hematuria in association with penile voiding pain to a urologist.

Foreign Body. Immediately consult a urologist.

Posterior Urethritis. Treat with 1 week of antibiotics (<8 years: ampicillin 250 mg qid; >8 years: trimethoprim-sulfamethoxazole, 8 mg/kg/day of TMP divided bid). There is a high rate of recurrence and bulbar urethral stricture can result, so refer the patient to a urologist.

Sexually Transmitted Urethritis. Treat with tetracycline 500 mg qid or doxycycline 100 mg bid, for 7 days (see p 242).

INDICATIONS FOR ADMISSION

- Inability to void
- Urethral foreign body

REFERENCES
1. Bowie WR: Urol Clin North Am 7:17, 1980
2. Jacobs NF Jr, Kraus ST: Ann Intern Med 82:7, 1975

Urinary Retention

INTRODUCTION

Ninety percent of all newborns void within the first 24 hours of life, and 99% do so by 48 hours of age. In the male infant, posterior urethral valves are the most common cause of retention, but a urethral polyp, urethral stricture, anterior urethral valve, urethral diverticulum, and meatal stenosis are other etiologies. In the female infant, retention is most often secondary to a prolapsing ureterocele.

Infections (cystitis, urethritis, meatitis), iatrogenic or self-instrumentation, spinal cord lesions, medications (anticholinergics and sympathomimetics), and psychogenic retention are other causes of urinary retention.

CLINICAL PRESENTATION AND DIAGNOSIS

Urinary retention in a newborn male presents as dribbling, or a poor stream. In the female, a *ureterocele* causes dribbling on urination and a bulging introital mass. In either sex, the bladder may be persistently palpable.

In older patients, urinary retention may be associated with urgency, hesitancy, frequency, dribbling, a poor stream, or recurrent urinary tract infections. Dysuria (*cystitis* or *urethritis*), a urethral discharge (urethritis), or an inflamed, swollen urethral meatus (*meatitis*) may be present. The patient may be taking an *antihistamine, decongestant, bronchodilator,* or *anticholinergic* (tricyclic antidepressant, probantheline).

Patients with *spinal cord abnormalities* usually have visible deformities of the back. On neurologic examination, there may be altered lower extremity reflexes, decreased anal sphincter tone, a sensory level, or differential responses to sensory testing in the lower extremities.

Psychosomatic retention usually occurs in females with no previous history of voiding abnormalities. The initiating stress factor is often unrecognized by the patient and parents, and no other congenital or acquired etiology can be found.

ER MANAGEMENT

Immediately refer all infants with dribbling, poor stream, or failure to void within 48 hours of birth to a urologist. Obtain blood for BUN test creatinine and urine for urinalysis and culture.

The management of cystitis (p 224), urethritis (p 477), and meatitis (p 212) is discussed elsewhere.

For retention secondary to urinary tract instrumentation, recommend sitz baths tid and give Pyridium (12 mg/kg/day), but warn the family that the urine will turn orange. Discontinue any medication causing retention.

If a spinal cord lesion is suspected, consult with a neurologist. However, intermittent catheterization or an indwelling catheter may be required as a temporizing measure.

If psychosomatic retention is suspected, immediately refer the patient to a psychiatrist. Once again, temporary intermittent catheterization or an indwelling catheter may be required.

INDICATION FOR ADMISSION

- Urinary retention that cannot be relieved in the ER

REFERENCES

1. Cremin BJ: Br J Urol 48:113, 1975
2. Tsingoglou S, Dickson JAS: Arch Dis Child 47:215, 1972

10

Gynecologic Emergencies

Breast Lesions

INTRODUCTION

The most common breast disorders are neonatal hypertrophy, premature thelarche in prepubertal girls, gynecomastia in adolescent boys, and breast abscesses in newborns and teenaged girls.

CLINICAL PRESENTATION

Neonatal Breast Hypertrophy. Neonatal breast hypertrophy occurs in up to two-thirds of normal newborns of both sexes. It presents as palpable breast tissue, present from birth, in an otherwise healthy infant. Occasionally, there is also galactorrhea, clitoral hypertrophy, and a bloody vaginal discharge. Most cases resolve within 4 weeks, but the condition occasionally persists for several months.

Premature Thelarche. Premature thelarche is isolated unilateral or bilateral breast enlargement without other signs of puberty. It occurs in girls 1–5 years old and either regresses or does not progress. There is no associated nipple change, growth spurt, axillary or pubic hair, clitoral enlargement, acne, or nipple discharge. Pathologic causes include true precocious puberty, central nervous system (CNS) disorders, ovarian tumors, and exogenous estrogens.

Gynecomastia. Gynecomastia, or enlargement of the male breast, is seen in 60–90% of teenaged boys, but is rare in preadolescents. It occurs at 12–15 years of age in otherwise healthy, often obese, boys who are experiencing a normal male puberty. The enlargement is unilateral or bilateral, tenderness may be present, but the nipple remains normal. The enlargement regresses spontaneously. Prepubertal and pathologic adolescent gynecomastia may be caused by drugs (cimetidine, digitalis, tricyclic antidepressants, marijuana), liver disease, testicular tumors, anorchia, Kleinfelter syndrome (XXY karyotype and small testes), and adrenal disease.

Breast Abscess. Breast abscesses occur in newborns and adolescent females as a result of breast tissue hypertrophy. Staphylococci and streptococci are the usual organisms. They present as warm, erythematous, tender masses which may be fluctuant.

DIAGNOSIS

Premature Thelarche. Perform a thorough physical examination, looking for other secondary sexual characteristics, café-au-lait spots (neurofibromatosis, McCune-Albright syndrome) or ash leaf macules (tuberous sclerosis), abdominal mass, ovarian mass (perform a rectal examination), and visual field disturbances.

Gynecomastia. Palpate the abdomen for hepatomegaly and examine the testicles to evaluate the size and rule out a mass.

Abscess. The diagnosis is usually evident upon inspection.

Papillomatosis. Bleeding from the nipple in association with a breast mass suggests a tumor (papillomatosis, rarely carcinoma).

ER MANAGEMENT

Neonatal Breast Hypertrophy. Reassurance, cool compresses, and avoidance of breast massaging are all that is necessary. Refer the patient to a primary care provider.

Gynecomastia. Reassure the adolescent and if obese, prescribe a weight reduction regimen. Arrange for primary care follow-up within 6 months. Immediately refer prepubertal boys to a pediatric endocrinologist for further evaluation.

Premature Thelarche. Immediately refer these girls to a primary care physician for further evaluation.

Benign Papillomatosis. This usually resolves spontaneously, but refer the patient immediately to a surgeon.

Breast Abscesses. Treat neonates with oral dicloxacillin (50 mg/kg/day divided qid) and warm soaks. If the baby has a temperature over 101°F or looks "toxic" perform a complete sepsis work-up (including lumbar puncture) and treat with intravenous oxacillin (100 mg/kg/day). Refer adolescent girls to an experienced surgeon for incision and drainage. If the infection is not yet fluctuant, treat with dicloxacillin (500 mg q6h) and warm compresses (q2h), and see the patient daily.

INDICATION FOR ADMISSION

- Febrile or toxic neonate with a breast abscess

REFERENCE

1. Capraro VJ, Dewhurst CS: Clin Obstet Gynecol 18:25–50, 1975

Dysfunctional Uterine Bleeding

INTRODUCTION

Normal menstrual bleeding does not occur more often than every 21 days, the flow lasts no more than 8 days, and no more than six well-soaked pads or 10 well-soaked tampons are used in 24 hours.

Dysfunctional uterine bleeding (DUB) is irregular, painless bleeding of endometrial origin. Most cases are secondary to anovulation, which is common during the first two years after menarche. However, abnormal vaginal bleeding may signify serious local or systemic disease and must be evaluated carefully.

CLINICAL PRESENTATION

A typical pattern of DUB is prolonged or excessive flow alternating with periods of amenorrhea. In contrast to adults, intermenstrual spotting is infrequent. Pain, fever, chills, and vaginal discharge are absent.

With *mild DUB* the menses may be somewhat prolonged or the cycle shortened for 2–3 months. The hematocrit is normal (>37–

38%). *Moderate DUB* is characterized by gross irregularity with prolonged periods, moderately increased flow, and polymenorrhea severe enough to cause a decrease in hematocrit (>28%). *Severe DUB* results in a hematocrit <28%, with clinical signs of acute blood loss (tachycardia, orthostatic vital sign changes).

DIAGNOSIS

DUB is a diagnosis of exclusion: causes of irregular or excessive vaginal bleeding are summarized in Table 10-1.

Inquire about the age of menarche, date of last menstrual period, frequency and regularity of menses, length of flow, and the number of pads or tampons used. Ask about bleeding manifestations, sexual activity (including genital trauma), vaginal or uterine foreign bodies, medication use, endocrine disorders, exposure to DES in utero, emotional stress, and chronic illnesses. Obtain a family history of abnormal bleeding (epistaxis, easy bruising, bleeding gums).

On physical examination, look for orthostatic hypotension, tachycardia, petechiae, ecchymoses, bradycardia (hypothyroidism), or evidence of a chronic illness. Examine the breasts for signs of pregnancy (fullness, tenderness, enlarged and darkened areolae, galactor-

TABLE 10-1. CAUSES OF IRREGULAR VAGINAL BLEEDING

Dysfunctional uterine bleeding	Genital trauma
Complications of pregnancy	First intercourse
Abortion	Rape
Ectopic	Foreign body
Bleeding disorder	IUD
Congenital or acquired	Diaphragm
Salpingitis	Tampon
Endocrine disorders	Anatomical abnormality
Hypo- or hyperthyroidism	Ovarian cyst
Adrenal disorders	Tumor
Diabetes mellitus	DES exposure in utero
Medication use	Chronic illness
Coumadin	Stress
Birth control pills	

rhea) and the abdomen for an enlarged uterus (palpable abdominally at 12 weeks), mass, or tenderness (suggesting pelvic inflammation).

A gynecologic exam is indicated for any teenager with moderate or severe DUB. Inspect the external genitalia for signs of trauma or bleeding sources. Next, perform a speculum exam looking for evidence of trauma, exposure to DES (vaginal adenosis, cock's comb cervix), pregnancy (bluish color to the cervix), abortion (opening of the os), or infection (cervical discharge). Upon bimanual (or rectoabdominal) examination, check the cervix for softness (pregnancy) and tenderness on motion (salpingitis). Palpate the uterus to determine size and tenderness, and examine the adnexae for masses and tenderness.

For all patients obtain a complete blood count (CBC) with differential, platelet count, and urinalysis. Obtain a Pap smear, gonorrhea and chlamydia cultures, and a pregnancy test for all sexually active girls. Clotting studies (PT, PTT), bleeding time, and thyroid function studies are indicated for severe or prolonged bleeding or if there is excessive bleeding at menarche.

Pregnancy (p 234) is suggested by a history of fatigue, nausea, vomiting, and urinary frequency. Breast tenderness and an enlarged uterus may be noted. *Salpingitis* (p 238) may be present with a vaginal discharge, lower abdominal pain, fever, chills, and cervical motion tenderness. With a *bleeding disorder* (p 256), there may be other bleeding manifestations, such as petechiae, ecchymoses, epistaxis, bleeding gums, hematuria, and rarely, hematochezia.

ER MANAGEMENT

Observation and reassurance are all that are needed for adolescents with *mild DUB*. Iron supplementation (300 mg/day of ferrous sulfate) may be necessary, but the majority of these patients spontaneously convert to normal menstrual cycles within several months.

Treat *moderate DUB* with intensive hormonal therapy. Use a high ratio progesterone:estrogen pill, such as Enovid 5 mg, one tablet q6h until the bleeding stops (2–3 days), then bid to complete the week, then qd for 2 weeks. Compazine (10 mg PO q 6h or 25 mg PO bid) may be needed for the accompanying nausea. Iron therapy (300 mg tid of ferrous sulfate) is also indicated. Arrange a follow-up appointment for 1–2 days to ensure that the bleeding has ceased. If the bleeding does not stop within 2–3 days after the start of therapy, refer the patient to a gynecologist. See the patient weekly for 1 month to ensure compliance with medical therapy. After the intensive hormonal therapy, give a low dose oral contraceptive (Norinyl 1 + 35, Lo-Ovral) for 2–3 months, beginning on day 5 of the withdrawal bleed.

The priority in managing adolescents with *severe DUB* is restoration of adequate perfusion (see shock, p 11) with 20 cc/kg of normal saline followed by a packed red cell transfusion (10 cc/kg) if the patient remains orthostatic or symptomatic at rest (tachycardia, dizziness). Admit the patient for high dose intravenous conjugated estrogen (Premarin, 25 mg q 4h for up to six doses) until the bleeding has stopped. Concurrently, start Enovid 5 mg, as for moderate DUB (above). Continued bleeding for 24 hours is rare. It may signal an anatomical abnormality and is an indication for gynecologic consultation to consider examination under general anesthesia with possible dilatation and curettage. Iron therapy and ongoing hormonal therapy are given as for patients with moderate DUB.

INDICATION FOR ADMISSION

- Severe DUB (hematocrit <28%, postural hypotension)

REFERENCES

1. Claessens EA, Cowell CA: Pediatr Clin North Am 28:369–378, 1981
2. Litt IF: Pediatr in Rev 4:203–212, 1983

Dysmenorrhea

INTRODUCTION

Dysmenorrhea (painful menstrual periods) is common in teenagers and may be a response to elevated levels of F2-alpha prostaglandin. The majority of cases are primary, present within 2 years of menarche, and have no significant associated pelvic pathology. Secondary dysmenorrhea, on the other hand, most often occurs in conjunction with the presence of an intrauterine device (IUD), salpingitis, endometriosis, or genital tract obstruction.

CLINICAL PRESENTATION

Typically, there is colicky suprapubic pain that radiates to the back or down the thighs. Nausea, vomiting, diarrhea, irritability, and muscle cramps may also occur. These symptoms appear with the onset of menses and abate by the end of the period.

DIAGNOSIS

Ascertain the age of menarche and the frequency and severity of the pain and its relation to the periods. Ask about a history of vaginal discharge, sexual activity, and IUD use. Perform a pelvic examination, looking for cervical motion tenderness, pelvic tenderness and nodularity, and adnexal or uterine enlargement. Normal findings confirm the diagnosis of primary dysmenorrhea.

The pain of *salpingitis* may exacerbate during periods. On examination, fever, a vaginal discharge, cervical motion tenderness, and adnexal enlargement may be found. The pain of *endometriosis* typically starts before the period and persists after the bleeding has stopped. The uterus or ovaries may be tender or enlarged, and the uterus may be nodular and sensitive to motion. *Genital tract obstruction* presents with cyclical lower abdominal pain in an amenorrheic patient. On examination, uterine enlargement is found.

ER MANAGEMENT

The treatment of primary dysmenorrhea has been revolutionized by the advent of the prostaglandin synthetase inhibitors. Aspirin, the weakest antiprostaglandin, is not effective for 48 hours, so begin treatment 2 days prior to the start of the menses. For mild cases (less than 6 hours of pain), aspirin (2 tablets q 4–6h) may suffice. For more severe pain, treat with stronger medications at the onset of the period. These include ibuprofen (Motrin 400 mg q 4–6h), naproxen (Naprosyn 500 mg to start, then 250 mg q 6–8h), naproxen sodium (Anaprox 550 mg to start, then 275 mg q 6–8h), and mefenamic acid (Ponstel 500 mg to start, then 250 mg q 6h). Side effects include nausea, dyspepsia, dizziness, and gastric irritation. These medications are contraindicated in patients with ulcers and aspirin allergy, and should be used with caution in patients taking anticoagulants or with liver or kidney disease.

Suppression of ovulation by oral contraceptives is effective, but reserve this therapy for the office setting, where the patient's needs can be better assessed.

Consult a gynecologist to remove an IUD or if endometriosis or genital tract obstruction is suspected. The management of salpingitis is discussed on p 238.

REFERENCE

1. Gantt PA, McDonough PC: Pediatric Clin North Am 28:389–395, 1981

Pregnancy and Complications

INTRODUCTION

It is estimated that one out of ten teenage girls becomes pregnant each year. Spontaneous abortions complicate 10–15% of pregnancies, while ectopic pregnancies occur in 1 of every 125–300 pregnancies.

CLINICAL PRESENTATION

Knowing whether a patient may be pregnant is essential in evaluating her complaints and determining management. The first step is to interview the teenager privately and assure her that your discussion is confidential. Often the pregnant patient presents with vague complaints of "abdominal pain" or "not feeling right" because she does not want her parents to suspect the truth. The patient herself may not realize it or may be trying to deny the possibility of pregnancy. Also, she may not volunteer the information that she has missed a period or had unprotected intercourse.

During early pregnancy, a teenager may report "missing" her period or that it is "different" (longer or shorter than usual). Breast tenderness may be noted within 1 week of conception. Fatigue, dizziness, syncope, nausea and vomiting, urinary frequency, and weight gain may be noted by 2 weeks. Nipple discharge (colostrum) can occur at 6 weeks.

On examination, the breasts have darkened areolae and enlarged nipples. Often, there is protrusion of Montgomery glands. Findings on pelvic examination depend on the time elapsed since the last normal period. At 5 weeks the examination may be normal; at 6 weeks there may be softening of the upper cervix (Hegar sign); at 8 weeks the cervix and vaginal mucosa may have a bluish tinge (Chadwick sign) and the uterus may be soft and slightly enlarged. At 12 weeks, the globular uterus can be palpated at the level of the symphysis pubis and, after 12–14 weeks, the fetal heart may be heard.

Threatened and Imminent Abortions. With a threatened abortion, the history is compatible with early pregnancy. There is vaginal bleeding with or without cramps, and the cervical os is closed. With an imminent abortion the cervix becomes shortened and dilated.

Inevitable and Complete Abortion. An inevitable abortion resembles an imminent abortion, except that tissue is seen protruding from the dilated effaced cervix. The embryo and placenta are completely expelled in a complete abortion.

Incomplete Abortion. An incomplete abortion implies that fragments of placenta remain in the uterus with persistent cramps, bleeding, and cervical dilation.

Missed Abortion. A missed abortion is a fetal death in utero before the 20th week, but with the pregnancy retained. Patients have amenorrhea without uterine growth. They present with vaginal bleeding and cramps—the start of an abortion.

Ectopic Pregnancy. An ectopic pregnancy is more likely if there is preexisting chronic salpingitis, adhesions, anomalies, fibroids, or an IUD in place. The classic presentation is amenorrhea with symptoms of early pregnancy, followed by vaginal bleeding. After several hours (to days), there is sudden onset of abdominal pain secondary to rupture and bleeding into the peritoneum. Initially the pain is unilateral and pelvic. Later, it becomes generalized with abdominal, vaginal, and cervical motion tenderness, shoulder pain (as blood accumulates under the diaphragm), and a tender adnexal mass (50% of patients). Although only 15% of patients have the classic ectopic presentation, approximately 90% complain of mild pelvic discomfort and 80% have abnormal vaginal bleeding, often mild and intermittent. However, the history or physical examination can be normal. The patient usually is afebrile with a normal to slightly elevated white blood cell count.

DIAGNOSIS

Pregnancy tests detect the presence of human chorionic gonadotropin (hCG) in the blood or urine. The beta subunit by radioimmunoassay is extremely sensitive. It can be positive within 7 days of conception and detect the small amounts of hormone present with ectopic and abnormal (hydatidiform mole) pregnancies. Do not use the less sensitive blood or urine assays and do-it-yourself slide tests if these are suspected.

The standard urine immunoassay is not positive until 25–28 days after conception (2 weeks after the missed period). It is 95–98% sensitive, especially if the first morning urine is used, and takes 2–3 hours to run. The do-it-yourself slide tests are faster (2–3 minutes) but less sensitive, so early pregnancies can be missed.

Regardless of which pregnancy test is used, consider a laboratory error when the test results are incompatible with the history and physical examination findings. False-positive urine tests may be caused by drug ingestion (methadone, chlorpromazine, promethazine, haldoperidol), proteinuria (1 gm/24 hr), and gross hematuria. False-negative results occur during early pregnancy, abnormal pregnancies (ectopic, molar, missed abortion, imminent abortion), or with dilute urine specimens.

Not all patients present early in pregnancy, so the diagnosis can sometimes be made on physical examination, especially if an enlarged uterus or fetal heart sounds are appreciated. Pregnancy can be confirmed and the length of gestation estimated by ultrasound.

The diagnosis of the various types of spontaneous abortion is usually evident on pelvic examination.

The differential diagnosis of an ectopic pregnancy includes a normal pregnancy with another cause of pain (*ruptured corpus luteum, stretched ligaments, ovarian* or *tubal torsion, appendicitis, renal stone*), threatened abortion, *intrauterine pregnancy with implantation bleeding, pelvic inflammatory disease* (PID), and complications of a *tumor* or *cyst*.

ER MANAGEMENT

The priority is the expedient diagnosis and management of an *ectopic pregnancy*. Suspect an ectopic in any pubertal female with vaginal bleeding and/or lower abdominal pain, especially if her period is late, and perform a pelvic examination. If the findings are consistent with a possible ectopic (cervical motion tenderness, shoulder pain, adnexal mass), *immediately* obtain gynecologic consultation, which will determine further management (ultrasound, culdocentesis, surgery). Insert a large bore intravenous (IV) and monitor the patient carefully, with frequent vital signs and serial hematocrits. Obtain blood for a CBC, type and cross-match and beta subunit. If an ectopic is likely (rebound tenderness, orthostatic vital sign changes, falling hematocrit) the treatment is immediate *surgical exploration.* If an ectopic cannot be ruled out, admit the patient for close observation.

If an ectopic is unlikely (stable vital signs and hematocrit, soft abdomen), the patient can be discharged with "ectopic precautions." That is, she should return if there is dizziness, fainting, increasing abdominal pain, or shoulder pain.

Manage *threatened* and *imminent abortions* expectantly, with complete bedrest and no intercourse. If bleeding continues, hospitalize the patient and obtain a type and cross-match in case a transfusion becomes necessary.

Admit patients with *inevitable* and *incomplete abortions* and consult with a gynecologist for oxytocin infusion (10 units/500 cc D5 NS) and suction dilation and curettage. Obtain a CBC, spun hematocrit, and type and cross-match in the ER, and give packed red cell transfusions to maintain the hematocrit over 35%.

Send home the patient with a *complete abortion,* unless there are signs of significant blood loss (orthostatic vital sign changes, respiratory distress). In these cases obtain a CBC, spun hematocrit, and type and cross-match and transfuse to a hematocrit of 35%.

If a *normal intrauterine pregnancy* is diagnosed, make an appointment for the teenager (and her boyfriend) to be seen within the next few days in an adolescent gynecology or family-planning clinic for appropriate counseling and management. In addition, social work referral may be indicated.

INDICATIONS FOR ADMISSION

- Ectopic pregnancy
- Incomplete and inevitable abortions
- Severe acute blood loss causing symptoms, for blood transfusion

REFERENCES

1. Kitchin JD, Wein RM, Nunley WC, et al: Am J Obstet Gynecol 134:870, 1979
2. Saxena BB, Pediatr Clin North Am 28:437, 1981

Salpingitis, Urethritis, and Syphilis

INTRODUCTION

Neisseria gonorrhea and *Chlamydia trachomatis* are responsible for most cases of salpingitis. *Chlamydia* and *Ureaplasma urealyticum* cause at least 70% of the cases of nongonococcal urethritis. *Treponema pallidum,* the agent responsible for syphilis, can cause severe systemic disease.

CLINICAL PRESENTATION

Salpingitis. Salpingitis can be acute, subacute, or chronic, and the clinical picture does not help identify the causitive organism. Classic acute salpingitis typically presents within 1 week of the onset of a menstrual period with vaginal discharge, high fever, shaking chills, and severe unilateral or bilateral lower abdominal pain. On abdominal examination, there is marked lower abdominal tenderness, guarding, and rebound. On pelvic examination, a purulent cervical discharge with cervical motion tenderness (especially side-to-side), tender adnexae, and a normal-sized uterus are noted. The white blood count (WBC) is usually greater than 10,000–15,000/mm³, and the erythrocyte sedimentation rate (ESR) is markedly elevated (>50 mm/hr).

Just as often, the presentation can be subacute with lower abdominal pain without fever, with or without a vaginal discharge.

Fitzhugh-Curtis Syndrome. The Fitzhugh-Curtis syndrome, perihepatitis in association with salpingitis, presents with right upper quadrant (RUQ) pain, occasionally accompanied by pleuritic pain at the right lung base.

Urethritis. Urethritis is the most common sexually transmitted disease in males. Dysuria and a urethral discharge are noted, occasionally in association with epididymitis (p 218). In females, *Chlamydia* commonly causes the *acute urethral syndrome* with dysuria, urgency, suprapubic tenderness, pyuria without hematuria, and a negative routine urine culture.

Syphilis. The hallmark of primary syphilis is the chancre that develops 3–4 weeks after exposure. It appears as a painless ulcer with a smooth clean base, raised indurated borders, and a scanty yellow discharge. In males, the chancre is most frequently seen on the penis, scrotum, anus, or in the mouth. In females, it occurs on the vulva, vagina, cervix, urethra, or in the mouth. Fifty percent of patients have more than one chancre, and enlarged, firm regional lymph nodes are seen in 60–80% of patients. Untreated, the chancre resolves in 3–6 weeks, followed in 6–8 weeks by the signs of secondary syphilis.

Several skin (and mucous membrane) eruptions are typical of secondary syphilis. Nonpruritic, well-demarcated, brownish-red macules and papules are symmetrically distributed on the trunk and extremities. Papules arising in moist areas become flattened and are known as condylomata lata. When the maculopapules involve the mucous membranes in the mouth, they appear as shallow grey ulcers called mucous patches. Other signs of secondary syphilis include "moth-eaten" alopecia and nontender, firm or rubbery lymphadenopathy. Constitutional symptoms, including low grade fever, headache, fatigue, sore throat, weight loss, arthralgias, and myalgias occasionally accompany the above findings.

DIAGNOSIS

Salpingitis. The priorities are to identify salpingitis and rule out an ectopic pregnancy. Have the parent leave the room and ask about intercourse (including anal), number of partners, oral-genital contact, IUD use, and a history of salpingitis or other sexually transmitted disease (STD). The risk of salpingitis increases with IUD use (3–5 times increased risk), multiple partners (4–5 times the risk), and previous episodes. Obtain anal and pharyngeal gonococcal (GC) cultures from patients with extragenital contact, since some of the treatment regimens may be ineffective for infection in these sites. Ask when menarche began, and note the regularity and duration of menses and the dates of the previous period as well as the one before. Symptoms beginning within 1 to 2 weeks of the last period suggest salpingitis.

Also inquire about a history of recurrent *urinary tract infections* (UTI), inflammatory bowel disease, known *ovarian pathology*, or *previous abdominal surgery*. Positive responses might suggest other etiologies for the abdominal or pelvic pain.

On physical examination, look for evidence of *pregnancy*, surgical scars on the abdomen, and signs of respiratory distress (tachypnea, retractions), since *pneumonia* can present with severe lower abdominal pain. Examine the abdomen carefully for tenderness, rebound, guarding, and the presence and quality of bowel sounds.

Perform a pelvic examination if a postmenarchal female complains of vaginal discharge, abdominal pain, or menstrual abnormalities, or has physical signs of pregnancy (see pp 234–235). On speculum exam, obtain endocervical cultures for gonorrhea (Thayer-Martin medium, Transgrow bottles) and a *Chlamydia* culture or slide test (MicroTrak), if available. Prepare a slide for Gram stain and perform a Papanicolaou smear as well. *Neisseria* species are normally found in the female genital tract. However, the presence of gram-negative intracellular diplococci on the Gram stain of a purulent endocervical discharge is highly suggestive of gonococcal infection. After the speculum exam, perform a bimanual exam, attempting to elicit horizontal cervical motion tenderness suggestive of tubular pathology. Examine the adnexae for the presence of a mass or bogginess (ovarian mass, tuboovarian abscess). Finally, obtain a clean catch urine for culture and urinalysis (and pregnancy test, if indicated), and culture the pharynx and rectum for gonococcus. Obtain blood for a CBC, ESR, blood urea nitrogen (BUN), and creatinine if pyelonephritis is suspected, or a beta HCG and type and cross-match if an ectopic pregnancy cannot be ruled out.

In the differential diagnosis of salpingitis, consider *gastroenteritis* (diarrhea), *inflammatory bowel disease* (weight loss, bloody stools, change in bowel pattern), *acute appendicitis* (periumbilical pain localizing to the right lower quadrant (RLQ)), *UTI* (suprapubic or flank pain, bacteriuria in association with pyuria), right lower lobe *pneumonia* (cough, tachypnea, rales, RLQ pain), and, rarely, *cholecystitis* (RUQ pain, fatty food intolerance). In all of these, the pelvic examination is normal. Always consider an *ectopic pregnancy* when there has been amenorrhea or abnormal menses preceding the episode. There may be pregnancy symptoms and a positive urine or serum pregnancy test (see p 236), but fever and leukocytosis are absent. In many females, the diagnosis is not certain from the history and physical examination. Consult a gynecologist, who may recommend abdominal ultrasound, culdocentesis, or laparoscopy. A large bore IV must be in place for all patients who leave the ER for diagnostic tests or who may have an ectopic pregnancy.

Urethritis. Obtain a urinalysis and urine culture if there are symptoms of urethritis. Ask sexually active males to try to express any discharge, which must be cultured for gonococcus (and *Chlamydia,* if possible). If the patient has noticed a discharge previously, but none is present at the time of examination, insert a Calgiswab 2.5 cm into the urethra to obtain a specimen for culture and Gram stain. Assume that an asymptomatic male has urethritis if there are >4 WBC/hpf on Gram stain of an intraurethral smear. If gram-negative intracellular diplococci are seen on the Gram stain of the discharge in a male, the diagnosis is *gonococcal urethritis,* and treatment can be started without waiting for the culture results.

Syphilis. Suspect all genital lesions of being syphilitic. Chancres can be confused with *chancroid* (multiple soft, tender ulcers with tender contiguous adenopathy), *granuloma inguinale* (soft, smooth granulating painless lesion), *lymphogranuloma venerum* (transient vesicular ulceration with nearby tender nodes) or *lichen planus* (annular flat-topped papules). They can also look like *herpes* (multiple, superficial, painful lesions), a *pyogenic granuloma* (single, painful, erythematous, history of trauma or surgery), *Molluscum contagiosum* (grouped, umbilicated, flesh-colored papules, similar lesions elsewhere on body), and *condyloma accuminata* (dry, single or clustered warty lesions). The skin lesions of *pityriasis rosea* look similar, but they are absent from the palms and soles, and *psoriasis* can be associated with scaly plaques on the penis but there should be lesions elsewhere on the body.

Send wet smears from lesions for darkfield microscopy, and obtain a VDRL or other nontreponemal serologic test for syphilis (STS). A newly positive test or a fourfold rise in titer of the STS from its previous level is diagnostic. These tests are reactive within 3 weeks of the appearance of the chancre. If the VDRL is positive, the fluorescent treponemal antibody-absorption test (FTA) should also be positive. False-positive VDRL (usually low titer) occur with hepatitis,

TABLE 10-2. TREATMENT OF SEXUALLY TRANSMITTED DISEASES

Gonorrhea			
STAGE	MALE	FEMALE	TREATMENT
Asymptomatic			1. Aqueous procaine penicillin G 4.8 mill units IM *plus* probenecid 1 g PO, or 2. Ampicillin 3.5 g or amoxicillin 3 g PO *plus* probenecid 1 g PO,[a] or 3. Tetracycline 500 mg PO qid or doxycycline 100 mg PO bid, for 7 days,[b] or 4. Spectinomycin 2 g IM (penicillinase producing species)[c]
Uncomplicated	Afebrile Discharge Dysuria	Afebrile Discharge Dyspareunia Cervical friability but no cervical motion tenderness	Same as above
Complicated	Prostatitis Epididymitis Orchitis	Cervical or adnexal tenderness (ie, salpingitis)	*Males:* No. 1 above, followed by tetracycline 500 mg qid or doxycycline 100 mg bid × 10 days *Females:* Doxycycline 100 mg IV q 12h *plus* cefoxitin 2 g IV q 6h

Syphilis

STAGE	TREATMENT
Primary Secondary (<1 year)	1. Benzathine penicillin G 2.4 mill units IM, or 2. Tetracycline 500 mg PO qid × 15 days
Duration unknown or >1 year[e]	1. Benzathine penicillin G 2.4 mill units IM weekly for 3 weeks, or 2. Tetracycline 500 mg PO qid × 30 days

Nongonococcal Infections[d]

MALES	FEMALES	TREATMENT
Urethritis	Urethritis Endocervitis	1. Tetracycline 500 mg PO qid or doxycycline 100 mg PO bid for at least 7 days, or 2. Erythromycin 500 mg PO qid for at least 7 days
	Salpingitis	As for gonorrhea salpingitis

[a]Often ineffective against anorectal and pharyngeal gonorrhea.
[b]Often ineffective against anorectal gonorrhea.
[c]Often ineffective against pharyngeal gonorrhea.
[d]Often associated with gonoccal infections.
[e]Perform lumbar puncture prior to treatment.
(From Sexually Transmitted Diseases Summary 1982. Atlanta, Ga: C.D.C., U.S. Dept. of Health and Human Services.)

mononucleosis, collagen vascular disease, tuburculosis, viral pneumonia, malaria, varicella, measles, and narcotics abuse.

ER MANAGEMENT

Antibiotic treatment is summarized in Table 10-2. Obtain a VDRL in all sexually active patients who might have an STD. Remind the patient that the sexual partner(s) must be examined and treated, and arrange a follow-up visit with a primary care provider for a test-of-cure evaluation.

Obtain a CBC and liver function tests and secure an IV if there are signs and symptoms of acute *salpingitis.* Because of the tremendous risk of subsequent infertility, ectopic pregnancy, and chronic pelvic pain, admit all adolescents suspected of having salpingitis for IV therapy.

Treat afebrile patients with *cervicitis* (cervical discharge and friability but no cervical motion tenderness) on an outpatient basis with oral medications. If the patient has an IUD, remove it. Schedule a follow-up office visit within a week of completing therapy, and emphasize both the avoidance of intercourse until the patient's partner is cultured and treated and the use of condoms to prevent both future infections and pregnancy. Oral contraception may be started in the ER if the patient is within a week of the end of her last period.

Treat males with presumptive or definite *urethritis,* and schedule one revisit within 48–72 hours to evaluate progress and another within a week of completing the medication for repeat cultures. Until the patient's sexual partner is cultured and treated, intercourse must be avoided.

Treat females with *acute urethral syndrome* for *Chlamydia* urethritis, and schedule a follow-up office visit within a week.

Treat patients with primary or secondary *syphilis,* and refer them for follow-up serologic testing 3, 6, 12, and 24 months after treatment. Evaluate and treat sexual partners, and remind the patient to avoid sexual activity until that time.

INDICATION FOR ADMISSION

- Acute salpingitis

REFERENCES
1. Wald ER: Pediatr Infect Dis 3:510–513, 1984
2. Bell TA: Pediatr Infect Dis 2:153–161, 1983
3. Flumara NJ, Finegold J: Infections in Surgery 359–371, 1984
4. Rosenfeld WD, Litman N: PIR 4:257–265, 1983
5. Shafer MB, Irwin CE, Sweet RL: J Pediatr 100:339–350, 1982
6. The Medical Letter 26:5–10, 1984

Vulvovaginitis

INTRODUCTION

The etiologies of prepubertal vulvovaginitis differ from pubertal causes. The thin epithelium and labia, neutral to alkaline pH, and lack of estrogenic stimulation make the prepubertal vagina a good culture medium. Also, younger girls are more likely to manipulate themselves with dirty hands or insert foreign objects. Sexual activity is the major etiologic factor in pubertal vulvovaginitis.

CLINICAL PRESENTATION IN PREPUBERTAL GIRLS

Nonspecific Vaginitis. Eighty percent of prepubertal vulvovaginitis is "nonspecific," ie, a routine bacterial culture is negative and there is no obvious etiology. Included in this group are girls who have been using bubble bath or wearing tight synthetic underpants. The inflammation is generally low grade, yet persistent, and may be associated with dysuria and pruritis.

Gonorrhea and Chlamydia. In this age group, gonorrhea and chlamydia are vaginal, not cervical, infections. Often a definite history of sexual contact is lacking, although nonsexual acquisition of these infections is exceedingly rare. In fact, suspect sexual abuse whenever a sexually transmitted disease is diagnosed in a prepubertal child.

They present with a copious, yellowish, purulent discharge with labial swelling, dysuria, and genital pruritis. The vagina is often very inflamed and excoriated.

Other Bacterial Infections. An overgrowth of normal vaginal *coliform* bacteria can occur secondary to poor hygiene and lead to a low grade, foul-smelling discharge. Other organisms, such as *Staphylococcus aureus, Pneumococcus,* and *Proteus* can be transferred to the vagina and cause an acute purulent discharge.

Seven to 10 days after an upper respiratory infection, *group A beta-hemolytic Streptococcus* infection can cause hyperemia and irritation of the vulva and vagina. Symptoms include dysuria, pruritis, and discomfort when walking. *Shigella* can cause a bloody discharge in girls who have recently had gastroenteritis.

Foreign Body. A vaginal foreign body produces a foul-smelling discharge which is often bloody. Toilet paper remnants are most common.

CLINICAL PRESENTATION IN PUBERTAL GIRLS

In addition to the discharge, dysuria is a very common complaint, often in association with ''sterile'' pyuria.

Infestations. Vulvitis may be caused by infestations such as *pediculosis pubis* (''crabs'', p 81). The lice resemble moving dandruff and pruritis can be intense. *Scabies* (p 86) can involve the genitalia, and often intensely pruritic, excoriated erythematous papules are seen.

Viral Infections. The flesh-colored, warty tags of *condylomata acuminata* (veneral warts, p 96) and the small, ulcerating blisters of *herpes simplex* (p 77) can cause a vulvitis (or vaginitis).

Candida Albicans. Monilia (p 66) is a common cause of vaginitis. The infection is often associated with antibiotic or oral contraceptive use and diabetes mellitus; it can be sexually transmitted as well. A thick, white, cheesy discharge is seen along with extreme pruritis and inflammation.

Trichomonas Vaginalis. This infection is usually acquired by sexual contact. A grey, bubbly, malodorous discharge occurs, often associated with pruritis or dyspareunia.

Gardnerella Vaginalis. This organism, a normal inhabitant of the vagina, is thought to be responsible for ''nonspecific vaginitis.'' Infection usually presents with a greyish, malodorous discharge.

Gonorrhea or Chlamydia. Adolescents may occasionally complain of a vaginal discharge, although they usually have an infection higher in the genital tract (cervicitis, endometritis, salpingitis, p 238).

Foreign Body. Most often a forgotten tampon or the remnant of a masturbation aid (candle, vegetable) causes a discharge which is purulent, brownish, and malodorous.

Contact Reaction. A contact vaginitis may be caused by bubble bath, deodorant, or contraceptive foam or jelly.

Physiologic Leukorrhea. Adolescents may sometimes complain of a clear or mucoid "discharge," either prior to menses or at midcycle. The "discharge" is normal, composed of epithelial cells and endocervical mucus.

Psychosocial Etiologies. In the rare case when the patient's complaints are not consistent with the objective findings, consider *psychosomatic illness, sexual molestation,* and *school phobia.*

DIAGNOSIS

Perform a brief physical examination, focusing on the breasts (Tanner stage, signs of pregnancy), abdomen (pregnancy, mass, tenderness), and inguinal area (lymphadenopathy). Next, inspect the introitus for Tanner stage, inflammation, signs of trauma, or other abnormality.

The vaginal examination of the prepubertal child is easily performed with the girl lying prone, in a knee-chest position, with the buttocks in the air and the legs 6–8 inches apart. Instruct her to relax and let her belly sag downward, then gently spread the labia to view the vagina. It is helpful to have the patient's mother in the room, possibly assisting by spreading the labia. Specimens can then be obtained with a sterile medicine dropper or Q-tip moistened with saline. Perform a Gram stain (looking for gram-negative intracellular diplococci–gonorrhea), and culture for routine bacteria, gonorrhea and chlamydia. If the discharge is bloody or particularly foul smelling, inspect the vagina for a foreign body. Solid objects can often be palpated on rectal exam.

Perform a wet prep on a sample of all vaginal discharges. After the specimen is obtained with a Q-tip, place it in a test tube containing a small amount of saline. Place several drops of this solution on a slide and observe under high power. Budding yeast are seen with a monilial infection; pseudohyphae can be seen after 10% KOH is added and the slide is gently heated. Trichomonads appear as live, flagellated, motile organisms. With *Gardnerella,* the wet prep reveals clue cells—epithelial cells stippled with dark granules (bacteria); the odor becomes "fishy" with the addition of KOH.

Do not assume that an adolescent with dysuria has a urinary tract infection, even if pyuria is noted. If a sexually active female has dysuria associated with a vaginal discharge, pruritis, or foul odor, perform a pelvic examination. Obtain endocervical cultures for gonorrhea and *Chlamydia,* and evaluate for vulvovaginitis, in addition to obtaining a urine culture.

ER MANAGEMENT

Prepubertal Girls

Nonspecific Vaginitis. Treat with plain water sitz baths, tid. Teach the parents proper hygienic techniques and have the girl avoid tight fitting pants (cotton underpants preferred). If symptoms persist for a month, prescribe a topical antibiotic cream (triple sulfa, Vagitrol, AVC), bid for 1 week.

Gonorrhea and Chlamydia. In this age group, a positive Gram stain or culture is indicative of sexual abuse (p 439). Obtain cultures of the pharynx and rectum, and treat the child with amoxicillin (50 mg/kg up to 3 g) *and* probenecid (25 mg/kg up to 1 g) for gonorrhea, erythromycin (50 mg/kg/day divided qid for 7–10 days) for chlamydia. Report the case to the child protection services.

Other Bacterial Etiologies. If the culture is positive, treat with a culture-specific antibiotic. Ampicillin (100 mg/kg/day, divided q 6h) is indicated for *coliforms* and *Shigella,* and penicillin (50,000 units/kg/day divided q 6h) for *group A Streptococcus* and *Pneumococcus.*

Foreign Body. Usually, removal can be accomplished with a forceps. On occasion, sedation or general anesthesia is required.

Pubertal Girls

The treatment of infectious vulvovaginitis is summarized in Table 10-3.

TABLE 10-3. TREATMENT OF INFECTIOUS VULVOVAGINITIS IN PUBERTAL GIRLS

Diagnosis	Treatment	Comment
Monilia	Miconazole cream/supp qhs × 1 wk or Clotrimazole cream/supp qhs × 1–2 weeks or Nystatin supp bid × 2 weeks	Treat during menses Avoid pantyhose and tight jeans No need to treat partner unless patient becomes reinfected quickly
Trichomonas	Metronidazole 2 g PO, once	Same dose for partner No alcohol for 2 days Do not use if pregnant
Gardnerella	Metronidazole 250 mg PO bid × 1 week	No need to treat partner
Pediculosis pubis	Lindane 1% × 8 hours	Wash off thoroughly
Scabies	Lindane 1%, from neck down, × 12 hours or crotamiton (Eurax), from neck down and again 48 hours later. Bathe 48 hours after last application	Wash off thoroughly; repeat 1 week later prn
Condyloma acuminatum	Podophyllin 10–25%	Refer to dermatologist or gynecologist for treatment
Herpes genitalis	Acyclovir ointment q 3h (6× 1 day) × 1 week or capsules q4h (5 daily) × 10 days	Refer to gynecologist

Foreign Bodies. These can usually be removed with a forceps in the ER, although younger patients may require sedation or possibly, general anesthesia.

Contact Reaction. Avoidance of the offending agent is usually all that is required. Treat severe pruritis with hydroxyzine (2 mg/kg/day divided q 6h).

Physiologic Leukorrhea. No treatment is necessary, although panty liners may be helpful.

Psychosocial Etiologies. Have an experienced interviewer speak with the patient. Attempt to ascertain if *sexual molestation* occurred. Refer all patients without a definite organic etiology to a primary care provider.

INDICATIONS FOR ADMISSION

- Suspected sexually transmitted disease in a prepubertal girl
- Severe vulvovaginitis with urinary retention or systemic signs (fever, toxicity)

REFERENCES

1. Altchek A: J Reprod Med 29:359, 1984
2. Rein MF: Sex Transm Dis 8:316, 1981

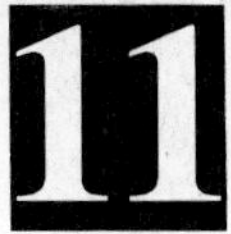

Hematologic Emergencies

Anemia

INTRODUCTION

The definition of anemia varies with age (Table 11-1), with the lower limits of a normal hemoglobin ranging from 10–11 g/dl at 3 months of age to 13 g/dl in the teenager. Anemia is never a final diagnosis, but a sign of some underlying disorder. As such, it requires an appropriate investigation to determine the cause.

The many disease processes associated with anemia can be divided into three general categories (Table 11-2). Decreased red cell production, frequently secondary to nutritional iron deficiency, is particularly prevalent in infants, adolescents, and pregnant females. The second category is ineffective erythropoiesis with red cell destruction within the marrow. The third group is decreased red cell survival (blood loss, hemolysis). Blood loss can be acute or chronic and hemolytic disorders can be inherited or acquired.

CLINICAL PRESENTATION

The signs and symptoms of anemia are caused by the decreased oxygen-carrying capacity of the blood and depend on the degree and rapidity of onset. Exercise intolerance, tachycardia, fatigue, and systolic murmurs occur with moderate anemia. Severe or rapidly developing anemia causes pallor, nonexertional dyspnea, dizziness, orthostatic vital sign changes, cardiac gallop, syncope, hypotension, and heart failure.

TABLE 11-1. VALUES (NORMAL MEAN AND LOWER LIMITS OF NORMAL) FOR HEMOGLOBIN, HEMATOCRIT, AND MCV DETERMINATIONS

Age (yr)	Hemoglobin (g/dl)		Hematocrit (%)		MCV (μ^3)	
	MEAN	LOWER LIMIT	MEAN	LOWER LIMIT	MEAN	LOWER LIMIT
0.5–1.9	12.5	11.0	37	33	77	70
2–4	12.5	11.0	38	34	79	73
5–7	13.0	11.5	39	35	81	75
8–11	13.5	12.0	40	36	83	76
12–14						
Female	13.5	12.0	41	36	85	78
Male	14.0	12.5	43	37	84	77
15–17						
Female	14.0	12.0	41	36	87	79
Male	15.0	13.0	46	38	86	78
18–49						
Female	14.0	12.0	42	37	90	80
Male	16.0	14.0	47	40	90	80

(Adapted from Dallman PR, Siimes MA. J Pediatr 94:26, 1979.)

TABLE 11-2. CAUSES OF ANEMIA

Decreased red cell production	
Nutritional iron deficiency	
Other nutritional deficiencies: folate, B_{12}	
Drugs: chloramphenicol, cancer chemotherapeutic agents	
Chronic inflammation	
Chronic disease	
Toxins: lead	
Infections	
Marrow failure—aplastic anemia	
Bone marrow replacement:	leukemia, lymphoma, neuroblastoma, storage disorders
Ineffective erythropoiesis	
Thalassemia	
Megaloblastic anemia	
Decreased red cell survivial	
Blood loss:	trauma, coagulopathies, platelet disorders, milk intolerance, menorrhagia, hookworm infestation
Hemolysis:	sickle cell disease, thalassemia, G-6-PD deficiency, hereditary spherocytosis, infections, autoimmune processes, drugs, toxins, microangiopathic anemias

DIAGNOSIS

The history can be very helpful, including diet, recent infections, pica, trauma, menstrual irregularities, and ongoing medical problems. Patients with hemolytic disorders often have positive family histories for anemia, cholecystectomy, or splenectomy (hereditary spherocytosis).

On examination, a healthy, vigorous child is more likely to have *iron deficiency anemia;* a patient with a *malignancy,* severe *malnutrition,* severe *chronic disease,* or *bone marrow infiltration* appears ill. Jaundice, often accompanied by splenomegaly and dark urine, is seen in *hemolytic processes. Thalassemia major* is associated with frontal bossing, malar prominence, hepatosplenomegaly, and dental malocclusion. Generalized lymphadenopathy and hepatosplenomegaly are frequently features of *malignancies* and *myeloproliferative disorders.* Petechiae, purpura, and multiple ecchymoses occur in *hemostatic disorders.* Orthopedic anomalies may suggest *Fanconi anemia* (abnormal radii or thumbs) or *Blackfan-Diamond syndrome* (triphalangeal or bifid thumbs).

In the ER, anemia is often discovered when a complete blood count (CBC) is obtained during the evaluation of some other problem. Despite the diverse etiologies, a CBC with red cell indices, a reticulocyte count, and examination of the peripheral smear help narrow the differential diagnosis and guide further laboratory examinations (Fig. 11-1).

Since iron deficiency is the most likely diagnosis in an otherwise well child with mild-to-moderate microcytic, hypochromic anemia, a diagnostic and therapeutic trial of oral iron supplementation prior to any further laboratory work-up is acceptable. An increasing hemoglobin and hematocrit and a reticulocytosis after 1 week confirms the diagnosis of iron deficiency. If the mean corpuscular volume (MCV) is available, the Menser index (MCV in μ^3 divided by the number of red blood cells (RBC) in millions: MCV/RBC) can help differentiate among the microcytic anemias. If the ratio is under 11, then thalassemia minor is likely, while ratios over 14 suggest iron deficiency, lead intoxication, or the anemia of chronic disease.

ER MANAGEMENT

Treat *iron deficiency* with oral ferrous sulfate, 6 mg/kg/day of elemental iron divided tid between meals. This can be given with juice (vitamin C enhances iron absorption), but never with milk (impairs iron absorption). A rise in hemoglobin and reticulocyte count 1 week later confirms both the diagnosis and compliance with the regimen. Lack of response suggests a wrong diagnosis, ongoing blood loss, incorrect dose, or noncompliance. Warn the patient or parents that constipation and darkening of the stools may result from the iron therapy. For occasional epigastric pain, divide the doses into smaller volumes at more frequent intervals or give the iron with food (not milk).

Treat anemia secondary to *blood loss* with a packed red cell transfusion (10 cc/kg) if the patient is symptomatic (tachycardia, orthostatic hypotension, syncope). As a rough estimate, 1 cc/kg of packed cells will raise the hematocrit 1%. For symptomatic anemias of other etiologies, consult a pediatric hematologist before giving blood.

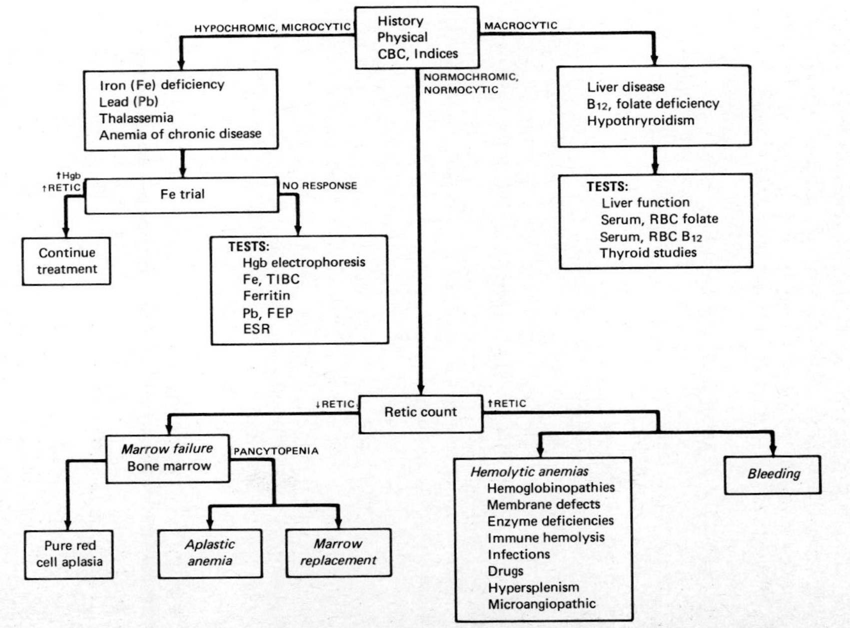

Figure 11-1. Evaluation of anemia

Treat *autoimmune hemolytic anemia* with prednisone (2 mg/kg/day), after consultation with a pediatric hematologist.

Institute specific therapy for any underlying conditions. However, therapy of most hematologic etiologies of anemia other than iron deficiency, lead intoxication, and bleeding, requires consultation with a hematologist/oncologist.

INDICATIONS FOR ADMISSION

- Significant cardiovascular or cerebral symptomatology (fainting, tachycardia, heart failure)
- Acute blood loss requiring transfusion
- Pancytopenia or suspicion of a malignancy
- Acute Coombs-positive or extrinsic hemolytic anemia with hemoglobin under 8 g/dl
- Chronic hemolytic disease with acute reticulocytopenia and fall in hematocrit (sickle cell aplastic crisis)
- Severe G-6-PD deficiency with exposure to oxidant stress (eg, moth balls, sulfonamides, antimalarials)
- Hgb<6g/dl

REFERENCES

1. Wolfe LC, Lux S: Pediatr Ann 8:435, 1979
2. Oski FA, Stockman JA: Pediatr Clin North Am 27:237, 1980

Bleeding Disorders

INTRODUCTION

Hemostasis is dependent on a complex interaction among circulating platelets, coagulation proteins, and vascular endothelium. Any of these systems may be dysfunctional and lead to abnormal bleeding.

Thrombocyte disorders usually involve a decrease in the number of circulating platelets, secondary to underproduction as in marrow failure (aplasia, infections, or drugs) or marrow replacement (leukemia), increased peripheral destruction (idiopathic thrombocytopenic purpura [ITP], hypersplenism, hemangiomas), or microangiopathic processes (hemolytic-uremic syndrome, disseminated intravascular coagulation [DIC]). Less common are disorders of platelet function which can be acquired (uremia, aspirin ingestion) or inherited (von Willebrand disease).

Coagulation factors are necessary for the formation of fibrin strands at bleeding sites. Hemorrhage can occur when any of them are either decreased in amount or dysfunctional. Decreased factor activity is present in the normal newborn, and with inherited deficiencies (von Willebrand disease), vitamin K deficiency (newborns, coumadin therapy, prolonged oral antibiotic therapy), liver failure, and DIC. Abnormal proteins with markedly diminished or absent function, as in hemophilia and dysfibrinogenemia, are less common.

The endothelium is responsible for the production of factor VIII and prostacyclin (a platelet inhibitor) and the insulation of coagulation factors and platelets from exposure to underlying collagen. Dysfunction of the endothelial system is observed in vasculitis (lupus, Henoch-Schönlein purpura) and infections (meningococcemia, rickettsia).

CLINICAL PRESENTATION

The presenting complaint varies greatly, depending on the location, rapidity, and severity of bleeding. *Platelet abnormalities* cause petechial or mucosal bleeding which occurs immediately after the trauma and usually responds to local pressure. With *ITP*, skin and mucosal bleeding often follows a benign viral illness. Patients with *coagulation factor abnormalities* may have delayed, posttraumatic deep tissue hemorrhages into muscles and joints. Abrasions and tooth extractions respond poorly to local pressure. Bleeding secondary to *vasculitis* usually presents as purpura.

DIAGNOSIS

A family history of bleeding disorders can be very helpful, as in *hemophilia A and B* (x-linked) and *von Willebrand disease* (autosomal dominant). A seriously ill child may have leukemia (pallor, fever, fatigue, hepatomegaly, lymphadenopathy), hemolytic-uremic syndrome (lethargy, diarrhea, oliguria), hepatitis (vomiting, jaundice, hepatomegaly, dark urine, acholic stools), or DIC.

The final identification of the underlying disease can be facilitated by a few simple screening tests: platelet count (normal, 150,000–300,000/mm^3); prothrombin time (PT), which tests the extrinsic clotting system (factors I, II, V, VII, X; normal within 2 seconds of control); partial thromboplastin time (PTT), which tests the intrinsic system (factors I, II, V, VIII, IX, X, XI, XII; normal within 5 seconds of control, or less than 35–40 seconds); and bleeding time, which assesses the platelet-endothelium interaction (normal under 7–8 minutes). As shown in Table 11-3, the results of these tests suggest the most likely diagnosis.

ER MANAGEMENT

For the patient with vitamin K deficiency who is actively bleeding, give 5–10 mg of vitamin K by slow intravenous (IV) infusion. Correction of coagulation factor levels begins within hours, with marked improvement by 24 hours. If there is a history of coumadin ingestion, a repeat administration of vitamin K might be necessary.

Treat thrombocytopenic conditions with local pressure to superficial bleeding sites. If this is unsuccessful, or the platelet count is under 50,000/mm^3, obtain a type and cross-match and consult a hematologist.

The management of coagulopathies is summarized in Table 11-4. In addition, avoid giving nonsteroidal antiinflammatory agents, including aspirin, to all children with a bleeding diathesis.

INDICATIONS FOR ADMISSION

- Massive bleeding that causes hypovolemic symptomatology or requires transfusion of packed red blood cells.
- Suspected or proven intracranial hemorrhage and hemophiliacs with any significant head trauma
- Significant hematemesis and hematochezia
- Newly diagnosed thrombocytopenia (platelet count under 50,000/mm^3)
- Severe inherited coagulopathy with gross hematuria, significant trauma, large laceration, or severe abdominal pain

TABLE 11-3. DIFFERENTIAL DIAGNOSIS OF THE BLEEDING CHILD

Platelet Count	Prothrombin Time	Partial Thromboplastin Time	Diagnoses
Normal	Prolonged	Normal	Moderate liver disease Coumarin ingestion Factor VII deficiency
Normal	Normal	Prolonged	Von Willebrand disease Heparin effect Factors VIII, IX, XI, or XII deficiency
Decreased	Prolonged	Prolonged	DIC Giant hemangioma Congenital heart disease
Decreased	Normal	Normal	Thrombocytopenia
Normal	Prolonged	Prolonged	Severe liver disease Vitamin K deficiency High dose heparin or coumarin therapy Factor II, V, or X deficiency Dysfibrinogenemia
Normal	Normal	Normal	(Obtain Bleeding Time) Von Willebrand disease Platelet dysfunction Factor XIII deficiency Henoch-Schönlein purpura Connective tissue disease

TABLE 11-4. OUTPATIENT MANAGEMENT OF COAGUALTION DISORDERS

Coagulopathy	Type of Hemorrhage	Blood Products of Choice	Dose and Length of Therapy	Advantages	Disadvantages
Hemophilia A (Factor VIII) * = Mild, moderate Δ = Severe	Early joint or muscle bleed; moderate mucosal bleed[a]	*FFP	10–15 cc/kg × 1 dose	Small risk of hepatitis, readily available	Large volumes; transfusion reactions
		*,ΔCryoprecipitate	0.2 bag/kg × 1 dose	Moderate hepatitis risk, less expensive than concentrate	Highly variable amounts of factor VIII
		Factor VIII concentrate	20 U/kg × 1 dose	Convenient and accurate dosage	Hepatitis; hemolytic reactions; expensive
	Significant joint[b] or muscle bleed; mild, moderate hematuria	*,ΔCryoprecipitate	0.2 bag/kg qd × 2–3 days	As above	As above
		ΔFactor VIII concentrate	30 U/kg qd × 2–3 days		

Hemophilia B (Factor IX); Factor II, VII, or X deficiencies	Early joint or muscle bleed; moderate mucosal bleed[a]	FFP	10–15 cc/kg × 1 dose	As above	As above
		Factor IX concentrate	40 U/kg × 1 dose	Convenient, accurate administration	Hepatitis, expensive, venous thrombosis
Factor II, VII, or X deficiencies	Significant joint[b] or muscle bleed; mild, moderate hematuria	Factor IX concentrate	100 U/kg qd × 2–3 days for VII, IX, X 100 U/kg × 1 for II	As above	As above
Von Willebrand disease	Early joint or muscle bleed; moderate mucosal bleed[a]	FFP	10–15 cc/kg × 1 dose	As above	As above
		Cryprecipitate	0.2 bag/kg × 1 dose		
Fibrinogen deficiency or dysfibrinogenemia	Significant joint or muscle bleed; hematuria or mild menorrhagia	Cryoprecipitate	0.2 bag/kg qd × 2–3 days	As above	As above
Factor V, XI, or XIII deficiencies	Any mild to moderate bleeding	FFP	10–15 cc/kg	As above	As above

[a]For oral mucosa bleeding, follow blood product infusion with Amicar 100 mg/kg PO q 6hr for 5–7 days to inhibit clot lysis.
[b]For significant hemarthroses, give prednisone 1–2 mg/kg/day for 3 days (do not taper).

- Clinical features suspicious for marrow replacement, DIC, hemolytic-uremic syndrome, or hepatic failure
- Generalized petechial or purpuric eruption in an acutely ill child with fever

REFERENCES

1. Montgomery RR, Hathaway WE: Pediatr Clin North Am 27:327–344, 1980
2. Abilgaard CF: Semin Hematol 12:223–232, 1975

Infection and the Immunocompromised Host

INTRODUCTION

After the first few months of life, most infants will have the ability to resist serious infections. The hallmark of an immunocompromised patient, however, is an increased susceptibility to infection, including increased frequency, duration, and severity, as well as infection caused by unusual pathogens.

CLINICAL PRESENTATION

Although symptoms will vary with the organism and site of infection, these patients often have recurrent respiratory infections and repeated severe bacterial illnesses (sepsis, pneumonia, meningitis). Persistent lymphadenopathy and hepatosplenomegaly are common findings. Many patients have chronic diarrhea with some form of malabsorption and failure to thrive (IgA deficiency, exocrine pancreatic insufficiency). A variety of skin lesions may be seen, including eczema (Wiscott-Aldrich syndrome), pyoderma (cyclic neutropenia, Job syndrome), and diffuse dermatitis (chronic granulomatous disease). A variety of symptom complexes might suggest specific disorders.

SYMPTOM COMPLEXES SUGGESTING IMMUNODEFICIENCIES

1. An infant with eczema, thrombocytopenia, and frequent pyogenic infections: Wiscott-Aldrich syndrome

2. Bacterial infections appearing with regularity every 3 (range 2–4) weeks: cyclic neutropenia
3. Black child with frequent bouts of bone pain, leukocytosis, and a chronic hemolytic anemia: sickle cell disease (SCD)
4. Recurrent bacterial infections in a child with oculocutaneous albinism and leukocytes with large intracytoplasmic granules: Chédiak-Higashi syndrome
5. An adolescent with cervical adenopathy, fever, weight loss, splenomegaly, and herpes zoster or prolonged varicella infection: Hodgkin disease
6. A young male with lymphadenopathy, hepatosplenomegaly, pneumonia, dermatitis, and frequent infections with *Staphylococcus* and gram-negative enteric organisms: chronic granulomatous disease
7. A child with persistent, severe fungal infections of the skin, fingernails, and oral mucosa, with dysphagia and hypothyroidism: chronic mucocutaneous candidiasis
8. Infant with bilateral simian creases, Brushfield spots, prominent epicanthal folds, developmental delay, and frequent infections: Down syndrome
9. The infant of an IV drug abuser with lymphadenopathy, hepatospenomegaly, and failure to thrive, or a hemophiliac with severe interstitial pneumonia: acquired immune deficiency syndrome *(AIDS)*

DIAGNOSIS

Prior to proceeding with an extensive immunologic evaluation, try to distinguish the immunodeficient child from the one with frequent colds and *normal immunologic function.* Many children have up to 8–10 respiratory infections in any given year, but these are usually mild, self-limited, unaccompanied by fever, with complete recovery between bouts. *Allergy* is more likely in children with repeated or persistent infections limited to the upper respiratory tract. Likewise, infections limited to a particular organ suggest specific disease entities: *cystic fibrosis, foreign body, collagen vascular disease, bronchiectasis* with recurrent pneumonia, or *cow's milk sensitivity, celiac disease,* and *inflammatory bowel disease* with chronic diarrhea and failure to thrive. Finally, many *chronic diseases* predispose patients to frequent infections (rheumatic disorders, chronic renal disease, sickle cell disease, diabetes, nutritional deficiencies, and malignancies).

ER MANAGEMENT

If the child has either two or more serious infections (pneumonia, meningitis, sepsis) in a short period of time or an infection with an unusual pathogen, obtain a CBC with differential platelet count, ESR, and quantitative immunoglobulins. In addition, evaluate cell-mediated immunity with skin testing (*Candida*, streptokinase / streptodornase, mumps, and purified protein derivative [PPD]). Further evaluation requires the assistance of an immunologist or hematologist.

Treatment of children with chronic immunodeficiencies and granulocyte disorders is usually supervised by a pediatric hematologist or immunologist. However, these children may occasionally be seen in an ER. When a child with a known immunodeficiency or neutrophil disorder presents with a fever (>101°F), a very conservative approach is mandatory. Obtain a CBC and cultures of the blood, urine, and any wound prior to initiating treatment. The child with central nervous system (CNS) symptoms must have a lumbar puncture with the fluid evaluated for unusual organisms (tuberculosis, india ink stain for *Cryptococcus*) in addition to the standard cultures and Gram stain.

Treat neutropenic patients with broad-spectrum antibiotics, including gentamicin (7.5 mg/kg/day divided q 8h), cephalothin (160 mg/kg/day divided q 4h), and carbenicillin (500 mg/kg/day divided q 4h). Give children with defective cell-mediated immunity who have fever and respiratory symptoms trimethoprim-sulfa (20 mg/kg/day of trimethoprim [TMP] divided q 6h) along with broad-spectrum antibiotics. Consider granulocyte transfusions for patients with neutrophil disorders who have serious infections. Treat patients with splenic dysfunction with ampicillin (100 mg/kg/day divided q 4–6h) along with a second drug active against *Pneumococcus* and *Haemophilus influenzae* (chloramphenicol, 75 mg/kg/day, or a third-generation cephalosporin).

INDICATIONS FOR ADMISSION

- Fever (>101°F) in a patient with a granulocyte count under 500/mm^3, a documented phagocytic defect, or other immunodeficiency.
- Immunocompromised patient with pneumonia, an abscess, or localized infection (eg, otitis, cellulitis) not responding to initial antibiotic therapy

- Child under 2 years of age with sickle cell disease and high fever (>102°F)
- Suspected malignancy
- Varicella or herpes zoster infections in a child with defective cell-mediated immunity

REFERENCES

1. Pennington JE: Semin Inf Dis 1:142, 1978
2. Frazier JP, Kramer WG, Pickering LK, et al: Pediatr Inf Dis 3:40, 1984
3. Pizzo PA: J Pediatr 98:341, 513, 1981
4. Allegretta GJ, Weisman SJ, Altman AJ: Pediatr Clin North Am 32:613–624, 1985

Leukemia and Lymphoma

INTRODUCTION

The most common pediatric malignancy is acute lymphoblastic leukemia (ALL), while lymphomas are the second most common solid tumors. Early recognition of these diseases is imperative so that effective therapy can be instituted as soon as possible.

CLINICAL PRESENTATION

Leukemia. The presentation of ALL usually results from the absence of the normal hematopoietic elements. Clinical findings are related to the degree of anemia (pallor, fatigue, light-headedness, palpitations), thrombocytopenia (petechiae, purpura, epistaxis), and neutropenia (infections). Other findings include joint or bone pain, hepatosplenomegaly, lymphadenopathy, skin nodules, and gingival hypertrophy. CNS involvement can be asymptomatic; alternatively, there can be symptoms related to increased intracranial pressure (headache, vomiting, irritability, visual disturbances) or unusual constellations of findings such as an isolated cranial nerve paresis or the "hypothalamic syndrome" (marked hyperphagia with weight gain, personality changes). Leukemic infiltration in organs such as the testes and ovaries can lead to firm, painless enlargement.

Hodgkin Disease. Hodgkin disease most commonly presents with either firm, nontender, asymptomatic lymphadenopathy (particularly the cervical, mediastinal, and paraaortic nodes) or constitutional symptoms (fever, night sweats, weight loss). Pruritis rarely occurs in children and complications such as jaundice and superior vena cava obstruction are uncommon. Prolonged varicella or a history of herpes zoster are often reported.

Non-Hodgkin Lymphomas. The non-Hodgkin lymphomas may also present with isolated, nontender, firm lymphadenopathy, but children more frequently have widespread disease. A primary mediastinal mass causes dyspnea, cough, pleural effusion, and superior vena cava obstruction (respiratory distress; distended neck veins; edema of face, neck, and arms). Children can have primary tumors in Waldeyer's ring, presenting with tonsillar involvement misdiagnosed as a peritonsillar abscess. Primary gastrointestinal lymphomas (Peyer's patches of distal ileum) can cause asymptomatic abdominal distention, vomiting and diarrhea, intussusception, or intestinal obstruction. Burkitt lymphoma can present with retroperitoneal or mesenteric tumors and occasionally with involvement of the maxillary sinus, but jaw masses are uncommon in the United States.

DIAGNOSIS

The hallmark of *ALL,* in addition to cytopenias, is the presence of large numbers of primitive leukocytes (blasts) in the blood and bone marrow. Rarely, *neuroblastoma* may replace the bone marrow with primitive cells, but these do not appear in the peripheral blood.

Most often confused with ALL and lymphomas are *infectious mononucleosis* and *mono-like syndromes* (cytomegalovirus, toxoplasmosis) which can present with fever, lymphadenopathy, hepatosplenomegaly, cytopenias, and immature leukocytes on blood smear. However, these cells can usually be distinguished from blasts. *Pertussis* can induce a profound leukocytosis ($>50,000/mm^3$), but the cells are mature and there is no anemia. Children with ITP do not appear chronically ill, the platelets are large, and other cytopenias are absent. *Storage disorders* (Gaucher disease) may present with hepatosplenomegaly and pancytopenia, necessitating a bone marrow or liver biopsy for differentiation.

A lymphoma-like picture can be seen with *sinus histiocytosis, di-*

phenylhydantoin therapy, and rarely, in *Kawasaki disease (KD).* A node biopsy is indicated if there is weight loss, supraclavicular lymphadenopathy, or the node is firm and progressively enlarging.

ER MANAGEMENT

If ALL or a lymphoma is suspected, obtain a CBC with differential, platelet count, reticulocyte count, heterophile antibody or monospot test, electrolytes, liver function tests, a blood culture, and chest x-ray. Consult with a pediatric hematologist-oncologist and admit patients with blasts on peripheral smear, pancytopenia, or lymphadenopathy that meets the criteria for biopsy (see p 269). Refer other patients to a primary care setting for follow-up.

INDICATIONS FOR ADMISSION

- Newly diagnosed or suspected malignancy
- Pancytopenia

REFERENCES

1. Canellos GP: PIR 6:3–9, 1984
2. Bleyer WA: Pediatr Ann 12:277–292, 1983
3. Gardner RV, Graham-Pole J: Pediatr Ann 12:322–335, 1983
4. Poplack DG: Pediatr Clin North Am 32:669–698, 1985

Lymphadenopathy

INTRODUCTION

Palpable lymph nodes may be a normal finding or a sign of disease, either minor or life-threatening. Lymph nodes are not usually palpable until a few months of age. Afterwards there is a steady increase in the body's normal lymphoid tissue, so that by puberty nearly 100% of children will have at least some palpable nodes, most commonly in the cervical and inguinal areas. Therefore a variety of factors must be considered when deciding whether to pursue a work-up for enlarged nodes.

CLINICAL PRESENTATION

Generalized Lymphadenopathy. Generalized lymphadenopathy is enlargement in at least three noncontiguous lymph node regions. It is always abnormal and usually nonlymphoid features of the primary disease process are evident (fever, rash, pharyngitis, arthritis, arthralgia, bruising, pallor, hepatosplenomegaly, etc). The most common cause is an infection, particularly *infectious mononucleosis* or a *mono-like illness* (cytomegalovims, toxoplasmosis). Other infectious etiologies include the exanthemous viral infections of childhood (measles, rubella, varicella), enteroviruses (echo, Coxsackie), tuberculosis, hepatitis B, syphilis, and malaria. Noninfectious causes include rheumatoid diseases (juvenile rheumatoid arthritis, systemic lupus erythematosus), serum sickness, drug reactions (Dilantin), sarcoidosis, storage diseases, and eczema. Malignancies to consider are leukemia, lymphoma, and histiocytosis. Finally, generalized lymphadenopathy, failure to thrive, and splenomegaly suggest AIDS.

Localized Lymphadenopathy. Localized lymphadenopathy is most often a response to a nearby infection (*reactive lymphadenopathy*). The location often suggests the primary infection. For example, occipital lymphadenopathy occurs in response to scalp conditions such as seborrhea, tinea capitis, and pediculosis; preauricular enlargement is secondary to conjunctivitis; and submandibular and submental nodes may enlarge with infection of the gingiva, teeth, buccal mucosa, and tongue. Axillary lymphadenopathy can be caused by cat scratch fever, rat bite fever, or a recent immunization, while inguinal involvement occurs with venereal diseases (syphilis, gonorrhea, lymphogranuloma venereum, chancroid). Reactive cervical enlargement is most common, frequently secondary to a viral upper respiratory infection (URI), and is discussed on pp 102–105. Since the supraclavicular nodes drain from the lungs and mediastinum, enlargement here is always a concern. Etiologies include infections (tuberculosis, histoplasmosis, coccidioidomycosis), neoplasms (lymphomas), and sarcoidosis. For any node site, a nearby cellulitis or local pyogenic infection will cause reactive enlargement.

A second category of local lymphadenopathy is primary infection of the node, or *adenitis*. Most often this is bacterial in origin, with the most common organisms being *S. aureus* and group A *Streptococcus* although anaerobes, and *Haemophilus influenzae* have been implicated. Tuberculosis and atypical mycobacteria are other etiologies.

DIAGNOSIS

A complete history and physical examination are necessary to locate a primary infection, document a local adenitis, or diagnose a disease causing generalized lymphadenopathy. Particularly important are fever, weight loss, rash, jaundice, arthritis, arthralgias, bruising, pallor, pharyngitis or upper respiratory symptoms, hepatosplenomegaly, contact with contagious diseases, history of a cat scratch or rat bite, and sexual activity.

When examining the involved node(s) there are six features to consider:

Location. Generalized enlargement always warrants further investigation, as does supraclavicular adenopathy. Isolated cervical, inguinal, and occipital nodes are not commonly pathologic.

Size. Generally, nodes larger than 1 cm in diameter should be considered abnormal, but particularly in the cervical area, nodes may be 2–3 cm without disease.

Rate of Enlargement. Rapid enlargement is generally caused by an infection, either an adenitis or a reactive hyperplasia. Slow growth suggests a malignancy or a systemic disease.

Mobility. A node fixed to adjacent structures or matted to other nodes suggests an infiltrative disease that demands further evaluation. A freely mobile node is generally benign.

Consistency. Soft, shotty nodes are usually normal or represent reactive enlargement. Adenitis causes fluctuance, while malignancy is associated with hard, rubbery nodes.

Overlying Skin. Bacterial adenitis causes erythema and warmth of the overlying skin. Adherence of the skin to the node occurs in cat scratch fever and atypical *Mycobacterium* infection. A reactive node does not affect the overlying skin.

ER MANAGEMENT

Generalized Lymphadenopathy. If *infectious mononucleosis* is suggested by the clinical findings (fever, pharyngitis, hepatosplenomegaly), a CBC with differential showing atypical lymphocytosis and a positive monospot or heterophile antibody test will confirm the diagnosis. (In a child <4 years old, the heterophile is likely to be negative, but specific EBV serologies are available). Treatment is supportive (bedrest, acetaminophen) and the patient should be instructed to avoid contact sports because of the risk of splenic rupture.

For all other cases, the clinical picture should guide the work-up, although in general a CBC with differential, erythrocyte sedimentation rate (ESR), liver function tests, VDRL, hepatitis B antigen, heterophile antibody, PPD, and chest x-ray are indicated.

Localized Lymphadenopathy. In most cases a contiguous infection will be found and *reactive adenopathy* diagnosed. The primary infection should be appropriately treated—the reactive node(s) will shrink as the infection resolves.

Treat an *adenitis* with dicloxacillin (50 mg/kg/day divided qid), erythromycin (40 mg/kg/day divided qid), or cephadrine (25 mg/kg/day divided qid). Warm compresses applied for 15–30 minutes every 3–4 hours are an important adjunct. Reevaluate the patient in 48–72 hours—if there has been a response, continue the antibiotic for a full 10-day course. If the node does not respond, consider other etiologies or drug resistance. Adding clindamycin (40 mg/kg/day divided qid) or ampicillin (100 mg/kg/day divided qid) may result in improvement. If at follow-up (24–48 hrs) there is no change, obtain a CBC and blood culture and admit the patient for further evaluation and parenteral antibiotics (oxacillin 100 mg/kg/day and/or clindamycin 40 mg/kg/day).

INDICATIONS FOR ADMISSION

- Systemic toxicity
- Suspicion of a malignancy or AIDS, to facilitate the work-up and management
- Adenitis unresponsive to oral antibiotics

REFERENCES

1. Zuelzer WW, Kaplan J: Sem Hematol 12:323–333, 1975
2. Knight PJ, Mulne AF, Vassy LE: Pediatrics 69:391–396, 1982

Oncologic Emergencies

INTRODUCTION

Although a child being treated for a malignancy is under the care of an oncologist, he or she may be brought in the ER if the family notices an acute change in his or her condition. The most common problems are fever, acute neurologic symptomatology, superior vena cava obstruction, and metabolic derangements.

CLINICAL PRESENTATION

Since malignant diseases and their treatments lead to defective immunity, patients are particularly susceptible to *infectious* complications, as manifested by fever >101°F. The patient with *pneumonia* is at risk for opportunistic infections (*pneumocystis, Aspergillus,* Legionnaire disease). If the child is exposed to varicella and has a negative history for the disease, he or she is at great risk for disseminated infection.

Acute neurologic symptomatology may include spinal cord compression and CNS involvement. *Spinal cord compression* causes back pain, lower extremity weakness and sensory loss, and bladder and bowel dysfunction. Headache, vomiting, and isolated cranial nerve paresis can occur with *CNS involvement.*

Uncommonly, *superior vena cava obstruction* can occur, manifested by dyspnea, edema of the head and neck, and prominent superficial veins on the upper body.

These children are also at risk for significant *metabolic derangements,* including hyperuricemia (oliguria), hyperkalemia (ECG changes), and hypocalcemia (tetany, laryngospasm, carpopedal spasm, seizures).

DIAGNOSIS AND ER MANAGEMENT

For all oncology patients with fever (>101°F), obtain a CBC with differential, urinalysis, chest x-ray (if there are respiratory symptoms), and cultures of the throat, blood, urine, and wound (if any). If there is granulocytopenia (<1000/mm^3), consult the oncologist and admit the patient for IV antibiotics pending culture results. Give ticarcillin (250 mg/kg/day) and gentamicin (6 mg/kg/day) with or without a cephalosporin (100 mg/kg/day). If there is evidence of pneumonia, add trimethroprim-sulfamethoxazole (TMP-SMX) (20 mg/kg/day of trimethoprim). The treatment of varicella exposure in a patient with a negative history (and no titers) is zoster-immune globulin, 10 cc/kg given within 4 days of exposure. If clinical varicella develops, admit and treat with IV acyclovir.

If spinal cord compression is suspected, obtain plain films of the spine and consult the oncologist and neurologist immediately. Children with signs of CNS involvement require an emergency CTT. If a mass lesion is found, immediately consult with a neurologist and an oncologist. In the absence of a mass, CNS leukemia is likely, for which radiation and intrathecal chemotherapy are usually indicated.

The diagnosis of superior vena cava obstruction is confirmed by finding an anterior mediastinal mass on chext x-ray or chest CT. Obtain a CBC with differential, platelet count, and reticulocyte count while awaiting consultation with an oncologist. The treatment is radiation or chemotherapy.

Treat elevation of the uric acid (>10 mg%) with hydration (twice maintenance), allopurinol (250 mg/M^2/day), and alkalinization of the urine with sodium bicarbonate (1–2 mEq/kg). Treat hyperkalemia (>6 mEq/L) with kayexelate enemas (1 g/kg) or (if >7 mEq/L), insulin (0.1 unit/kg), glucose (0.5 g/kg) and calcium (50–100 mg/kg). Alternatively, peritoneal dialysis can be performed. Treat hypocalcemia (<7.5 mEq) with 500 mg/kg/day of calcium gluconate, PO (see pp 143–145) and reduction of the phosphorous with amphojel 500 mg PO.

INDICATIONS FOR ADMISSION

- Fever (>101°F) and granulocytopenia (<1000/mm^3), pneumonia, or serious infection
- Clinical varicella
- Spinal cord compression, CNS leukemia, superior vena cava obstruction, airway obstruction
- Significant complication of therapy or serious metabolic derangement (uric acid >10 mg%; potassium >6 mEq/L; calcium <7.5 mEq/L).

REFERENCES

1. Byrd RL: Pediatr Ann 12:450–460, 1983
2. Bruckman JE, Bloomer WD: Semin Oncol 5:135–140, 1978

3. Lolich JJ, Goodman R: JAMA 231:58–61, 1975
4. Allegretta GJ, Weisman SJ, Altman AS: Pediatr Clin North Am 32:601–612, 1985

Sickle Cell Disease

INTRODUCTION

The sickle cell syndromes are inherited disorders characterized by a chronic hemolytic anemia of variable severity, as well as recurrent obstruction of the microvasculature.

CLINICAL PRESENTATION

Children with sickle cell disease (SCD) may present with a constellation of signs and symptoms, termed *crises*. The most common type is the *vasoocclusive crisis,* which is secondary to stasis of sickled red blood cells in capillaries. Multiple organ systems are frequently involved, with severe pain, fever, and symptoms that can mimic many infectious and inflammatory disorders. A common finding is bone pain in multiple sites, particularly the extremities and back. In children under 2 years of age, vasoocclusive crises often take the form of dactylitis, or the ''hand-foot'' syndrome, with pain and swelling in the hands, feet, fingers, and toes. Other presentations may include priapism, pneumonia, limp, hematuria, acute hemiplegia (stroke), acute visual impairment caused by retinal vein occlusion or proliferative retinopathy, and leg ulcers. Right upper quadrant pain and jaundice occur in older children secondary to cholelithiasis from chronic hemolysis.

In addition to the vasoocclusive events, several other ''crises'' are seen in children with SCD. *Aplastic crises* are manifested by worsening anemia and reticulocytopenia. These crises usually follow viral infections that transiently suppress the bone marrow. Patients present with fatigue, light-headedness, tachycardia, and palpitations.

Splenic *sequestration crises,* with pooling of red blood cells in a rapidly enlarging spleen, are most often seen in young patients with sickle thalassemia (S-Thal) and S-C disease. These children have cold clammy skin, marked tachycardia, and profound hypotension, as well as a large left-sided abdominal mass (spleen). If unrecognized, deterioration can be rapid with a fatal outcome.

Hyperhemolytic crises, with a falling hematocrit, increasing jaundice, and markedly elevated reticulocyte counts (>20%), are rare and may in reality be the resolving phase of aplastic crises. Increased hemolysis with a rise in bilirubin can also be seen in blacks with concurrent *G-6-PD deficiency.*

Megaloblastic crises, due to folate depletion are rare and may be diagnosed by finding hypersegmented polys and pancytopenia.

Infections account for many of the serious problems in patients with SCD. Hyposplenism (initially functional, then anatomical) in conjunction with decreased antibody production, decreased serum-opsonizing activity, vasoocclusion, and defective neutrophil function, places these children at great risk for fulminant overwhelming sepsis, particularly with encapsulated organisms such as *Pneumococcus* and *H. influenzae.* They are also at increased risk for meningitis, pneumonia, pyelonephritis, and osteomyelitis (particularly *Salmonella*). Unfortunately, Pneumovax vaccine does not reliably prevent all serious pneumococcal infections, while *H. influenzae* type B vaccine is less effective under two years of age.

DIAGNOSIS

Test all black children who present with any of the classic sickle cell symptomatology noted above for SCD. This is accomplished with one of the readily available screening tests (Sickle-Dex) and subsequently confirmed with hemoglobin electrophoresis to determine the particular form of the disease (S-S, S-C, S-Thal). Suspect the diagnosis in an asymptomatic child whose peripheral blood smear reveals sickled cells and reticulocytosis (>5%). In addition, the smear will often contain target cells, "helmet" cells, polychromatophilia, and Howell-Jolly bodies.

The major diagnostic problem is to identify the cause of the current symptomatology. A vasoocclusive crisis is a diagnosis of exclusion. Leukocytosis (>18,000–20,000/mm^3) is typical in SCD, and fever is not helpful in distinguishing the different entities. Particular difficulties are seen with:

Bone Pain. Differentiating between bone *infarcts* and *osteomyelitis* can be very difficult, particularly when only one site is involved. X-rays and bone scans are often unreliable, necessitating needle aspiration to obtain a specimen for culture. An elevated ESR and an increased number of bands (>10% of the total white count) on peripheral smear may indicate an infection. *Aseptic necrosis* of the head of the femur or humerus presents with bone pain, and in most cases abnormal radiographs of the affected limb.

Right Upper Quadrant Abdominal Pain. Consider *hepatitis* (especially for patients on chronic transfusion therapy), *hepatic infarction,* and *cholelithiasis,* all of which can cause severe pain, fever, and elevated bilirubin. With hepatic infarcts, abnormal liver chemistries return to baseline in a much shorter amount of time (days) than with hepatitis, while an abdominal sonogram often detects biliary stones. To further confuse the picture, however, *right lower lobe pneumonia, rib infarcts,* and *renal disorders* (pyelonephritis and papillary necrosis) can all cause pain in a similar location, although other physical and laboratory findings help to differentiate among these.

Chest Pain and Respiratory Distress. The major differential is between vasoocclusion (*pulmonary infarct*) and infection (*pneumonia*). Fever, leukocytosis, and similar radiographic and auscultatory findings occur with both diseases. In addition, either illness can lead to the other, so it is prudent to treat for both entities. A ventilation-perfusion scan may differentiate between the two, although treatment will not be altered. Finally, chest pain can be secondary to *rib infarcts* and *abdominal disorders.*

ER MANAGEMENT

Vasoocclusive Crises. Since no antisickling agent is available, therapy consists of supportive care to alleviate symptoms and treatment of the triggering event and potentiating factors.

1. *Vigorous hydration*: The patient often presents with decreased plasma volume secondary to fever, vomiting, and chronic hyposthenuria. In addition to ad lib oral intake, administer several hours of intravenous hydration at twice-maintenance rate. The type of fluid is controversial, but D5 1/4NS or D5 1/2NS is satisfactory.

2. *Sodium bicarbonate*: Add sodium bicarbonate (1 mEq/kg) to the solution only if marked acidosis is present (pH <7.20).
3. *Analgesics*: For mild vasoocclusive crises, give aspirin or acetaminophen with codeine every 3–4 hours. Occasionally, a single injection of meperidine (1–2 mg/kg) in conjunction with a few hours of vigorous hydration can prevent hospital admission.
4. *Antipyretics*: Fever leads to further dehydration and sickling, so treat with aspirin or acetaminophen.
5. *Bedrest*: Muscular activity can produce lactate and worsen the acidosis.
6. *X-ray*: If the patient is limping, a radiograph of the hip must be obtained to rule out aseptic necrosis of the femoral head. If positive, immediately institute bedrest and consult with an orthopedist.

Fever. For patients older than 2 years in no distress, with temperature less than 102°F, and no apparent source, obtain a blood culture, CBC, ESR, urinalysis, and urine culture. If there is no marked left shift and the absolute band count is under 3000/mm³, the patient may be sent home to take oral antibiotics. Give children under 12 years of age amoxicillin (40 mg/kg/day) and treat adolescents with penicillin VK (250 mg qid); give the first dose IM. Follow-up is in 24 hours, or sooner if the temperature goes higher.

Admit the patient with T>102°F. Also admit toxic appearing patients and children <2 years of age with T>101°F. Treat with IV ampicillin (100 mg/kg/day) and chloramphenicol (75 mg/kg/day).

In addition to the basic fever work-up, if there are any respiratory symptoms, obtain a chest x-ray, regardless of the auscultatory findings. Treat any peripheral density as a pneumonia, with amoxicillin (40 mg/kg/day) and oxygen, if necessary. Children with fever and a single bone with point tenderness require a needle aspiration for Gram stain, cell count, and culture. A lumbar puncture is indicated for all febrile irritable infants under 2 years of age and all older patients with temperatures over 105°F and no fever source.

Sequestration Crisis. If the patient is hypotensive, immediately infuse plasmanate (10–20 cc/kg), followed by a transfusion of packed red cells (5–10 cc/kg slowly).

Megaloblastic Crisis. If the hematocrit is greater than 20, the absolute granulocyte count above 1000/mm³, and the platelet count above

75,000/mm^3, administer 1 mg/day of folic acid. Repeat the blood count in 4–7 days.

INDICATIONS FOR ADMISSION

- Serious symptoms, including acute hemiplegia, gross hematuria, acute visual disturbance, severe right upper quadrant pain, or respiratory distress
- Splenic sequestration or aplastic crisis
- Patient under 2 years old with temperature over 101°F, older child with sudden temperature over 102°F with or without an identifiable source
- Severe or prolonged vasoocclusive crisis with pain unresponsive to usual therapeutic measures
- Irritable infant with hand-foot syndrome
- Severe megaloblastic crisis (hematocrit $<$20%, platelet count $<$50,000/mm^3, or granulocyte count $<$1000/mm^3

REFERENCES

1. Vichinsky EP, Lubin BH: Pediatr Clin North Am 27:429–447, 1980
2. Mentzer WC, Wang WC: Pediatr Ann 9:23–28, 1980

Splenomegaly

INTRODUCTION

Splenomegaly is usually secondary to a *benign viral infection* (Epstein-Barr virus, cytomegalovirus). However, other possible *infectious* causes include bacteria (subacute bacterial endocarditis, tuberculosis), fungi (histoplasmosis), rickettsia (Rocky Mountain spotted fever), or parasites (malaria, *Leishmania*). Other etiologies include *neoplasms* (leukemia, lymphomas), congestion secondary to outflow obstruction (cirrhosis, cystic fibrosis, Budd-Chiari syndrome, portal vein thrombosis), *storage diseases* (sarcoid, histiocytosis, Hurler syndrome, Gaucher disease), and *generalized inflammation* (lupus, juvenile rheumatoid arthritis). In addition, splenomegaly occurs if there is *extramedullary hematopoiesis* (thalassemia, myelofibrosis, osteopetrosis) or a *hemolytic anemia* (SCD, autoimmune hemolytic anemia, hereditary spherocytosis).

CLINICAL PRESENTATION

A palpable spleen tip that is slightly below the costal margin is a frequent finding on routine physical examination in normal infants up to 1 year of age, as well as in patients with fevers or colds. Associated clinical findings depend on the primary disease. Regardless of etiology, massive splenomegaly can cause anemia (pallor, tachycardia, weakness), neutropenia, and thrombocytopenia (petechiae, purpura, frank bleeding).

DIAGNOSIS

Inquire about recent travel to endemic areas of disease (*malaria, Leishmania, histoplasmosis*) and family histories of inherited disorders (*thalassemia, sickle hemoglobinopathies, Gaucher disease, Hurler disease*), or splenectomy (*thalassemia, hereditary spherocytosis*). Ask about fevers (*infection, inflammation*), easy bruising or bleeding (*leukemia, lymphoma, marrow replacement*), hematemesis (*cirrhosis*), and transfusions (*hemoglobinopathy*).

On physical examination, look for evidence of infection (adenopathy, exanthem, pharyngitis), storage disorder (asymptomatic organ enlargement), malignancy (weight loss, bruising, bleeding, adenopathy, hepatomegaly, fever), or a connective tissue disorder (arthritis).

Although generalized adenopathy and hepatomegaly might be significant findings, they are found with splenomegaly of many etiologies, and therefore are usually not helpful in making the diagnosis. One of the most common constellations is fatigue, fever, pharyngitis, generalized adenopathy, and hepatosplenomegaly consistent with infectious mononucleosis, a mono-like syndrome (cytomegalovirus), and rarely, a more serious illnesses (leukemia).

ER MANAGEMENT

Laboratory examination is usually not immediately necessary in an infant or child who appears well and has a palpable spleen tip. Follow the patient and repeat the abdominal examination. Undertake further evaluation if the spleen remains palpable for more than 2 months, enlarges to more than 2 cm below the costal margin, or becomes associated with other signs or symptoms.

If the child presents with fatigue, upper respiratory congestion, and pharyngitis, a CBC with differential and a monospot or heterophile antibody usually confirm the diagnosis of infectious mononucleosis.

A more thorough laboratory evaluation is indicated for the child who exhibits any serious signs and symptoms such as pallor, ecchymoses, arthritis, or a toxic appearance, or has a history of weight loss or persistent splenomegaly. Obtain a CBC with differential, platelet and reticulocyte counts, an ESR, blood chemistries, and a chest x-ray, and place a 5TU PPD. If the clinical picture is suggestive of an infection, obtain a blood culture, and specific antibody titers. Admit these patients to facilitate the work-up.

Isolated splenomegaly usually does not cause significant problems, except for cytopenias and rupture following trauma. Patients may attend school (if otherwise well) but caution them about participating in contact sports and other activities that place them at risk for abdominal injury. Otherwise, management depends on the underlying etiology.

INDICATIONS FOR ADMISSION

- Suspected malignancy
- Splenomegaly and neutropenia ($<1{,}000/mm^3$) with associated fever, thrombocytopenia ($<50{,}000/mm^3$), or hematemesis
- Massive, unexplained splenomegaly for work-up
- Splenomegaly with anemia and abdominal pain, particularly with a history of abdominal trauma

REFERENCE

1. McMillian J, Neiberg P, Oski F: The Whole Pediatrician Catalog. Philadelphia, Saunders, 1977, pp 20–22

12

Infectious Disease Emergencies

Evaluation of the Febrile Child

INTRODUCTION

In the evaluation and management of the febrile child, decisions are based on clinical impression and physical examination, reinforced by the results of selectively ordered laboratory tests. The guidelines here are strict, intended for house officers at various levels of training, who cannot be assured of close patient follow-up. The pediatrician in private practice, with confidence in his or her clinical impression and the opportunity for close telephone and office follow-up, can order fewer laboratory tests and hospitalize patients less frequently.

Fever is one of the most common causes for a visit to the ER. It may be the presenting sign for a viral illness, a minor bacterial infection, or a life-threatening bacterial process. Although children can have sepsis without fever, it is more likely that seriously ill children have some elevation in their temperature. In fact, with the exception of very young infants, the incidence of sepsis increases with rising temperature.

CLINICAL PRESENTATION

The priority is the identification of the child with a serious bacterial infection. Clinical impression is based on the child's alertness, playfulness, interaction with the environment, color, state of hydration, quality of cry, and ability to be consoled. The older the child, the more reliable clinical impression becomes as a predictor of serious underlying illness.

Young infants (< 8 weeks) may have sepsis without many clinical findings. There may be a history of excessive crying, irritability, lethargy, or decreased feeding. Unfortunately, infants are at highest risk for sepsis in the first few days of life, when there has been little time for behavior patterns to develop. Therefore, the history is often not helpful. However, a history of a cyanotic episode or a seizure in an infant with fever is extremely worrisome, and mandates a full evaluation for sepsis.

On physical examination, the young infant may be pale or mottled, tachypneic, or tachycardic, with a weak cry and grunting respirations. Alternatively, he or she may simply be sleeping and difficult to arouse. Focal infections typically do not present with localized findings. Meningeal signs may be absent despite meningitis, and there is no ear tugging with otitis media. The infant with a urinary tract infection (UTI) may only have fever and vomiting or diarrhea, and there may not be rales associated with pneumonia.

With the older child, clinical impression becomes more accurate: the child with sepsis does not smile and is not interested in his or her surroundings. The parent often reports that there is a definite change in the child's behavior. Moreover, localized infections are often associated with focal complaints. The older child (toddler age) with meningitis usually has nuchal rigidity and positive Kernig sign (passive knee extension with a flexed hip is painful) and Brudzinski sign (passive neck flexion causes hip flexion).

"Occult" bacteremia may occur in 5% of children 6–24 months of age with fever greater than 102°F; it has been noted in younger infants as well. The patient is usually somewhat irritable, with symptoms of a upper respiratory infection (URI) or pharyngitis but no other detectable etiology for the fever.

A temperature >106°F is very unusual; 10% of children with such fever may have meningitis.

DIAGNOSIS AND ER MANAGEMENT

Clinical impression and the physical examination are the mainstays of diagnosing serious illness in the febrile child. Certain specific laboratory tests may help predict the risk of serious infection when the results of the clinical evaluation are ambivalent. White blood cell count (WBC) >15,000/mm^3 or erythrocyte sedimentation rate (ESR)

>30mm/hr have been shown to correlate with serious bacterial illness or a risk of occult bacteremia.

The management of febrile infants and children is summarized below. Modifications should be made if unusual pathogens are suspected (immunocompromised host, cerebrospinal fluid [CSF] shunt, recent course of parenteral antibiotics).

1. *Infants under 8 weeks of age with T > 100.6°F*
   Since clinical impression is difficult to apply in young infants, perform a full evaluation for sepsis including a complete blood count (CBC), ESR, blood and urine cultures, urinalysis, chest x-ray, and lumbar puncture for cell count, chemistries (glucose, protein), Gram stain, and culture. The urine must be obtained by catheter or suprapubic aspiration.
   a. *Under 4 weeks:* Treat with ampicillin (100 mg/kg/day) and gentamicin (5 mg/kg/day <1 week; 7.5 mg/kg/day >1 week), unless there is evidence of meningitis (bulging fontanelle, >10 polymorphonuclear neotrophil leukocytes (PMN)/mm^3 in non-bloody spinal fluid, organisms on Gram stain). If meningitis seems likely, use cefotaxime (<1 wk, 100 mg/kg/day divided q 12h; 1–4 wks, 150 mg/kg/day divided q 8h) in place of gentamicin, which does not reliably cross the blood-brain barrier.
   b. *Four to 8 weeks:* After 1 month of age, *Haemophilus influenza* replaces the gram-negative enterics as an important cause of sepsis. Treat with ampicillin (100 mg/kg/day) and chloramphenicol (75 mg/kg/day). If meningitis is suspected, increase the ampicillin dose to 300 mg/kg/day divided q 4h, and give 150 mg/kg as the first dose in the ER. Alternatively, use cefuroxime (100 mg/kg/first dose). Treat a UTI with ampicillin and gentamicin (7.5 mg/day).
2. *Infants 8 weeks to 6 months with T > 101°F*
   It is easier to apply clinical impression in this group. Give acetamenophen (10 mg/kg/dose) to lower the temperature and then observe the patient in his or her mother's lap, feeding or playing. An infant who smiles or takes a bottle eagerly is unlikely to be seriously ill. Look for a focus of infection (examine the urine if no other fever source can be found). If none is identified, and the patient looks well, he or she may be discharged, to return the next day for follow-up. Examine the ears carefully at each visit since otitis media is frequently associated with persistent URI.

Irritable patients require a CBC, ESR, blood and urine cultures, a chest x-ray, a stool culture (if there is diarrhea), and a lumbar puncture, in addition to a careful physical examination. If there is no evidence of meningitis on physical examination (bulging fontanelle, nucchal rigidity) or analysis of the spinal fluid, and the WBC and ESR are not elevated, clinical impression determines further management. Admit patients who appear toxic (lethargic, unconsolable, grunting) or have any focus other than otitis media, for parenteral ampicillin and chloramphenicol or cefuroxime. Infants who are consolable and feed well in the ER can be discharged home to return the next day for a follow-up examination.

3. *Children 6 to 24 months of age with T > 103°F*
   Perform a complete clinical evaluation including a lumbar puncture if the patient is lethargic or not consolable (even if a fever source has been identified). See the approprite sections for the treatment of specific infections. Occult bacteremia is prevalent in this group. The consolable patient without a focus of infection requires a blood and urine culture, a CBC, ESR, and a chest x-ray. If the WBC or the ESR is elevated, treat with amoxicillin (40 mg/kg/day) and schedule a follow-up visit for the next day.

   A 6- to 24-month old infant who looks well requires no laboratory studies or treatment, but must be rechecked the following day. If he or she remains febrile (>103°F) or becomes irritable, obtain a blood and urine culture, a CBC, ESR, and a chest x-ray, and treat, if the child is at risk for occult bacteremia (see above).

   Some of these patients will have positive blood cultures. Admit and treat them with IV antibiotics (patients with *Salmonella* may be treated orally). The only exceptions are patients with pneumococcus who have been afebrile > 24 hours and patients with *Salmonella* or *H. influenzae* who have been afebrile > 48 hours. Treat them with oral penicillin VK (50 mg/kg/day), trimethoprim-sulfamethoxazole (TMP-SMX) (8 mg/kg/day TMP), and amoxicillin (40 mg/kg/day) respectively.
4. *Patients > 24 months with T > 102°F*
   Localizing findings are reliable. Look for meningeal signs, evidence of focal infection or petechiae. In patients with lower abdominal pain, examine and culture the urine, although screening for occult bacteremia is not indicated.
5. *Patients with temperature > 106°F*
   Perform a complete evaluation for sepsis, including a lumbar

puncture, and admit the patient for parenteral antibiotics regardless of the child's appearance or the presence of an identifiable focus.

INDICATIONS FOR ADMISSION

- All infants < 8 weeks of age with temperature > 100.6°F
- Toxic appearance regardless of age or degree of fever
- Temperature > 106°F
- Patient afebrile < 24 hours recalled for pneumococcus in the blood; patient afebrile < 48 hours with *H. influenzae* or *Salmonella* in the blood
- Fever and profoundly abnormal laboratory tests (WBC > 40,000/ mm^3, ESR > 100 mm/hr (relative indication depending on age and presence or absence of an identifiable source)
- Parents unable to follow your instructions

REFERENCES

1. Klein JO: PID Supplement 3:55–58, 1984
2. Crain EF, Shelov SP: J Pediatr 101:686–689, 1982
3. Carroll WL, Farrell MK, Singer JI, et al: Pediatrics 72:608, 1983

Acute Bacterial Meningitis

INTRODUCTION

Bacterial meningitis is an inflammation of the leptomeninges, usually caused by blood-borne organisms. Uncommonly, meningitis occurs via direct extension from a nearby focus (mastoiditis, sinusitis).

In the neonate, group B *Streptococcus,* gram-negative enteric organisms, and *Listeria* are common pathogens, while in older patients *H. influenzae,* pneumococcus, and meningococcus are isolated most frequently. Patients with ventricular shunts or penetrating head wounds are at particular risk for staphylococcal infections.

CLINICAL PRESENTATION

Neonates and infants usually present with nonspecific signs such as irritability, lethargy, and poor feeding. Nuchal rigidity, Kernig sign (with the hip flexed, passive knee extension produces pain), Brudzinski sign (passive neck flexion causes hip flexion), and fever are not necessarily present. The anterior fontanelle, if still open, may be bulging.

The older child usually presents with high fever, nuchal rigidity, positive Kernig and Brudzinski signs, and central nervous system (CNS) symptoms (headache, lethargy). Patients of any age may present with seizures.

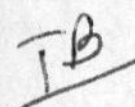

DIAGNOSIS AND ER MANAGEMENT

Since meningitis can be devastating and life threatening, maintain a high index of suspicion in a child with any of the presenting signs and symptoms. Especially in infants, the disease is not readily apparent on clinical grounds. Check for a bulging fontanelle or meningeal signs in all febrile, irritable, or lethargic patients. If there is any suspicion of meningitis, perform a lumbar puncture as quickly as possible. The only contraindication is increased intracranial pressure. If papilledema or focal neurologic signs are present, consult a neurologist (or obtain a CTT scan) prior to the lumbar puncture.

Obtain a CBC with differential, blood cultures, an ESR, a blood glucose, and other appropriate cultures (urine, etc) prior to antibiotic therapy. Place a 5 TU PPD on the forearm of all patients with meningitis. Evaluate the spinal fluid for cells, protein, and glucose, and obtain a specimen for culture, Gram stain, and, if available, counterimmunoelectrophoresis and C-reactive protein (CRP). In bacterial meningitis, the CSF shows a pleocytosis with PMN predominance, decreased glucose, and elevated protein (Table 12-1).

Whenever bacterial meningitis cannot be definitely ruled out, start intravenous antibiotic treatment immediately. For neonates, use ampicillin (300 mg/kg/day) and cefotaxime (100 mg/kg/day divided q 12h in the first week; 150 mg/kg/day divided q 8h, 1–4 weeks). Treat infants over 1 month of age with cefuroxime (100 mg/kg to 2g stat). If Staphylococcus infection is suspected, use oxacillin (200 mg/kg/day). Limit intravenous fluids to ⅔ daily maintenance, as these patients are at risk for inappropriate antidiuretic hormone (ADH) secretion. Corticosteroids are of no value.

During summertime enterovirus epidemics, older children with *viral meningitis* can have fever, headache, and photophobia, occasionally accompanied by myalgias or a nonpetechial exanthem, but with mini-

TABLE 12-1. CSF WBC, PROTEIN AND GLUCOSE: TYPICAL VALUES

	Infant > 2 Wks and Child	Bacterial Meningitis	Viral Meningitis	Tuberculous Meningitis
WBC	<5	50–5000	20–2000	100–500
% PMN	0	95	<30[a]	<30[a]
Protein	<30	>60	30–80	50–80
Glucose	>50	0–50	>60	<40
Glucose as % of serum glucose	>50	<40	>50	<40

[a]Early in the course there may be a PMN predominance.

mal or no nuchal rigidity. A bacterial etiology must be ruled out (lumbar puncture performed) if the patient is an infant, appears toxic, has a petechial rash, or does not present during a summertime epidemic. In viral meningitis the spinal fluid has a mononuclear pleocytosis, normal glucose, and slightly elevated (30–80 mg/dl) protein. There can be a polymorphonuclear predominance early in the course; a repeat lumbar puncture 4–6 hours later should reveal a monocytic predominance.

Tuberculous meningitis presents with low grade fever, vomiting, and meningeal signs. The spinal fluid has a mononuclear predominance with an elevated protein.

INDICATION FOR ADMISSION

- Possible bacterial or tuberculous meningitis

REFERENCES

1. McCracken,GH: Pediatr Infect Dis 2: 551–555, 1983
2. Kaplan SL, Feigen RD: Pediatr Clin North Am 30:259–270, 1983

Acute Rheumatic Fever

INTRODUCTION

Acute rheumatic fever (ARF), a nonsuppurative sequela of a group A streptococcal respiratory infection, occurs most commonly in children 6–15 years old. The incidence has fallen in the last decade, and ARF is now relatively uncommon.

CLINICAL PRESENTATION AND DIAGNOSIS

Because signs and symptoms are diverse and no laboratory test is diagnostic, the diagnosis of ARF is based upon fulfilling certain clinical criteria. A diagnosis is made if either two major manifestations or one major and two minor manifestations are present, along with evidence of a recent streptococcal infection (Table 12-2). Since Sydenham chorea may occur weeks to months after the streptococcal

TABLE 12-2. JONES CRITERIA (REVISED) FOR GUIDANCE IN THE DIAGNOSIS OF RHEUMATIC FEVER[a]

Major Manifestations	Minor Manifestations
	CLINICAL
Carditis	Previous rheumatic fever or rheumatic heart disease
Polyarthritis	Arthralgia
Chorea	Fever
Erythema marginatum	LABORATORY
Subcutaneous nodules	*Acute phase reactants:* Erythrocyte sedimentation rate, C-reactive protein, leukocytosis
	Prolonged P-R interval

Supporting evidence of streptococcal infection: increased titer of anti-streptococcal antibodies, ASO (anti-streptolysin O), others; positive throat culture for group A *Streptococcus;* recent scarlet fever

[a]The presence of two major criteria, or of one major and two minor criteria, indicates a high probability of acute rheumatic fever, *if supported by evidence of preceding Group A streptococcal infection.*

(Reproduced with permission. Jones Criteria [Revised] for Guidance in the Diagnosis of Rheumatic Fever, 1982, American Heart Association.)

illness, there may no longer be any evidence of the streptococcal infection.

Consideration of the major manifestations helps to differentiate ARF from other conditions in which one or more of these signs may also occur. The arthritis involves large joints, especially the knees, ankles, and wrists, and is migratory. Symptoms subside in the affected joints over 3–5 days while other joints become involved, and typically, the pain is far greater than the objective findings. Since even small doses of aspirin can significantly alter the arthritis, ask about a history of salicylate usage in a patient with an atypical presentation.

Juvenile rheumatoid arthritis (JRA) (p 416) and *septic arthritis* (p 316) are not migratory and do not respond dramatically to salicylates. *Gonoccal arthritis* (p 317) may be migratory at first, but it is usually accompanied by a papular rash.

The diagnosis of carditis is based on the presence of a significant new murmur, especially one of mitral or aortic insufficiency, with negative blood cultures. Less frequently there is heart failure, cardiac enlargement, or pericardial effusion, without a previous history of heart disease. Electrocardiographic changes associated with, but not pathognomonic of ARF, include a prolonged P-R interval (50–75% of patients with carditis) and evidence of myocarditis or pericarditis.

Subacute bacterial endocarditis (SBE) occurs in patients with a previous history of cardiac disease (ARF, VSD, PDA, valvular lesions). It is associated with recurrent fevers and malaise. Other manifestations include splenomegaly, Roth spots, splinter hemorrhages, Osler nodes, positive blood cultures, and hematuria. *Viral myocarditis* does not usually present with a significant new murmur.

Erythema marginatum, subcutaneous nodules, and Sydenham's chorea are rarely seen in the United States today. Erythema marginatum is evanescent; it begins as a faintly erythematous macular rash that becomes serpiginous with clear centers and sharp margins. Subcutaneous nodules are painless, hard, freely movable swellings found over the extensor surfaces of joints, along the spine, and in the scalp. They occur only with long standing, active carditis. Sydenham chorea is marked by purposeless, jerky movements, especially of the hands and face, associated with incoordination and behavior changes. When the patient (usually female) is asked to extend her arms and hands, the fingers hyperextend and wrists flex in a writhing manner. Patients tend to be embarrassed by the spontaneous movements and keep their hands at their sides or in their pockets.

ER MANAGEMENT

Hospitalize all children suspected of having ARF, as 75% of patients who develop carditis have symptoms within 7 days of onset of the clinical illness.

Obtain a throat culture, and give 1.2 million units of benzathine penicillin IM, or 250 mg PO qid for 10 days of Penicillin VK or erythromycin (penicillin-allergic patients) to eliminate residual group A *streptococcus* from the nasopharynx. Do not delay treatment while awaiting the results, and continue therapy despite a negative culture.

Salicylates and corticosteroids shorten the course of the illness but do not prevent long-term cardiac disease. Salicylates have a dramatic effect on the pain and swelling of rheumatic arthritis. Give 100 mg/kg/day, divided q 6h, for the first week, then reduce the dose to 65 mg/kg/day to complete a 3–4-week course. Corticosteroids are indicated for severe cardiac involvement (congestive failure, life-threatening pericarditis) or inadequate response to aspirin (resting tachycardia). The dose is 2 mg/kg/day of prednisone, divided q 6h.

TABLE 12-3. PROPHYLAXIS OF CARDIAC CONDITIONS

Endocardititis prophylaxis recommended:
- Prosthetic cardiac valve (including biosynthetic valves)
- Most congenital cardiac malformations
- Surgically constructed systemic-pulmonary shunts
- Rheumatic and other acquired valvular dysfunction
- Idiopathic hypertrophic subaortic stenosis (IHSS)
- Previous history of bacterial endocarditis
- Mitral valve prolapse with insufficiency

Endocarditis prophylaxis not recommended:
- Isolated secundum atrial septal defect
- Secundum atrial septal defect repaired without a patch 6 or more months earlier
- Patient ductus arteriosus ligated and divided 6 or more months earlier
- Postoperative coronary artery bypass graft (CABG) surgery

(From Shulman ST, et al: Pediatrics 75: 604, 1985. Reproduced by Permission of Pediatrics.)

All patients with a diagnosis of ARF must receive prophylactic antibiotics, since the disease has a tendency to recur with subsequent group A *Streptococcus* infections. "Once carditis, always carditis" is the rule; in addition, 10–20% of patients who present with arthritis may develop carditis subsequently. Effective prophylactic drugs include IM benzathine Penicillin (1.2 million units q 28 days), oral Penicillin VK (200,000 units or 125 mg bid), oral erythromycin (250 mg bid), and oral sulfadiazine (500 mg/day under 60 pounds, 1 g/day over 60 pounds).

Antibiotic regimens to prevent the recurrence of ARF are not adequate for the prevention of SBE. Patients who have had rheumatic carditis as well as those with certain congenital or acquired cardiac lesions (see Table 12-3) require SBE prophylaxis when undergoing dental procedures or abdominal or genitourinary surgery (see Table 12-4). The dosing and duration of prophylaxis is summarized in Table 12-5.

INDICATIONS FOR ADMISSION

- Suspected acute rheumatic fever
- Congestive heart failure, pericarditis, or a new murmur in a patient with previously diagnosed ARF

TABLE 12-4. PROCEDURES FOR WHICH ENDOCARDITIS PROPHYLAXIS IS INDICATED

All dental procedures likely to induce gingival bleeding (not simple adjustment of orthodontic appliances or shedding of deciduous teeth)
Tonsillectomy and adenoidectomy[a]
Surgical procedures or biopsy involving respiratory mucosa.
Bronchoscopy, especially with a rigid bronchoscope.[b]
Incision and drainage of infected tissue.
Genitourinary and gastrointestinal procedures including urethral catheterization, surgery, and endoscopy.

[a]Endocarditis has not been reported with myringotomy and tube placement, but the risk of bacteremia is not known.
[b]The risk with flexible bronchoscopy is low, but the neccesity for prophylaxis is not yet defined.
(Adapted from Shulman ST, et al: Pediatrics 75: 604, 1985. Reproduced by Permission of Pediatrics.)

TABLE 12-5. RECOMMENDED ANTIBIOTIC REGIMENS[a]

Dental/Respiratory Tract Procedure	
Standard regimen	
For dental procedures that cause gingival bleeding, and oral/respiratory tract surgery	Penicillin V, 2 g orally 1 h before, then 1 g 6 h later; for patients unable to take oral medications, 2 million U of aqueous penicillin G IV or IM 30–60 min before a procedure, and 1 million U 6 h later may be substituted.
Special regimens	
Parenteral regimen for use when maximal protection desired; eg, for patients with prosthetic valves	Ampicillin, 1–2 g IM or IV plus gentamicin 1.5 mg/kg IM or IV, ½ h before procedure, followed by 1 g oral penicillin V 6 h later; alternatively, parenteral regimen may be repeated once 8 h later.
Oral regimen for penicillin-allergic patients	Erythromycin 1 g orally 1 h before, then 500 mg 6 h later.
Parenteral regimen for pencillin-allergic patients	Vancomycin, 1 g IV slowly over 1 h, starting 1 h before; no repeat dose is necessary.
Standard regimen	
For genitournary/gastrointestinal tract procedures	Ampicllin 2 g IM or IV plus gentamicin, 1.5 mg/kg IM or

TABLE 12-5. CONTINUED

GI/GU Procedures	
	IV, given ½ to 1 h before procedure; 1 follow-up dose may be given 8 h later.
Special regimens	
Oral regimen for minor or repetitive procedures in low-risk patients	Amoxicillin, 3 g orally 1 h before procedure and 1.5 g 6 h later.
Penicillin-allergic patients	Vancomycin, 1 g IV slowly over 1 h, plus gentamicin 1.5 mg/kg IM or IV given 1 h before procedure; may be repeated once 8–12 h later.

[a]Pediatric doses: ampicillin, 50 mg/kg/dose; erythromycin, 20 mg/kg first dose, then 10 mg/kg; gentamicin, 2 mg/kg/dose; Pen V, full adult dose if >27 kg, ½ adult dose <27 kg; aq. Pen G, 50,000 U/kg (25,000 U/kg for follow-up); vancomycin, 20 mg/kg/dose. Total doses not to exceed adult doses.

(Adapted from Schulman ST, et al: Pediatrics 75: 604, 606, 1985. Reproduced by Permission of Pediatrics.)

REFERENCES

1. Kaplan EL: Pediatr Clin North Am 25:817–829, 1978
2. Commission on Rheumatic Fever and Bacterial Endocarditis of the Council on Cardiovascular Diseases in the Young. Pediatrics 75:603–607, 1985

Botulism

INTRODUCTION

Botulism is usually caused by ingestion of preformed toxin from contaminated preserved foods. Infant botulism occurs generally within the first 4–6 months of life, however, as a result of ingestion of live organisms that then manufacture toxin in the gut. In some infants, honey and dark karo syrup have been implicated as the source of the infection, while in others the source is unknown. The toxin prevents the release of acetylcholine at neuronal synapses, producing anticholinergic symptoms.

CLINICAL PRESENTATION

Gastrointestinal symptoms such as ileus, constipation, and dry mouth are common, although nausea and vomiting occur in nearly one-third of patients. A descending, symmetrical paralysis develops usually after cranial nerve involvement (difficulty swallowing, drooling, diplopia, ptosis). Respiratory muscles are eventually affected.

In the infant, constipation precedes other signs and symptoms, probably reflective of the formation of toxin within the gastrointestinal tract. Progressive weakness ensues over several days, with decreased suck, weak cry, and hypotonia.

DIAGNOSIS

Other causes of paralysis to be considered include *Guillian-Barré syndrome* (ascending paralysis with an elevated CSF protein), *polio* (asymmetrical involvement, fever, and CSF pleocytosis), and *myasthenia gravis* (muscle fatigability with reversal of ptosis with Tensilon). In a febrile infant who is lethargic or feeding poorly, *bacterial sepsis* and *meningitis* must be ruled out.

ER MANAGEMENT

If botulism is suspected, admit the patient to an intensive care unit where respiratory support is available, as respiratory arrest can occur at any time. The diagnosis can be confirmed by analyzing blood, gastrointestinal contents, and recently ingested food for evidence of toxin or organisms. Botulinum antitoxin is available from the Center for Disease Control (CDC): (404) 329-3753 or 329-3644. However, antitoxin (and antibiotics) are ineffective for infant botulism.

Patients presenting with hypotonia, paralysis, or respiratory difficulty must have a complete evaluation for sepsis, including a CBC (with differential), blood culture, and lumbar puncture (culture, cytology, and chemistries). If sepsis cannot be ruled out, then age-dependent antibiotics are indicated (see pp 281–285).

INDICATION FOR ADMISSION

- Suspected botulism or infant botulism

REFERENCE

1. Long SS: Pediatr Infect Dis 3: 266–271, 1984

Encephalitis

INTRODUCTION

Encephalitis is inflammation of the brain; it often occurs with involvement of the meninges (meningoencephalitis). The majority of cases are caused by viruses (mumps, ECHO, Coxsackie, poliomyelitis, herpes simplex and zoster, measles, cytomegalovirus, and arthropod-borne viruses), although rickettsia, parasites, *Mycoplasma,* and postimmunization encephalitis are other etiologies.

CLINICAL PRESENTATION

The patient presents with irritability, fever, headache, and photophobia, with or without meningeal signs and an altered level of consciousness. Other findings may include vomiting, myalgias, and lethargy.

ECHO and *Coxsackie,* infections tend to occur in the summer and early fall, often associated with a rash. *Herpes* can present with fever, focal or generalized seizures, focal neurologic signs, and altered level of consciousness.

DIAGNOSIS

The priority is to rule out *bacterial meningitis.* Therefore, perform a lumbar puncture with opening pressure if the patient has fever associated with meningeal signs, altered level of consciousness, focal seizures, or a petechial rash. A lumbar puncture is also necessary for infants with fever and generalized seizures (see febrile seizures, p 385). If there are focal neurologic findings arrange for an immediate CTT scan prior to performing the lumbar puncture.

Obtain a CBC with differential, blood culture, serum glucose, urinalysis, and, if there have been seizures, electrolytes, BUN, and calcium.

A platelet count is necessary if there is a petechial rash. If the patient is febrile, do not delay performing the lumbar puncture until the platelet count is available, unless there are other manifestations of a bleeding diathesis (ecchymoses, epistaxis, hematuria, prolonged bleeding after venipuncture).

Newborns with fever, lethargy, and focal seizures or neurologic signs may have *herpes simplex* infection. Ask the mother whether she has had herpes genitalis. Obtain viral cultures of the blood, urine, throat, and stool. An immediate CTT and electroencephalogram (EEG) are indicated if herpes is suspected. If a viral infection is suspected, obtain an extra tube of CSF for viral culture. Also, culture the throat and stool for virus and send serum for antibody determination.

ER MANAGEMENT

Except for herpes, there is no specific treatment for a viral encephalitis or meningoencephalitis. Admit the patient to an intensive care setting, monitoring vital signs and fluid status carefully.

During the summer and fall, patients over 6 years who present with a typical *enterovirus* infection (nontoxic appearance, CSF monocyte pleocytosis with normal chemistries) may be sent home for bedrest, fluids, and aspirin or acetaminophen. Admit younger patients and those with unreliable parents.

The treatment of *herpes* is acyclovir (5 mg/kg q 8h).

INDICATION FOR ADMISSION

- Encephalitis or meningoencephalitis

REFERENCE

1. Nahmias AJ, Whitley RJ: Pediatr in Review 2:259–266, 1981

Infectious Diseases Associated with Exanthems

INTRODUCTION

The successful diagnosis of a febrile exanthematous disease requires a careful history and physical examination. The goal is to either make a definitive diagnosis or, at the very least, exclude a number of the more serious illnesses.

CLINICAL PRESENTATION

Erythema Infectiosum. Erythema infectiosum, also known as fifth disease, is manifested by a series of three rashes. The sudden appearance of berry red (''slapped'') cheeks is followed in 1–4 days by a fine maculopapular eruption on the extremities and trunk, which develops a characteristic lacy appearance. In the variable third phase, a recurring maculopapular rash may be elicited by heat (hot bath) or cold exposure. Fever is low grade at most and constitutional symptoms are not severe.

Roseola. Roseola, or exanthem subitum, is a disease of presumed viral etiology that occurs in children 6–36 months of age. The illness begins with an abrupt fever of 103–105°F in a previously healthy child. Although most patients look surprisingly well, some present with a febrile convulsion. After 3 or 4 days, the fever rapidly falls to normal. This is followed (in a few hours to 2 days) by an erythematous macular or maculopapular eruption on the trunk, and occasionally, the face and extremities. The rash lasts a few hours to a few days.

Measles. Measles (rubeola) is uncommon in this country, although miniepidemics continue to occur because infected patients enter from abroad and have contact with nonimmune individuals. A 3- to 4-day prodrome is characterized by fever, malaise, cough, coryza, and conjunctivitis. After 2 days, or 2 days before the onset of the rash, pathognomonic Koplik spots develop on the buccal mucosa or gingiva. These are small erythematous lesions with pinpoint white centers that disappear 2 days after the rash develops. The eruption begins with discrete maculopapules on the forehead and behind the ears. Over 3 days, the rash becomes confluent and spreads down over the entire body, and then begins to fade in the same direction as it spread, leaving a brownish discoloration. Fine desquamation, sparing the hands and feet, may occur. The temperature reaches 104–105°F at the peak of the rash and then becomes normal by the seventh day of the illness. Otitis media and pneumonia are frequent complications. Encephalitis develops in 1:1000 cases.

Rubella. Rubella, or German measles, in contrast to rubeola, is generally a mild illness. It consists of URI-like symptoms, low grade fever, lymphadenopathy (particularly occipital, retroauricular, and posterior cervical), and a measles-like rash that starts on the face, then spreads down the body and disappears within 3 days. "Rose spots" on the soft palate may appear just before the skin rash. The greatest threat of rubella is infection during the first trimester of pregnancy, which can lead to microcephaly, cataracts, deafness, and cardiac defects in the infant.

Varicella. Varicella, or chickenpox, is a highly contagious disease characterized by a 24-hour prodrome of fever and malaise, followed by the eruption of multiple crops of pink papules over the next 3–4 days. These pruritic papules almost immediately become teardrop vesicles that form a crust. The lesions, which can involve the mucous membranes, first appear on the trunk and then spread peripherally. The severity, which typically varies with the number of lesions, can range from virtually asymptomatic infection to severe, life-threatening disease with pneumonitis and hepatitis. Neonates whose mothers develop the rash between 5 days before and 2 days after delivery are at risk for disseminated disease, as are immunocompromised patients of any age.

Herpes Zoster. Herpes zoster is an acute infection caused by reactivation of the varicella virus. Pain and tenderness along a dermatome precede the eruption of classic chickenpox lesions clustered within one to three contiguous dermatomes. Pain, tenderness, and localized lymphadenopathy persist while the skin lesions are present (1–2 weeks).

Meningococcemia. Meningococcemia can cause a range of illnesses, from a mild URI to fulminant sepsis. The rash can be erythematous, papular, maculopapular, petechial, or asymmetric, palpable purpura. Disseminated intravascular coagulation and shock occur with severe illness.

Rocky Mountain Spotted Fever. Rocky Mountain spotted fever is caused by a rickettsia that is transmitted via the bite of a tick. One to 5 days after the onset of nonspecific symptoms of fever, malaise, arthralgias, myalgias, and headache, a maculopapular rash erupts on the wrists and ankles. The eruption spreads centrally and may become purpuric and petechial. Thrombocytopenia and vascular collapse can ensue.

DIAGNOSIS

The history must include the following questions: (1) prior exposure to a similar illness or unusual event (tick bite, rat bite, etc.), (2) the time elapsed between the exposure and the current illness, (3) a history of prior immunizations (measles, rubella), (4) a prior history of exanthematous diseases (measles, rubella, varicella, scarlet fever, Kawasaki disease [KD]), and (5) a medication history (particularly immunosuppressive drugs).

Certain diseases occur more commonly in particular *age* groups. Roseola infantum occurs primarily in 6-month to 3-year olds, fifth disease in 2- to 12-year olds, varicella and scarlet fever in school-age children and KD in children less than 2 years of age.

Other diseases are characterized by a pronounced *seasonal* predilection. Rocky Mountain spotted fever occurs primarily in the spring and summer months, varicella in the fall, late winter, and spring, and scarlet fever in the late winter and spring.

The *time elapsed* between the onset of the fever and the appearance of the rash also provides an important clue to the diagnosis. The rash in both rubella and varicella occurs simultaneously with the fever. Patients with scarlet fever generally are febrile for 12–24 hours prior to the onset of the rash. Patients with measles have 4–5 days of fever, coryza, conjunctivitis, and cough before to the development of a rash. Thus, a patient with the simultaneous occurrence of both a fever and rash is unlikely to have measles. Children with roseola infantum usually have 4–5 days of hectic fever but otherwise look well prior to the appearance of their rash. Patients with Rocky Mountain spotted fever are ill with fever, chills, and headache for 2–4 days before the development of the rash. While these relationships are not absolute, they do represent the norm and are therefore valuable adjuncts in making the proper diagnosis and in ruling out incorrect diagnoses.

A *description of the rash* as well as its *progression* and *distribution* are also of great significance. Rashes can be divided into three major groups; *maculopapular, vesicular,* and *purpuric.*

Maculopapular rashes are the most common and are usually associated with enteroviral infections (ECHO and Coxsackie). They can be further characterized as being either morbilliform (confluent, like measles) or the more common rubelliform (discrete, like rubella). *Vesicular* exanthems present either as single or localized lesions (herpes simplex, herpes zoster), generalized lesions with a centripetal distribution (varicella), generalized lesions with a centrifugal distribution (smallpox), or in a peripheral distribution (hand-foot-mouth syndrome and other enteroviral infections).

Although the enteroviruses are the most common cause of *petechial* rashes, assume that any child with fever and petechiae is bacteremic (usually *Neisseria meningitidis,* but occasionally *H. influenzae* type B, *Staphlococcus aureus,* or *Streptococcus pneumoniae*) until proven otherwise.

Pertinent physical findings include the patient's appearance, regional or generalized lymphadenopathy, conjunctivitis, hepatosplenomegaly, and gastrointestinal and pulmonary involvement.

Adenopathy is particularly important when considering the diagnosis of rubella (postauricular and suboccipital adenopathy), KD (cervical adenopathy), and mononucleosis (most commonly cervical adenopathy, but any chain may be involved). The appearance of an enanthem also suggests a specific diagnosis. Koplick spots first appear on the buccal mucosa 2 days prior to the rash in measles and increase in number by the first day of the exanthem. They appear as "grains of salt" on an erythematous base. Petechiae or red spots on the soft palate have been described in rubella, mononucleosis, and strep pharyngitis.

The first phase of erythema infectiosum resembles *scarlet fever,* but with fifth disease the child appears well and there is no evidence of streptococcal infection.

A roseola-like illness has been ascribed to an *enterovirus.* Many children with the prodromal fever of roseola are given antibiotics, so that the rash is occasionally misdiagnosed as a *drug allergy.*

Measles can be confused with *scarlet fever* (cough and conjunctivitis absent), *Kawasaki disease* (KD) (cracked lips present, rash does not spread down the body), and *rubella* (shorter prodrome and rash duration, patient appears much less sick). In none of these are Koplik spots seen.

Varicella has a typical appearance. However, mild eruptions can be confused with *bullous impetigo* and *insect bites,* although these lesions do not erupt in crops or go through a series of stages. Zoster may resemble a *contact dermatitis* or *cellulitis,* but pain is not as central a feature of these illnesses.

The rash of meningococcemia can be confused with other causes of *bacterial sepsis, viral infections, idiopathic thrombocytopenic purpura,* and *Rocky Mountain Spotted Fever.* Unroofing a skin lesion and Gram staining the contents may reveal the pathognomonic gram-negative intracellular diplococci. The diagnosis is confirmed by a positive blood culture.

Suspect Rocky Mountain spotted fever in a patient with a rash on the distal extremities, flu-like symptoms, and a history of tick bite or exposure to wooded areas. The diagnosis can be confirmed by the Weil-Felix agglutination test positive for OX-19 and OX-2 strains of proteus by the second or third week of the illness.

ER MANAGEMENT

There is no specific treatment for *roseola, erythema infectiosum,* or *rubella.* Once the diagnosis is made, reassure the parents as to the expected course and benign outcome of the illness. There is no need for antibiotics. If *rubella* is suspected, refer pregnant female contacts to their obstetricians immediately (for titers).

Similarly, there is no treatment for *measles* other than supportive measures (antipyretics, fluids). If the illness is complicated by an otitis, treat with an appropriate antibiotic (pp 79–101). Admit patients with pneumonia and treat with antibiotics to prevent a secondary bacterial infection. If the patient has any neurologic signs or symptoms (altered consciousness, seizures, focal findings), perform a lumbar puncture to rule out bacterial meningitis. With measles encephalitis there is an elevated protein and a lymphocytic pleocytosis (glucose is normal). Admit patients with encephalitis for observation. Notify public health officials of any suspected case of measles so that appropriate community measures can be instituted.

Treat *varicella* with acetaminophin (not aspirin) for the fever and oatmeal baths and antihistamines (hydroxyzine 2 mg/kg/day, divided q 6–8h) for the pruritis. The treatment of *zoster* is analgesia (acetaminophen with codeine, 1 mg/kg/dose) and wet compresses. Newborn exposure to varicella, congenital varicella, and varicella pneumonia or zoster in an immunosuppressed patient poses a serious risk of overwhelming infection. Admit these patients and consult with an infectious disease specialist regarding antiviral therapy.

If *meningococcemia* is suspected, immediately obtain blood and spinal fluid specimens and institute antibiotic therapy. Use ampicillin (100–300 mg/kg/day) and chloramphenicol (75–100 mg/kg/day) since other organisms (*H. influenzae*) can cause a similar clinical picture. Give prophylactic rifampin (10 mg/kg bid, to maximum of 600 mg bid, for 2 days) to household contacts and nonpregnant medical personnel who gave mouth-to-mouth resuscitation. For *H. influenzae* type B disease, prophylaxis is rifampin, 20 mg/kg once a day for 4 days. Treat *Rocky Mountain spotted fever* with tetracycline, 50 mg/kg over 8 years old or chloramphenicol, 75 mg/kg/day, divided q 6h, and cardiovascular support.

INDICATIONS FOR ADMISSION

- Measles, pneumonia or encephalitis
- Varicella or zoster in an immunocompromised patient
- Meningococcemia
- Rocky Mountain spotted fever
- Fever with petechiae

REFERENCES

1. Krugman S, Katz S: Infectious Diseases of Children, 7th ed. St. Louis, Mosby, 1981, pp 507–516
2. Leads from the MMWR, JAMA 251:1401–1413 1984

Infectious Mononucleosis

INTRODUCTION

Epstein-Barr virus (EBV) is the etiologic agent of infectious mononucleosis (IM). In most instances in the United States, infection leads to a classic, self-limited disorder that causes no long-term morbidity. Other organisms that can cause a mono-like illness include adenovirus, toxoplasmosis, and cytomegalovirus.

CLINICAL PRESENTATION

In the older child and adolescent, IM is characterized by several days to weeks of lethargy, fever, sore throat (usually exudative), lymphadenopathy of gradual onset (usually cervical, sometimes generalized), and splenomegaly. The onset of symptoms is preceded by a 4- to 7-day prodrome, and a prolonged convalescent period may follow. Hepatomegaly, maculopapular rash, bilateral eyelid edema, and rarely, CNS symptoms (Guillian-Barré syndrome, meningoencephalitis) can occur. In younger patients the disease is usually less severe, with pharyngitis, low grade fever, and mild hepatosplenomegaly. Occasionally it is asymptomatic.

Complications include upper airway obstruction secondary to lymphoid hyperplasia, autoimmune hemolytic anemia, hepatitis, splenic rupture, and myocarditis or pericarditis.

DIAGNOSIS

Streptococcal or *viral tonsillitis* can present with fever, sore throat, and cervical adenopathy. There is usually no hepatosplenomegaly or generalized lymphadenopathy. Cervical adenopathy and splenomegaly are often secondary to viral infections, especially *cytomegalovirus* (pharyngitis unusual). Similarly, primary acquired *toxoplasmosis* can cause generalized lymphadenopathy and fever. Early KD may resemble IM, although involvement of the lips, tongue, conjunctiva, and distal extremities is not typical of IM. Generalized lymphadenopathy and pharyngitis are not features of *viral hepatitis*.

A presentation of fever, weakness, hepatosplenomegaly, and generalized lymphadenopathy always raises the concern of a malignancy (*leukemia* or *lymphoma*). These patients usually appear ill, and may also have weight loss, pallor, high fever, and evidence of bleeding.

When the diagnosis is suspected, obtain a CBC with differential and either a slide test for IM (Monospot, Monosticon) or heterophile antibody test. A leukocytosis with an absolute lymphocytosis ($\geq$ 50%) and atypical lymphocytes ($\geq$ 10%) is frequently seen. Lymphoblasts, anemia, and thrombocytopenia are absent. Slide test agglutination is presumptive evidence of EBV infection. A heterophile antibody titer of 1:56, or 1:28 after guinea pig kidney adsorption, occurs in 80% of patients, but it is usually negative in young children. If diagnostic certainty is necessary, obtain acute and convalescent anti-EBV titers.

Other laboratory abnormalities include elevated liver transaminases (serum glutamic oxaloacetic transaminase (SGOT), serum glutamic pyruvic transaminase (SGPT)) in 20–40%, hyperbilirubinemia in 5%, and rarely, a positive Coombs test.

ER MANAGEMENT

Obtain a throat culture to rule out *Streptococcus* and prescribe supportive treatment (bedrest, fluids, acetaminophen). Warn the patient with a palpable spleen to avoid contact sports, because of the risk of splenic rupture. If the throat culture is positive, treat appropriately (p 117).

If the patient appears otherwise well, has not had any weight loss, and follow-up is assurred, hematologic work-up can be deferred for several weeks. At that time, continued symptoms or a worsening of the patient's condition are indications for a CBC with differential and either a slide test or heterophile antibody. Continue the supportive therapy if the results are consistent with the diagnosis of IM. Otherwise, refer the patient to a hematologist.

Acute upper airway obstruction is the *only* indication for steroids in IM. Insertion of a nasopharyngeal airway and 2 mg/kg/day of prednisone (for 7 days) provide dramatic relief.

INDICATIONS FOR ADMISSION

- Upper airway obstruction
- Neurologic complications

REFERENÇES

1. Shurin SB: Pediatr Clin North Am 26:315–326, 1979
2. Sumaya CV, Ench Y: Pediatrics 75:1003–1010, 1985.

Kawasaki Disease

INTRODUCTION

Kawasaki disease (KD), or the mucocutaneous lymph node syndrome, is a unique acute febrile exanthematous disease of childhood. Although the etiology is unknown, it probably is infectious.

CLINICAL PRESENTATION

KD usually occurs in children between 6 months and 4 years of age, with a peak in the second half of the first year of life. It has infrequently been reported in children over the age of 5 years.

The clinical course is divided into three distinct stages. During the first stage (days 1–10), a high fever precedes the onset of most of the following findings: conjunctival injection; cracked, swollen, red lips; erythema of the oral mucosa; cervical adenitis; and a polymorphous rash with erythema of the palms and soles and edema of the hands and feet.

In the second stage (days 11–24), there is resolution of the fever, rash, and lymphadenopathy, while desquamation of the distal extremities, thrombocytosis, and cardiovascular complications can occur. These include development of coronary artery aneurysms, coronary obstruction and thrombosis, and myocardial and endocardial inflammation.

In the final stage (after day 24), there is total resolution of the external findings and either resolution of the cardiovascular complications or progression to myocardial infarction and decompensation.

In addition to these major manifestations, occasional findings include urethritis and sterile pyuria (70%), arthralgias and arthritis (35%), aseptic meningitis with extreme irritability, abdominal pain and diarrhea, hepatitis, obstructive jaundice with hydrops of the gallbladder, and acute mitral insufficiency.

DIAGNOSIS

The diagnosis of KD is based on the presence of at least five of the following six major criteria:

1. Fever (≥ 104°F) of more than 5-day duration

2. Conjunctival injection (bilateral)
3. Changes in the mouth including erythema and fissuring of the lips; diffuse oropharyngeal erythema, and a strawberry tongue
4. Changes in the peripheral extremities, including induration of the hands and feet, erythema of the palms and soles, desquamation of the fingers and toetips approximately 2 weeks after onset, and transverse grooves across the fingernails 2–3 months after onset.
5. Erythematous rash
6. Enlarged lymph node mass, measuring more than 1.5 cm in diameter (unilateral, cervical)

Although there is no characteristic laboratory finding in KD, thrombocytosis frequently occurs. Elevation of the platelet count begins near the end of the first stage and peaks between 600,000 and 1,200,000/mm^3 during stage 2. However, the late onset precludes using thrombocytosis as a confirmatory test during the first stage. Nonspecific laboratory findings in the first stage include a leukocytosis (20,000–30,000/mm^3), elevated ESR and CRP and an acute rise in IgE level.

Early in the course, KD can resemble *scarlet fever* (pharyngitis, Pastia lines, no conjunctivitis), *viral exanthems* (less sick appearing, no distal extremity involvement), *Rocky Mountain spotted fever* (petechial and purpuric rash, no enanthem), *drug reactions* (use of presumptive agent, no fever), *staphylococcal toxic shock syndrome* (hypotensive, renal involvement with elevated BUN and creatinine), and *leptospirosis* (icterus, proteinuria).

ER MANAGEMENT

Consider KD in a child who presents with fever and at least four of the other five major manifestations. Obtain a CBC with differential, platelet count, ESR or CRP, blood culture, urinalysis, chest x-ray, and throat culture.

Because of the high rate of cardiac complications during stage 2, admit the patient and arrange M-mode and two-dimensional echocardiography to be performed in the latter part of stage 1, then weekly.

At the present time, there is no definitive treatment. However, give aspirin, 80–100 mg/kg/day through stage 1, then 10–20 mg/kg/day during stages 2 and 3. Aspirin is an effective anti-inflammatory agent (high dose), and it inhibits platelet aggregation (low dose).

INDICATION FOR ADMISSION

- Suspected Kawasaki disease

REFERENCES

1. Meade, RH, Brandt L: J Pediatr 100:588, 1982
2. Melish ME: Pediatr in Review 2:107, 1980

Osteomyelitis

INTRODUCTION

Osteomyelitis is a bacterial bone infection, caused by organisms introduced hematogenously or via direct spread from a contiguous local focus. *S. aureus* is by far the most common agent. Group B Strep and enterics are common in young infants, while children with sickle cell disease are at risk for *Salmonella* infections. The usual site is the metaphysis, especially of the distal femur and proximal tibia. In the newborn, the proximal humerus is a common location.

CLINICAL PRESENTATION

The usual presentation is pain and point tenderness at a long bone site, with swelling, erythema, and warmth. The patient is usually febrile and often refuses to bear weight on the limb, holding it as motionless as possible. With vertebral osteomyelitis, there is chronic back pain with spasm of the paraspinal muscles. Infants may have nonspecific signs, such as fever, irritability, and vomiting. Occasionally there is an area of cellulitis overlying the site.

DIAGNOSIS

The typical combination of fever, point tenderness, and unwillingness to use an extremity is not invariably seen, but when present is highly suggestive of osteomyelitis.

Trauma can cause pain, swelling, and limitation of movement.

Usually there is a positive history, the x-rays may be diagnostic (fracture), and the ESR and CBC are normal.

Cellulitis of a distal extremity can be mistaken for a manifestation of osteomyelitis. However, there is no point tenderness over the bone.

A sympathetic effusion in the contiguous joint can resemble a *septic arthritis*.

Sickle cell disease can cause pain which may be secondary to infection or vasoocclusive crisis. Distinguishing between the two may be difficult, although the pain of a crisis tends to recur in the same sites, it can be in several locations at once, and it often resolves with intravenous hydration.

Other considerations include *bone tumor, Caffey disease,* and *histiocytosis*. All of these can be ruled out by x-rays.

ER MANAGEMENT

When osteomyelitis is suspected, obtain multiple blood cultures, a CBC with differential, an ESR, and x-rays of the extremity. In general, the x-rays are normal for about 10 days, but there may be an increased white blood cell count (WBC) (with a shift to the left) and an elevated ESR. If available, a 99mTc phosphate bone scan usually confirms the diagnosis (increased uptake at the site) although it may be normal early in the illness. Needle aspiration is essential to drain the pus and provide specimens for culture and Gram stain. It will also rule out a sickle cell vasoocculive crisis when the clinical picture is unclear.

Appropriate antibiotic treatment is a penicillinase-resistant antistaphylococccal drug, such as oxacillin (100 mg/kg/day, IV, divided q 6h). Add *Salmonella* coverage for patients with sickle cell disease (ampicillin 100 mg/kg/day or chloramphenicol 75–100 mg/kg/day, divided q 6h), and gram-negative coverage for neonates.

INDICATION FOR ADMISSION

- Osteomyelitis

REFERENCES

1. Waldvogel FA, Vasey H: N Engl J Med 303:360, 1980
2. Kolyvas E, Ahronhein G, Marks I, et al: Pediatrics 65:867, 1980

Parasitic Infections

INTRODUCTION

Up to 20% of Americans are infected with nematodes and outbreaks of other parasitic infections are frequently reported. Immigrants from regions where parasites are endemic have high rates of infection, and travelers to endemic areas can become infested with a number of organisms.

CLINICAL PRESENTATION

Pinworm. Pinworm (*Enterobius vermicularis*) is the most common parasite in North America. Although pinworm infection can be asymptomatic, anal pruritis is the most common complaint. Cystitis, with microscopic hematuria, can occur in young girls if worms enter the urethra. There is no tissue migration of the larvae and no eosinophilia.

Roundworm. Giant roundworm (*Ascaris lumbricoides*) infestations are usually asymptomatic while the worm inhabits the intestine. However, larval migration through the lungs causes fever, cough, malaise, and eosinophilia. Occasionally a worm may be coughed out of the mouth or nose. Serious complications include intestinal obstruction or perforation, obstruction of the pancreatic or bile ducts, appendicitis, intussusception, and volvulus.

Hookworm. Hookworm (*Necator americanus* and *Ancyclostoma duodenale*) disease is most commonly found in the Southern United States. Larvae usually enter through the feet and cause a severely pruritic cutaneous eruption called "ground itch." Fever, headache, nausea, dyspnea, and cough result from pulmonary migration. While in the intestine, *Ancyclostoma* attaches to the mucosa and causes the loss of 0.2 cc of blood per day, leading to a hypochromic, microcytic iron deficiency anemia that can be accompanied by hypoalbuminemia.

Threadworm. Threadworm (*Strongyloides stercoralis*) is also found most often in the rural South. The life cycle is similar to the hookworm, and an urticarial rash, pneumonia, epigastric pain, and watery diarrhea with intestinal bleeding may be noted. Most patients, however, are asymptomatic. Overwhelming infection can occur in the immunocompromised host with fever, severe abdominal pain, gram negative sepsis, and shock.

Whipworm. Whipworm (*Trichuris trichiura*) infections are usually asymptomatic, although heavy infestations can cause nausea, vomiting, diarrhea, abdominal distention and tenderness, rectal prolapse, and occasionally intestinal bleeding.

Giardia Lamblia. *Giardia lamblia* is a major parasite of cosmopolitan environments. Within 3 weeks of ingestion of the cysts in contaminated food or water, there is the onset of diarrhea with watery, foul-smelling, steatorrheic stools. Nausea, anorexia, abdominal distention, and epigastric pain and tenderness are common. Eosinophilia does not occur and symptoms usually persist for days, but can linger for months. Fever and weight loss are uncommon, although a malabsorption syndrome resembling sprue can develop. Untreated, this form of the illness can last for months or years and be very debilitating.

Entamoeba Histolytica. *Entamoeba histolytica,* a protozoan found throughout the world, usually causes an asymptomatic infection. However, there may be diarrhea which can lead to mucosal ulceration and chronic bloody dysentery. *Amoeba* can cause metastatic disease with nonspecific symptoms such as fever and malaise. Right lobe liver abscess is most common, with right upper quadrant pain and hemidiaphragm elevation. Spread to the lungs, pleura, and skin can then occur by direct extension.

DIAGNOSIS

The diagnosis of a parasitic infection can only be made if the possibility is considered. Recent travel to or emigration from endemic areas makes infestation likely. Chronic or bloody diarrhea, dysentery, weight loss, cutaneous eruptions, or eosinophilia suggest the possibility of a parasitic infection. Occasionally the patient or parent will report seeing a worm in the stool, vomitus, sputum, or perianal region. *Viral* and *bacterial gastroenteritis, pneumonia, malabsorption syndromes, cystitis, hepatitis,* and *"nervous" disorders* can have similar presentations and courses.

Pinworm infestation is most easily confirmed by early morning application of transparent adhesive tape to the perianal region. The 50- to 60-micron eggs adhere to the tape and can then be visualized under the microscope.

Microscopic examination of a fresh stool specimen can confirm the diagnosis of a parasitic infection. Ninety percent of infections will be detected by the collection of samples on three successive mornings. Refrigerate stool that cannot be examined within 1 hour. However, stool identification requires patience and experience, and therefore is best performed by trained laboratory personnel.

Stool examination is negative in up to 50% of *Giardia* infections. If *Giardia* is still suspected after negative stool examinations by a parasitology laboratory, refer the patient to a gastroenterologist for a String test/enterotest. Extraintestinal amebic infections can be accurately diagnosed with indirect hemagglutination or indirect immunofluorescence antibody techniques.

Peripheral eosinophil counts may be helpful in the diagnosis of *Ascaris,* hookworms, *Strongyloides,* and *Trichuris.*

ER MANAGEMENT

Although a pinworm infection may be treated on the presumptive evidence of rectal itching in the absence of local pathology, treat other parasitic infections only if positive identification is available. Otherwise, arrange for the collection of specimens and refer the patient for primary care follow-up.

The management of parasitic infections has been revolutionized by safe, effective, broad-spectrum medications (Table 12-6). Appropriate follow-up includes repeat stool cultures 1–2 weeks after the completion of therapy. Refer patients with *Amoeba* and *Strongyloides* infections to a parasitology clinic or primary care center for treatment.

Mebendazole is possibly the most effective medication against nematodes, except for *Strongyloides.* It is the only safe, effective treatment for *Trichuris* and rarely causes any side effects (diarrhea, colicky pain). However, it has been shown to be teratogenic in animals and therefore should be avoided during pregnancy.

Pyrantel treats *Enterobius, Necator, Trichuris,* and *Ascaris.* Side effects (dizziness, headache) are rare. Piperazine is effective against *Ascaris,* but it cannot be used with pyrantel because of antagonistic actions.

TABLE 12-6. TREATMENT OF PARASITIC INFECTIONS

Parasite	Drug	Dose
E. vermicularis	Mebendozole	Single dose of 100 mg for children >2 years; repeat after 2 weeks
	Pyrantel pamoate	Single dose of 11 mg/kg (maximum of 1 g); repeat after 2 weeks
A. lumbricoides	Mebendazole	100 mg bid × 3 days
	Pyrantel pamoate	Single dose of 11 mg/kg (maximum of 1 g)
Hookworm	Mebendazole	100 mg bid × 3 days
	Pyrantel pamoate	Single dose of 11 mg/kg (maximum of 1 g)
S. stercoralis	Thiabendazole	25 mg/kg/bid × 2 days (maximum of 3 g/day); 5 days for disseminated disease
T. trichuria	Mebendazole	100 mg bid × 3 days
G. lamblia	Quinacrine HCl	6 mg/kg/day divided tid × 5 days (maximum of 300 mg/day)
	Metronidazole	15 mg/kg/day divided tid × 5 days (maximum of 750 mg/day)
E. histolytica	Diiodohydroxyquin (Iodoquinol)	30–40 mg/kg/day divided tid × 20 days (for asymptomatic cyst passers)
	Metronidazole	35–50 mg/kg/day divided tid × 10 days (for hepatic disease, intestinal disease and mild to moderate extraintestinal disease)
	Iodoquinol plus Metronidazole	For severe extraintestinal disease

Eighty percent of *Giardia* infections will be eradicated by quinacrine or metronidazole. If there is a therapeutic failure, a second course of the same medication may be successful. Quinacrine can cause yellowish skin discoloration, exacerbation of psoriasis, and insomnia, while metronidazole exerts a potent Antabuse effect, so advise the patient to avoid alcohol intake during treatment.

Thiabendazole is the drug of choice for *Strongyloides* (including disseminated disease), but its usefulness is limited by side effects (anorexia, nausea, vomiting, dizziness). Less commonly, reversible leukopenia, crystalluria, hallucinations, hypoglycemia, and hypotension occur.

The therapy of *Amoeba* depends on the location and severity of the disease. Treat intraluminal infestation and asymptomatic cyst carriers with diiodohydroxyquin, although prolonged use can rarely cause optic atrophy. Metronidazole is effective for colitis and hepatic infection. Treat nonhepatic extraintestinal disease with emetine hydrochloride, which is effective in all forms of amebiasis, but can cause cardiac arrhythmias as late as 2 weeks after the discontinuation of therapy.

INDICATIONS FOR ADMISSION

- Dehydration, severe weight loss, prostration
- Extraintestinal amebiasis

REFERENCES

1. Most H: N Engl J Med 310:298–304, 1984
2. The Medical Letter 26:27–34, 1984

Pertussis

INTRODUCTION

Pertussis (whooping cough) is an acute respiratory infection caused by *Bordetella pertussis*. As a result of immunization practices, the disease is relatively uncommon in this country.

CLINICAL PRESENTATION

The majority of patients are under 1 year of age and have received at most one diphtheria, pertussis, tetanus (DPT) immunization. There are three clinical stages. During the 1- to 3-week catarrahal stage, the illness resembles a nonspecific URI, with mild cough, rhinorrhea, and conjunctivitis. The second (paroxysmal) stage lasts 2–4 weeks and is marked by severe paroxysms of coughing followed by a sudden inspiratory whoop. During the paroxysms there may be facial redness, bubbling of mucus from the nose and mouth, vomiting, and afterwards the child appears exhausted. Cyanosis can occur during the episodes, but between the paroxysms the patient seems well. Gradual recovery occurs during the final convalescent stage (1–2 weeks).

DIAGNOSIS

The diagnosis is usually not suspected until the paroxysmal stage, when the characteristic whoop is first noticed. However, whooping does not occur in young infants. Suspect pertussis in any patient who vomits after an episode of paroxysmal coughing, especially if a primary DPT series has not been completed.

Obtain a CBC with differential, a blood culture, and a chest x-ray. A leukocytosis with an absolute lymphocytosis is characteristic of pertussis, but may not occur in the first 3–6 months of life. The chest x-ray may reveal perihilar infiltrates, a secondary bacterial pneumonia, or a "shaggy" heart border.

A pertussoid illness can be caused by *adenovirus* and *Bordetella parapertussis*, but confirming an etiologic diagnosis is not crucial to adequate patient management. *Chlamydia pneumonia* presents with a staccato cough in an afebrile, tachypneic infant under 12 weeks of age. Eosinophilia and bilateral patchy infiltrates on chest x-ray are characteristic of *Chlamydia* infection.

ER MANAGEMENT

To confirm the diagnosis of pertussis, obtain a nasopharyngeal swab for culture on Bordet-Gengou medium or immunofluorescence (results are available sooner, but less accurate).

Admit all young infants (< 6 months) and patients with cyanotic episodes, respiratory distress, or x-ray evidence of pneumonia. While there is no effective treatment, erythromycin (40 mg/kg/day) reduces the infectivity. Less severely affected patients older than 6 months can be sent home, with close follow-up arranged. Instruct the parents to not disturb the child during a paroxysm and to wait until the coughing has stopped to wipe away the mucus. Cyanosis during an episode is an indication to return immediately, for admission.

INDICATIONS FOR ADMISSION

- Cyanosis or respiratory distress
- Suspected pertussis in an infant < 6 months old

REFERENCE
1. Geller RJ: Pediatr Infect Dis 3:182–186, 1984

Rabies Prophylaxis

INTRODUCTION

Although the issue of rabies prophylaxis is raised most often after domestic animal (dog and cat) bites, wildlife (skunks, raccoons, bats, foxes) now constitute the major reservoir of the disease in the United States. Rodents (squirrels, hamsters, rats, mice, etc) and rabbits are rarely infected.

CLINICAL PRESENTATION AND DIAGNOSIS

An unprovoked attack, including a bite while attempting to feed an animal, indicates a risk of rabies. Exposure can be by bite (any penetration of the skin by the animal's teeth) or nonbite (scratch, abrasion, saliva). Petting alone does not constitute an exposure.

ER MANAGEMENT

Confine and observe healthy domestic animals for 10 days. If any signs of rabies develop, the animal must be sacrificed and the head sent to an appropriate laboratory. Similarly, sacrifice and submit the heads of all wild animals and unwanted or stray domestic animals.

Regardless of the nature of the attack, thorough cleansing of all wounds with soap and water is effective in preventing rabies. The indications for postexposure prophylaxis are summarized in Table 12-7. Give a 1 cc IM dose of human diploid cell rabies vaccine (HDCV), as soon as possible after exposure, then 3, 7, 14, and 28 days after the first dose. Also, give rabies immune globulin (RIG), 20 IU/kg, as soon as possible (within 8 days) after the start of the prophylaxis regimen. Try to infiltrate up to half the dose around the area of the wound and give the remainder IM at another site.

REFERENCES
1. Mann JM: Pediatr Infect Dis 2:162–167, 1983
2. Morbidity and Mortality Weekly Report, 33: July 20, 1984

TABLE 12-7. RABIES POSTEXPOSURE PROPHYLAXIS

Animal species	Condition at Time of Attack	Treatment
Dog, cat	Healthy (observed for 10 days)	None[a]
	Rabid or suspected rabid	RIG and HDCV
	Unknown (escaped)	Consult public health officials[b]
Skunk, bat, fox, coyote, raccoon, bobcat, other carnivores	Regard as rabid, until laboratory tests prove otherwise	RIG and HDCV
Livestock, rodents, rabbits, hares	Consider individually. Consult local public health officials. Bites of squirrels, hamsters, guinea pigs, gerbils, chipmunks, rats, mice, other rodents, rabbits, and hares almost never require antirabies prophylaxis.	

[a]During the holding period, immediately begin prophylaxis if the dog or cat develops any signs of rabies. Sacrifice the animal and test its brain.
[b]The incidence of rabies in the community determines the need for prophylaxis.
(Adapted from Morbidity and Mortality Weekly Report, Vol. 33, no. 28, July 1984.)

Septic Arthritis

INTRODUCTION

Septic arthritis is a bacterial infection of a joint, most commonly caused by *S. aureus, H. Influenzae* type-B (under 4 years), and group B streptococci (under 2 months). Children with functional or anatomical asplenia are at particular risk for encapsulated organisms, such as *Salmonella* and pneumococci. Other, less common, etiologies include gonococci (adolescents), gram-negative enteric rods (neonates), and mycobacteria. The infection most often spreads hematogenously, although direct extension from a contiguous site (osteomyelitis) can occur.

CLINICAL PRESENTATION

The symptomatology may be nonspecific in infants and younger children who often present with fever, irritability, and poor feeding. On occasion, the child may be noted to be unwilling to move or use the extremity. Limp, joint swelling, and inability to flex or extend a joint are the common presentations in older children.

On examination, the affected joint is swollen, tender, warm, and erythematous. There is limitation of range of motion and pain on movement. The patient usually holds the joint in a position of minimal hydrostatic pressure. For the hip this is moderate flexion with slight abduction and external rotation. The knee and elbow are held in flexion, the ankle in equinus position, and the shoulder abducted and rotated.

A gonococcal arthritis may present as a migratory polyarthritis which then settles in one large joint. There may be an associated rash (papular, vesicular, or hemorrhagic) or tenosynovitis.

DIAGNOSIS

Rapid diagnosis of septic arthritis is essential, as significant destruction of the joint may occur in a short period of time. A *monoarticular* arthritis is secondary to a bacterial infection until proven otherwise.

If there are signs of monoarticular arthritis (erythema, swelling, decreased range of motion) or polyarticular involvement associated with evidence of gonococcal infection (rash, tenosynovitis), immediately obtain anteroposterior (AP) and lateral x-rays of the involved joint. In septic arthritis there is an increase in the joint space with soft tissue swelling. If it is not clear whether a joint effusion is present, repeat the AP radiograph while axial traction is applied to the involved extremity. There is no effusion if a curvilinear lucency is seen within the joint space.

Although monoarticular joint involvement may also occur after *trauma,* there is usually a history of injury. *Toxic synovitis* rarely produces the same degree of joint findings on physical examination and the x-rays are usually normal.

Acute rheumatic fever classically causes a migratory polyarthritis with other features of the disease (see p 288), and the response to aspirin is dramatic. *Rheumatoid arthritis* (p 415) tends to have a more gradual onset with milder findings in more than one joint.

An *osteomyelitis* can cause a sympathetic effusion in the nearest joint. On examination, with osteomyelitis there is point tenderness, usually in the metaphysis, while with septic arthritis maximal pain is elicited in the joint.

Legg-Perthes disease and *slipped capital femoral epiphysis* cause limp with decreased hip range of motion. The patient is a febrile and nontoxic appearing.

ER MANAGEMENT

Immediate arthrocentesis is indicated if septic arthritis is suspected. Interpretation of the results is summarized in Table 12-8. In general, in bacterial disease the fluid is cloudy, with a high white cell count (over 80,000/mm^3), neutrophil predominance (>50%), decreased glucose (less than half of serum), and a poor mucin clot. Often the Gram stain reveals the offending organism.

Obtain a CBC with differential, ESR, glucose, and multiple blood cultures. Typically, the WBC is elevated (>15,000/mm^3) with a shift to the left and the ESR is increased (>30mm/hr). If gonococcal arthritis is suspected, culture the pharynx, rectum and cervix or urethra.

After the joint fluid is evaluated, admit the patient for intravenous antibiotics. Treat all patients with a semisynthetic antistaphylococcal drug (oxacillin 100 mg/kg/day divided q 6h). Use ampicillin (100 mg/kg/day) and chloramphenicol (75–100 mg/kg/day) if the patient is under 4 years old to provide coverage for *Hemophilus*.

If *gonococcal* infection is likely, use penicillin (10 million units/day IV) and oxacillin initially. When the diagnosis is confirmed and the patient is afebrile, change to ampicillin, 500 mg PO qid, to complete a 7-day course.

Aspiration of joint fluid is therapeutic as well as diagnostic. In general, arthrocentesis does not have to be repeated. However, a hip infection requires immediate drainage in the operating room. Do not instill antibiotics directly into the joint, as good levels are obtained via the intravenous route.

INDICATION FOR ADMISSION

- Suspected septic arthritis

REFERENCES

1. Petersen S, Knudsen FU, Anderson EA, et al: Acta Orthoped Scand 51: 451, 1980
2. Nelson JD: Pediatrics 50:437, 1972

TABLE 12-8. SYNOVIAL FLUID FINDINGS

Disease	Color	Clarity	Viscosity	Mucin Clot	Cell WBC/mm	% Polys
Normal	Straw	Transparent	High	Good	<200 WBC	<25
Traumatic arthritis	Straw to bloody to xantho-chromic	Transparent to turbid	High	Good	<2000 WBC, few to many RBC	<25
Rheumatic fever	Yellow	Slightly cloudy	Low	Good	10,000–12,000 WBC	50
Rheumatoid arthritis	Yellow to greenish	Cloudy	Low	Poor	15,000–20,000 WBC	75
Tuberculous arthritis	Yellow	Cloudy	Low	Poor	25,000 WBC	50–60
Septic arthritis	Grayish or bloody	Turbid or purulent	Low	Poor	80,000–200,000 WBC	75

(Adapted from Hollander JL, McCarthy DJ: Arthritis and Allied Conditions. 8th ed. Philadelphia, Lea & Febiger, 1972, p 72)

Toxic Shock Syndrome

INTRODUCTION

Toxic shock syndrome (TSS) is an acute febrile illness secondary to a toxin produced by *Staphylococcus aureus*.

CLINICAL PRESENTATION

The majority of cases have occurred in menstruating females using tampons, although there are reports of TSS in men and children with localized *S. aureus* infections.

The illness begins suddenly with high fever (>102°F), abdominal pain, vomiting, and diarrhea, often accompanied by sore throat, headache, and myalgias. Dizziness or syncope ensues, progressing to hypotension over 48 hours. A sunburn-like rash develops, followed by desquamation of the palms and soles (and often the digits) after 10–14 days. Hyperemia of the mucous membranes (oropharynx, vagina, conjunctiva), oliguria, and disorientation may occur.

Laboratory abnormalities may include sterile pyuria, thrombocytopenia, and increased BUN, creatinine, liver transaminases, creatine phosphokinase (CPK), and bilirubin.

DIAGNOSIS

The diagnostic criteria (CDC) for TSS are:

1. Temperature >102°F
2. Hypotension, syncope or dizziness
3. Rash with subsequent desquamation
4. Involvement of at least three of the following organ systems: gastrointestinal, muscular, mucous membrane, renal, hepatic, hematologic, and central nervous system
5. Negative throat and CSF cultures (blood can be positive only for *S. aureus*) and negative serologic tests for Rocky Mountain spotted fever, leptospirosis, and measles

Inquire about the patient's menstrual history and tampon use, and perform a careful, complete physical examination looking for sites of *Staphylococcus* infections.

The differential diagnosis include *measles* (cough, coryza, conjunctivitis, adenopathy, no immunization), *Rocky Mountain spotted fever* (history of tick bite, peripheral hemorrhagic rash), *scarlet fever* (strawberry tongue, Pastia lines, sandpaper-like rash), *infectious mononucleosis* (adenopathy, hepatosplenomegaly, exudative pharyngitis), *Kawasaki disease* (KD) (cervical adenopathy, strawberry tongue, swelling of hands and feet), *juvenile rheumatoid arthritis* (JRA) (splenomegaly, adenopathy, arthritis), scalded skin syndrome (positive Nikolsky sign, facial crusting and fissuring), and *bacterial sepsis* (petechial or purpuric rash).

ER MANAGEMENT

If toxic shock is suspected, obtain blood for culture, CBC with differential, platelet count, electrolytes, BUN and creatinine, liver function tests and CPK. Perform a urinalysis and obtain cultures of the throat, stool, and urine. If there is an alteration in consciousness, perform a lumbar puncture. A vaginal examination is necessary to remove a tampon, diaphragm, or intra-uterine device (IUD) and obtain cultures of the cervix and vagina for *S. aureus*.

Secure an IV and treat shock (p 11) with volume replacement and vasopressors (p 8). Start therapy with a penicillinase resistant antistaphylococcal antibiotic (oxacillin 100 mg/kg/day or clindamycin 40 mg/kg/day if allergic to penicillin).

INDICATION FOR ADMISSION

- Suspected toxic shock syndrome

REFERENCE

1. Wiesenthal AM, Todd JK: Pediatrics 74:112–117, 1984

Tuberculosis

INTRODUCTION

Tuberculosis remains a significant health problem, particularly in urban areas and among immigrants to this country. Despite the fact that more than 95% of primary infections are in the lungs, x-ray evidence of a primary complex is uncommon. Children generally acquire the infection from family members and others with whom they have had prolonged intimate contact. Transmission is by inhalation of respiratory droplets.

CLINICAL PRESENTATION

Most commonly, the patient is asymptomatic, but has a positive skin test (recent converter). Signs and symptoms, if present, usually involve the lungs, with cough, hilar adenopathy, infiltrates, or effusions. Uncommon presentations are systemic (failure to thrive, fever of unknown origin), neurologic (tuberculous meningitis or tuberculomas), bony (arthritis, osteomyelitis), and renal (sterile pyuria). Other findings may include lymphadenopathy, hepatosplenomegaly, and chronic otitis media.

DIAGNOSIS

Obtain a chest X-ray and place a 5TU PPD on the forearm of all children with chronic cough, persistent respiratory tract disease, pneumonia or pleural effusion, failure to thrive, fever of unknown origin, meningitis, or adenitis. If immunocompromise is suspected, an anergy screen (*Candida,* streptokinase (SK) streptodornase (SD), tetanus, etc) is required. A positive PPD is 10 mm or more of induration (not erythema) at 48–72 hours. If the skin test is positive, obtain a chest x-ray.

A *recent converter* is an asymptomatic patient with a newly positive skin test, but a normal chest x-ray.

ER MANAGEMENT

If the patient has a positive PPD, test all family members, unless they have a previous history of infection or positive skin test results.

Positive Chest X-Ray. Obtain at least three specimens of sputum, urine, and early morning gastric washings for acid-fast stain and culture. A CBC with differential and liver function tests are also necessary. When appropriate, culture other specimens (pleural fluid, bone marrow, lymph node), and if there are any CNS signs or symptoms, perform a lumbar puncture (with CSF culture).

Since culture results may take 3–10 weeks, begin antituberculous therapy empirically, if the suspicion is high. Admit patients who are symptomatic or suspected of having active disease, to facilitate the collection of specimens and institution of therapy. Treatment usually involves isoniazid (10–20 mg/kg/day) and rifampin (10 mg/kg/day).

Asymptomatic Recent Converter (Give isoniazid 10 mg/kg/day (300 mg maximum) for 9–12 months.

INDICATION FOR ADMISSION

- All patients with suspected tuberculosis, other than asymptomatic recent converters

REFERENCE

1. Lorin MI, Hso KHK, Jacob SC: Pediatr Clin North Am 30:333–348, 1983

13

Ingestions

Evaluation and Management of Poisoned Patients

INTRODUCTION

Among toddlers, most poisonings are accidental and usually involve household products or single drugs. Adolescent ingestions, on the other hand, typically involve multiple substances (usually drugs), often in the context of suicide attempts or gestures.

CLINICAL PRESENTATION

Although many patients appear asymptomatic, common signs of poisoning include lethargy, vomiting, drooling, coughing, agitation, and delirium.

Certain categories of poisons produce characteristic combinations of findings labeled "toxidromes" by Mofenson and Greensher (1974). The major toxicologic syndromes are listed in Table 13-1.

DIAGNOSIS

Many commercial products and plants are nontoxic (Table 13-2). For an ingestion to be considered nontoxic, the patient must be completely asymptomatic and the following additional conditions must be met: (1) the patient must have a phone available so that you can call the family and check on his or her status, (2) you must have the correct spelling of the product, and there must be no signal words on the container, (3) the parents must be certain of the amount ingested, and (4) the parents must be sure that only one substance was ingested. Only if all of these conditions are met may a child be discharged immediately from the ER.

Occasionally with a toddler, and more commonly with an adoles-

TABLE 13-1. POISONS

	Toxicologic Syndromes
Amphetamines	Excessive activity, argumentative, tremors, headache, hyperthermia, dilated reactive pupils, flushing, diaphoresis, dry mouth, hypertension, tachycardia, active bowel sounds, dysrhythmias
Anticholinergics	Agitation, seizures, hallucinations, flushing, dilated unreactive pupils, dry skin, hyperthermia, decreased bowel sounds, supraventricular or ventricular dysrhythmias
Barbiturates/ tranquilizers	Sleepy or comatose, slurred speech, ataxia, no alcohol odor on breath, miosis, vesicular skin lesions
Boric acid	Diffuse cutaneous erythema and desquamation ("boiled lobster"), coma, convulsions, acidosis, blue green diarrhea
Botulism	Epidemic, dysphagia, dysphonia, ptosis, ophthalmoplegia, descending paralysis, dilated pupils
Bromides	Acne, dementia/psychosis, hyperchloremic "cation gap"
Carbon monoxide	Epidemic, flu-like illness, metabolic acidosis, hemoglobin desaturation
Cocaine	Perforated nasal septum, psychosis, seizures, skin tracks, hyperthermia, dilated pupils (reactive)
Cyanide	Bitter almond odor, coma, convulsions, decreased (A-V) O_2 difference, ECG abnormalities
Digitalis	Visual disturbances, nausea, vomiting, delirium, ECG abnormalities
Ethylene glycol	Metabolic acidosis, osmolal gap, hypocalcemia, renal failure, oxalate crystalluria
Hydrocarbons	Pulmonary edema or hemorrhage, pneumonitis, ventricular dysrhythmias
Iron	Vomiting and diarrhea (bloody), coma, hepatomegaly, metabolic acidosis, pregnant female in house, radio-opaque material in gut
Lithium	Confusion, weakness, hyponatremia, dysrhythmias, QT prolongation, nephropathy
Mercury (mercuric salts)	Vomiting and diarrhea (bloody), acute tubular necrosis, coma
Methyl alcohol	Alcoholic, decreased visual acuity, metabolic acidosis, coma
Opiates	Track marks, coma, miosis, hypotension, bradycardia, hypothermia
Organophosphates/ carbamates	Salivation, lacrimation, urination, diarrhea, bronchorrhea, miosis, bradycardia, muscle fasciculations, garlic odor

TABLE 13-1. CONTINUED

Paraquat	Mucosal burns (pseudodiphtheria), vomiting and diarrhea, renal failure, ventilatory failure
Phencyclidine	Violence, schizophreniform psychosis, myoclonus, seizures, bidirectional nystagmus, hypertension
Phenothiazines/ butyrophenones	Oculogyric or torsion crisis, coma, tremor, miosis, hypo- or hyperthermia, increased ECG intervals, hypotension
Salicylates	Respiratory alkalosis and metabolic acidosis, fever, vomiting, coagulopathy, pulmonary edema
Strychnine	Extreme hypertonicity with meningismus, track marks, lactic acidosis

Coma Syndromes Due to Toxins

Depressed Reflexes, Hypotension	Hypotension, Pulmonary Edema
Barbiturates	Opiates
Benzodiazepines	Salicylates
Carbon monoxide	Sedative-Hypnotics
Clonidine	**Dysrhythmias, Seizures**
Ethyl alcohol	Arsenic
Isopropyl alcohol	Caffeine
Sedative-hypnotics	Cocaine
Myoclonus, Seizures, Mydriasis	Propranolol
Amphetamines	Theophylline
Anticholinergics	Tricyclics
Cocaine	**Seizures, Miosis**
Methaqualone	Codeine
Phencyclidine (sometimes miosis)	Meperidine (sometimes mydriasis)
Strychnine	Organophosphates
Theophylline	Propoxyphene

(From Mofenson HC, Greensher J: Pediatrics 54: 336–342, 1974. Reproduced by Permission of Pediatrics.)

cent, the poison is unknown. A specific toxicologic diagnosis rests on a thorough history and physical examination, appreciation of the role of the clinical and toxicology laboratories, and the use of up-to-date resources such as the Poison Control Center.

Some important questions to ask after the routine "what, how much, and when" include the following:

1. Where was the patient found?
2. Has he or she visited someone recently?

TABLE 13-2. NONTOXIC INGESTIONS

Abrasives	Iodophil disinfectant
Adhesives	Laxatives
Antacids	Lipstick
Antibiotics	Lubricant
Baby product cosmetics	Lubricating oils
Ballpoint pen inks	Lysol brand disinfectant (NOT toilet bowl cleaner)
Bathtub floating toys	Magic markers
Battery (dry cell)	Makeup (eye, liquid facial)
Bath oil (castor oil and perfume)	Mineral oil
Bleach (less than 5% sodium hypochlorite)	Motor oil
Body conditioners	Newspaper
Bubble bath soaps (detergents)	Paint—indoor or latex
Calamine lotion	Pencil (lead-graphite, coloring)
Candle (beeswax or paraffin)	Perfumes
Caps (toy pistols)	Petroleum jelly (Vaseline)
Chalk (calcium carbonate)	Phenolphthalein laxatives (Ex-Lax)
Cigarettes or cigars (nicotine)	Play-Doh
Clay (modeling)	Polaroid picture coating fluid
Colognes	Porous-tip ink marking pens
Contraceptives	Prussian blue (ferricyanide)
Corticosteroids	Putty (less than 2 oz)
Cosmetics	Rouge
Crayons (marked A.P., C.P.)	Rubber cement
Dehumidifying packets (silica or charcoal)	Sachets (essential oils, powder)
Detergents (phosphate type, anionic)	Shampoos
Deodorants	Shaving creams and lotions
Deodorizers (spray and refrigerator)	Shoe polish (most do not contain aniline dyes)
Elmer's Glue	Silly putty (99% silicones)
Etch-A-Sketch	Soap and soap products
Eye makeup	Spackles
Fabric softeners	Suntan preparations
Fertilizer (if no insecticides or herbicides added)	Sweetening agents (saccharin, cyclamate, aspartamine)
Fish bowl additives	Teething rings (water-sterility?)
Glues and pastes	Thermometers (mercury)
Golf ball (core may cause mechanical injury)	Thyroid hormone
Greases	Toilet water
Hair products (dyes, sprays, tonics)	Tooth paste (with and wthout fluoride)
Hand lotions and creams	Vaseline
Hydrogen peroxide (medicinal 3%)	Vitamins
Incense	Warfarin
Indelible markers	Water colors
Ink (black, blue)	Zinc oxide
	Zirconium oxide

TABLE 13-2. CONTINUED

Nontoxic House Plants[a]

African Violet (Saintpaulia ionantha)
Aluminum plant (Pilea)
Aralia False (Dizygotheca elegantissima)
Begonia (botanical name)
Bloodleaf Plant (Iresine)
Boston Fern (Nephrolepsis exata)
Cat Tail (Acalypha hispida)
Chinese Evergreen
Christmas Cactus (Zygocactus truncactus)
Coleus (botanical name)
Corn Plant (Draecaena)
Creeping Charlie (Pilea nummularifolia) or (Plectranthus australis)
Crocus (Spring blooming) Crocus Spp
Dandelion (Taraxacum officinale)
Devil's Walking Stick (Aralia)
Donkey Tail (Sedum morganianum)
Dracaena (Species) (Corn plant)
Dusty Miller (Cineraria)
Dwarf Cactus-Epiphyl. Hybrid-Elegantissimum
Dwarf Palm-Chamaedorea Elegans
Gardenia
Geranium (Pelargonium)
Grape Hyacinth
Hawaiian Ti (Cordyline terminalis)
Hens & Chicks (Escheveria or Sempervivum tectorus)
Hibiscus
Honeysuckle (Lonicera)
Impatiens
Jade Plant (Crassula argentea)
Kalanchoe (Pregnant plant)
Lady's Slipper
Lilac (Syringa)
Lipstick Plant (Aeschynanthus lobbianus)
Inch Plant (Tradescantai)
Magnolia Bush
Moses-in-a-Boat (Rhoea spathacea)
Mother-in-law's-tongue (Sanservieria trifascianta)
Monkey Plant (Rulla makoyana)
Palm
Patient Lucy
Peperomia (botanical name)
Piggy-Back Plant (Tolmiea menziestii)
Pilea (Botanical name)
Pink Polka Dot Plant (Hypoestes sanguinolenta)
Plectranthus (botanical name)
Prayer Plant (Maranta leuconeura kerchoveana)
Primula
Rattle Snake Plant (Calathea insignis)
Rose (Rosa species)
Rose Begonia (Begonia semperflorens)
Rose of Sharon
Rubber Plant (Ficus elastica)
Scheffelera (Brassaia actiniphylla—Umbrella plant)
Sensitive Plant (Mimosa pudica)
Snake Plant (Sanservieria)
Snapdragon (Antirrhinum)
Spider Plant (Anthericum or Chlorophytum cosmosum)
Swedish Ivy (Plectranthus australis)
Violets (Saintpaulia ionantha)
Wandering Jew (Zebrina pendula)
Wax Plant (Hoya)
Weeping Fig (Ficus benjamina)

[a]Plant identification is very difficult, but if the parent can identify the plant, and if it is listed in the nontoxic list, we advise simple observation.
(Adapted from the Nassau County Poison Control Center.)

3. Is the patient or anyone else in the house on medication—acutely, chronically, or intermittently?
4. Is anyone in the house ill now or was anyone ill recently?
5. Have there been any recent visitors in the house?
6. Were there any pills, pill bottles, or other open containers in the house (including the garbage) or were any unusual odors noticed?
7. Does anyone in the house have a hobby or use unusual chemicals?
8. Has the patient vomited or been given syrup of ipecac prior to arrival at the hospital?
9. Was the substance in the original container or was it transferred into another one?
10. Was there more than one substance in the container?

Finally, consider a nontoxicologic differential diagnosis (*head trauma, meningitis, cerebrovascular accident, postictal state, posthypoxia*), and ask if the patient has been ill or injured recently or has had headaches, seizures, or fever.

On physical examination (Table 13-3), check the vital signs, skin, eyes, neck, lungs, heart sounds, and abdomen (distention, tenderness, bowel sounds), and perform a brief neurologic survey (level of consciousness, focal signs, pupillary size and reflexes, gag reflex). Note any distinctive odors (Table 13-4).

Comatose patients (p 382) with symmetrical extraocular movements (EOM), pupillary reflexes, and motor responses most likely have a *toxic-metabolic* origin for their coma (although *hypoglycemia* can cause focal motor deficits). Assume that pupillary inequality signifies a *structural intracranial process*. Miosis, on the other hand, strongly suggests a toxic etiology.

A number of laboratory tests can help identify the specific poison or narrow the differential diagnosis. Perform a ferric chloride ($FeCl_3$) test in the ER using fresh urine and 10% ferric chloride mixed in a ratio of 2 ml of urine:0.5 ml $FeCl_3$. See Table 13-5 for the expected color reactions. Remember that false-positive reactions result from phosphates (brown, yellow, or white) or ketones (purple) in the urine.

"MUDPIES" is the mnemonic for conditions that give a metabolic acidosis with an elevated anion gap: methanol, uremia, diabetic ketoacidosis (DKA), phenformin or paraldehyde, idiopathic acidosis (hypoperfusion), iron, isoniazid, ethylene glycol, ethanol, and salicylates. Chronic toluene inhalation and acute chlorine gas inhalation

TABLE 13-3. PHYSICAL EXAMINATION FINDINGS

Vital Signs:

Increased temperature—salicylates, amphetamines, anticholinergics, cocaine, theophylline, phencyclidine

Decreased temperature—barbiturates, phenothiazines, opiates, ethanol, hypotension from any cause, hypoglycemia

Increased pulse rate—amphetamines, cocaine, caffeine, anticholinergics, theophylline, hypotension from any cause, hypoglycemia

Decreased pulse rate—opiates, barbiturates, digitalis, clonidine, beta blockers, cholinesterase-inhibitor pesticides, hypothermia, hypoglycemia, increased intracranial pressure

Increased respiratory rate—salicylates, theophylline, metabolic acidosis, Reye syndrome

Decreased respiratory rate—CNS depressants (many), clonidine (early)

Increased blood pressure—amphetamines, cocaine, anticholinergics, theophylline, phencyclidine, caffeine, increased intracranial pressure

Decreased blood pressure—CNS depressants (many), clonidine

Skin:

Cyanosis—methemoglobinemia, hypoxia

Flushing—anticholinergics, amphetamines

Diaphoresis—amphetamines, cocaine, cholinesterase-inhibitor pesticides

Hot, dry skin—anticholinergics

Piloerection—opiate withdrawal

Bullae—carbon monoxide, barbiturates, ethchlorvynol

Pruritis—vitamin A

Tracks, abscesses, lymphedema, acrocyanosis—parenteral drug abuse

Eyes:

Miosis—opiates, barbiturates, phenothiazines, cholinesterase-inhibitor pesticides

Mydriasis—amphetamines, cocaine, atropinics, methylalcohol, propoxyphene, opiate withdrawal

Conjunctival injection—direct irritants, cannabis

Nystagmus—phencyclidine, phenytoin

Visual disturbances—botulism, parathion, methanol, digitalis, vitamin A

Neck:

Rigidity—dystonia from phenothiazines and halopridol, phencyclidine, strychnine, meningitis

Breath Sounds:

Rhonchi, wheezes—petroleum distillate aspiration, toxic inhalants, cholinesterase-inhibitor pesticides

continued

TABLE 13-3. CONTINUED

Abdomen:

Distention, decreased bowel sounds—CNS depressants (many), anticholinergics,

Increased bowel sounds—amphetamines, cocaine, cholinesterase-inhibitor pesticides, drug withdrawal, food poisoning

Tenderness—alcoholic gastritis, corrosives

Distended bladder—anticholinergics

Neurologic:

Ataxia: Phenytoin, benzodiazepines, sedative hypnotics, solvents

Focal signs: Must r/o increased intracranial pressure due to mass lesion, hypoglycemia

Tremor: Carbon monoxide, parathion, phenothiazenes, mercury, ethanol, lithium, arsenic, solvents

TABLE 13-4. ODORS

Odor	Toxin
Ammoniacal	Uremia, ammonia
Garlic	Arsenic, phosphorus, thallium, organophosphates, selenium, dimethyl sulfoxide (DMSO)
Carrots	Cicutoxin
Bitter almonds	Cyanides (silver polish)
Acetone	Isopropyl alcohol, methanol, ASA, chloroform, ketoacidosis
Pungent aromatic (vinyl)	Ethchlorvynol (Placidyl)
Disinfectants	Phenol, Creosote
Violets (urine)	Turpentine
Shoe polish	Nitrobenzene, chlorinated hydrocarbons
Coal gas	Carbon monoxide
Moth balls	Camphor
Wintergreen	Methylsalicylate
Peanuts	N-pyridylmethylurea (Vacor), other rodenticides
Pear-like (acrid)	Chloral hydrate, paraldehyde
Eggs (rotten)	Hydrogen sulfide, mercaptans, Antabuse
Fish or raw liver (musty)	Hepatic failure, zinc phosphide
Fruit-like	Amylnitrite, ethanol, isopropyl alcohol
Petroleum	Petroleum distillates.

TABLE 13-5. URINE FERRIC CHLORIDE TEST

Salicylates	Purple
Phenothiazines	Blue
Isoniazid	Gray or yellow green

have also been reported to be causes of an elevated anion gap. The anion gap, or difference between the sums of the measurable cations and anions is calculated as follows:

$$[Na^+] - [Cl^- + HCO_3^-]$$

The upper limit of normal is approximately 12.

Order a serum osmolality to screen for significant amounts of ethyl alcohol, ethylene glycol, methyl alcohol, and isopropyl alcohol when specific assays are not available. In a toxic ingestion of one of these substances, the measured serum osmolality is higher than the calculated osmolality. Calculate the serum osmolality using the formula:

$$\text{Calculated osmolality} = 2[Na] + [Glucose]/18 + [BUN]/2.8$$

The normal measured serum osmolality is 280–300 mOsm. Ethanol is the most common toxic cause of an elevated osmolal gap in pediatric patients; every 100 mg/dl of ethanol raises the osmolality 25–30 mOsm/kg. Assuming, therefore, a baseline value of 280 mOsm/kg, an ethanol level of 200 mg/dl causes an osmolality of 330 mOsm/kg.

The mnemonic ''CHIPES'' refers to those toxins (tablets) that are radioopaque and may be seen on abdominal x-ray: chloral hydrate, carbon tetrachloride, heavy metals (lead, iron, arsenic), iodides, psychotropics (phenothiazines, tricyclic antidepressants), enteric-coated medications, and sodium and other elements (calcium, potassium, bismuth). Occasionally, an adolescent may conceal sealed bags or condoms with drugs (heroin, cocaine) by swallowing them. On x-ray, they appear as regular gas-density ''bubbles'' in the gut lumen.

When qualitative analysis is desired, urine is the best specimen, followed by gastric contents. Request specific blood levels for substances only when the information either predicts the seriousness of the ingestion or otherwise aids in management (indications for dialysis). Drug levels are available for a number of specific ingestions, although ''toxicology screens'' are usually not helpful. In general, requests for levels should be guided by the history and physical examination. The one exception is a request for an *acetaminophen level* which must be part of the evaluation of *every* adolescent poisoning victim. Acetaminophen overdose may be asymptomatic (see p 338) early and still lead to fulminant hepatic necrosis. Other substances for which levels may be useful include theophylline, salicylates, barbiturates, diphenylhydantoin, digoxin, ethyl alcohol and ethylene glycol, methyl alcohol, methemoglobin, lithium, and iron.

ER MANAGEMENT

The priorities are securing a patent airway, establishing adequate ventilation, and maintaining the hemodynamic status. Always consider the possibility of alternative diagnoses such as head trauma, central nervous system (CNS) infection, or hypoglycemia, that may mimic or occur in conjunction with an intoxication.

The Unconscious Patient

1. Assess the patient's respirations. If not adequate, perform a jaw-lift, insert an oral airway (if tolerated), and suction any secretions. If necessary, intubate the patient, preferably with a cuffed endotracheal tube.
2. Secure a large-bore IV line.
3. Measure the blood pressure and pulse. If the patient has clinical signs of hypoperfusion (poor capillary refill, pallor, cool extremities), give a rapid IV bolus (20 cc/kg) of Ringer's lactate or normal saline and raise the foot of the bed.
4. Obtain an electrocardiogram (ECG) and attach a cardiac monitor.
5. Although it may be clear that the patient is an overdose or ingestion victim, perform a careful neurologic examination to rule out an occult head injury.
6. Remove the patient's clothing to permit easier examination and to look for evidence of trauma.
7. Measure the temperature and, if possible, weigh the patient. A soft rectal thermometer probe measures extremes of temperature beyond the ranges of glass or digital thermometers.
8. Obtain an arterial blood gas (ABG) to assess the adequacy of ventilation and the acid–base status.
9. Obtain blood for a complete blood cell count (CBC), liver function tests, type and hold, pH electrolytes and glucose, dextrostix glucose determination, acetaminophen level, carboxyhemoglobin

(if CO poisoning cannot be ruled out by history), and an extra red top tube for other drug levels that may be needed.

10. Give 0.5 g/kg of glucose to *all* patients.
11. Give 0.01 mg/kg (IV, IM, SC, or ET) of naloxone (Narcan). If there is no response within 3–5 minutes, give a second dose of 0.1 mg/kg of Narcan. A positive response may last only 30 minutes so be prepared to give repeated doses or a continuous IV infusion (0.4–1.2 mg/hr). No response after the second dose usually rules out an opioid as the sole cause of the altered mental status, but complications of an opioid poisoning (hypoxia, postictal state), head trauma, CNS infection, or mixed drug overdose remain as possibilities.
12. Obtain urine by catheter for dipstick examination and ferric chloride testing.
13. Perform lavage with the patient in the left lateral position with an *orogastric hose,* not a nasogastric (NG) tube. An NG tube may be used only when a liquid toxin was ingested. Unconscious patients must be intubated first (see above), although lethargic patients who have a gag reflex do not require intubation. In patients less than 2 years of age, use an 18- to 28-gauge tube, use a 28- to 36-gauge tube in the 2- to 10-year old, and a 36- to 40-gauge tube in patients over 10 years of age. Attach a funnel to the orogastric hose and pour in 100 cc (toddler) to 200 cc (adolescent) aliquots of saline. Then lower the funnel to below the level of the patient and allow the fluid to drain by gravity. Continue this until no particles are seen and the lavage fluid is clear (2 or more liters).
14. When the lavage is completed, pour a slurry of activated charcoal (1 g/kg) down the tube.
15. Also instill 250 mg/kg (30 g max) of magnesium or sodium sulfate, 4 cc/kg of magnesium citrate, or 30 cc of milk of magnesia (do not use magnesium in patients with renal failure; avoid sodium cathartics in congestive heart failure). Then pinch off the tube and remove it. Contraindications to the use of cathartics include adynamic ileus, suspected abdominal trauma, intestinal obstruction, severe diarrhea, or significant electrolyte disturbances.

The Conscious Patient

1. First, measure the vital signs, including temperature and weight.
2. If the patient is alert and stable, try to determine the substance(s) and amounts ingested as well as time since the ingestion.

TABLE 13-6. CONTRAINDICATIONS TO REMOVAL OF TOXINS FROM THE GI TRACT

General:
- Most hydrocarbon ingestions (nonhalogenated, nonaromatic, not containing another toxic substance)
- Caustic ingestion
- Prior vomiting (relative)

By induced emesis (vs lavage):
- Coma
- Worsening level of consciousness
- No gag reflex
- Seizures
- Hematemesis, bleeding diathesis
- Prior vomiting (relative)
- Infant <6 months of age

3. Remove the poison from the gastrointestinal (GI) tract regardless of the time elapsed since the ingestion, unless removal is specifically contraindicated (Table 13-6). Syrup of ipecac (10 cc in the 6- to 12-month old, 15 cc <5 years old, 30 cc >5 years old) followed by 250 cc of water or juice (not milk) causes emesis in 90% of patients within 20–30 minutes. A second dose may be given if the patient has not vomited by this time, but if emesis does not occur, perform lavage to remove the poison. Do not give ipecac to a patient with a depressed mental status, since its use demands that the patient remain awake for at least half an hour. Give ipecac to an uncooperative patient by instilling it through a small bore nasogastric tube with water and then removing the tube to allow the patient to vomit.
4. Fifteen to 20 minutes after the emesis, give the patient (to drink or via NG tube) a slurry of activated charcoal (1 g/kg) and cathartic. Although there are some poisons whose elimination is not enhanced by charcoal, the only relative contraindication to its use is an acetaminophen ingestion, since the antidote, n-acetylcysteine (Mucomyst), is adsorbed to a variable extent by the charcoal. However, the charcoal can be removed from the GI tract prior to giving the Mucomyst (see p 338). Since activated charcoal is efficacious in binding many substances (including acetaminophen) that may be taken in a mixed overdose, give it unless it is certain that

acetaminophen was the *only* substance ingested. Repeated (q 2h) administrations of charcoal are indicated for barbiturate, theophylline, and tricyclic ingestions.

Perform *skin decontamination* if the patient is a victim of poisoning by organophosphate or carbamate insecticides, caustics, mace, or gasoline. Hospital staff should wear gowns and gloves, remove all the patient's clothing and place it in plastic bags, and wash the patient twice with soap and water, regardless of how much time has elapsed since the exposure.

Ocular decontamination is essential whenever the eye has been exposed to a toxin. Apply an ophthalmic anesthetic to the eye (2–3 drops) and retract the lids fully with retractors. Irrigate for 20 minutes or more with *at least* 1 full liter of normal saline or water run through IV tubing held a few inches from the patient's eye. Alternatively, hold the patient's eye(s) open under a running faucet or shower.

Further therapy can be tailored to the specific poison(s). Forced diuresis, performed in an intensive care setting, is indicated only for drugs that are excreted in the urine in significant amounts in their active form. Contraindications to forced diuresis include poisons with very large volumes of distribution or nonrenal mechanisms of excretion and patients who cannot tolerate large fluid loads or who have severe electrolyte abnormalities. The goal is a urine flow of 3–6 cc/kg/hr which is achieved by using an IV rate 2–3 times maintenance.

Alkaline diuresis may be helpful for weak acids such as salicylates, phenobarbital, and isoniazid. The goal is a urine pH of 7.5–8.0. Give 1–2 mEq/kg of sodium bicarbonate IV over 20– 30 minutes and then by continuous infusion to deliver approximately 0.5 mEq/kg/hr. Frequent monitoring of the serum potassium is essential. Do not use acetazolamide, which is potentially dangerous.

Although acid diuresis increases the renal clearance of phencyclidine (PCP), strychnine, and amphetamines, the potential dangers of inducing an acidemia in situations already associated with lactic acidosis and rhabdomyolysis far outweigh the benefits.

Extracorporeal drug extraction (hemodialysis, charcoal hemoperfusion) is indicated for all cases of methanol and ethylene glycol overdose as well as severe cases of salicylate, lithium, theophylline (charcoal hemoperfusion only), and barbiturate poisoning. Consider it for patients with renal failure who have taken drugs primarily excreted by the kidney and for patients who are deteriorating in the face of proper supportive care. Dialysis is contraindicated for drugs with very large volumes of distribution or high protein binding.

Toddlers who remain asymptomatic after 4–5 hours of observation may be discharged home if the parents are able to return to the ER if needed. Remind parents and other caretakers about safety precautions (keep medications and household products out of reach) and schedule a follow-up office visit for the next week to reinforce your teaching, answer any questions, and, if appropriate, provide and discuss the indications for ipecac. Unless a recent lead level can be documented, obtain one before the child leaves the ER, since toddlers who have ingested a nonfood substance may be at increased risk for pica.

INDICATIONS FOR ADMISSION

- All suicide gestures and attempts
- Symptomatic overdoses
- Any acid–base disturbance
- Any toddler ingestion suggestive of abuse or neglect

REFERENCES

1. Goldfrank LR: Toxicologic Emergencies, 3rd ed. Norwalk, CT: Appleton-Century-Crofts, 1986
2. Mofenson HC, Greensher J: Pediatr Clin North Am 17:583–593, 1970
3. Mofenson HC, Greensher J: Pediatrics 54:336–342, 1974
4. Cupit GC, Temple AR: Emerg Clin North Am 2:15–28, 1984
5. Easom JM, Lovejoy FH: Pediatr Clin North Am 26:827–836, 1979

Acetaminophen

INTRODUCTION

Acetaminophen overdose causes excessive amounts of hepatotoxic intermediate metabolites to be formed. The minimum toxic dose is 140 mg/kg (7.5 g for an adult), so that a 120 cc bottle of Tylenol elixir can poison up to a 27-kg child. However, the likelihood of significant poisoning is increased by concomitant ingestion of barbiturates, steroids, and antihistamines, or preexisting hepatic dysfunction or starvation. Since the elixir is 7% ethanol, concurrent alcohol intoxication can occur when a toddler ingests the elixir form.

CLINICAL PRESENTATION

The clinical course can be divided into three stages. In the first (within several hours of ingestion), diaphoresis and nonspecific gastrointestinal symptoms such as anorexia, nausea, vomiting, and abdominal pain are seen. This is followed, at 24–48 hours postingestion, by a latent stage during which the first stage symptoms resolve but subclinical hepatotoxicity begins. Occasionally, the patient has right upper quadrant (RUQ) pain and tenderness at this time. The bilirubin and liver transaminases are elevated and prothrombin time prolonged. During the third phase (3–4 days), jaundice, oliguria, hepatic failure, and encephalopathy with coma develop and death can occur.

DIAGNOSIS

Expedient diagnosis is necessary, as treatment must begin within 24 (ideally 12) hours of ingestion (prior to clinical hepatotoxicity) to be effective. Obtain an acetaminophen level at 4 hours postingestion, or if the timing is unclear, obtain two levels 4 hours apart. A nomogram (Fig. 13-1) that begins 4 hours postingestion facilitates accurate prediction of hepatotoxicity (acetaminophen level >200 mg% at 4 hours). The approximate half-life of acetaminophen in an overdose is 4 hours (assuming complete absorption).

For all adolescent overdose victims, obtain an acetaminophen level as these patients tend to take multiple drugs.

Other causes of acute hepatic insufficiency include various *drugs* (griseofulvin, valproic acid, isoniazid), *viral hepatitis* (exposure to a case or to blood products, IV drug use, positive serology), *Reye syndrome* (normal bilirubin and elevated ammonia, hepatic failure and encephalopathy occur simultaneously), and *Amanita phalloides mushroom poisoning* (history).

ER MANAGEMENT

Empty the stomach via induced emesis or gastric lavage. Obtain blood for a 4-hour acetaminophen level (see above), CBC, liver function tests, electrolytes, glucose, and prothrombin time (PT).

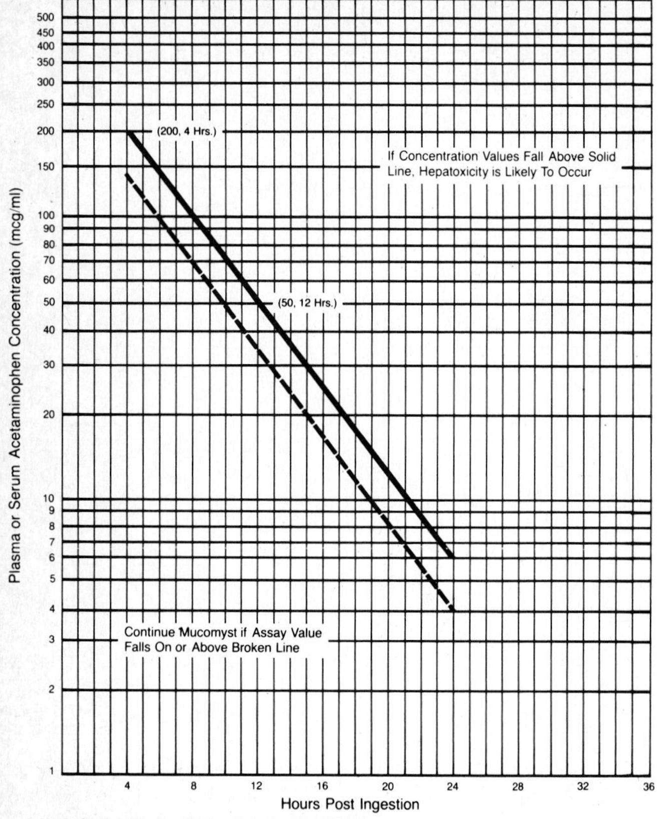

Figure 13-1. Nomogram for acetaminophen level. (*McNeil Consumer Products Company.*)

Oral n-acetylcysteine (Mucomyst) is the antidote. The loading dose is 140 mg/kg, followed by 70 mg/kg q 4h for 17 more doses. Mucomyst has an offensive odor and causes vomiting. Mix it in a 1:4 ratio with a soft drink or juice. If the patient cannot tolerate it orally, give it via a nasogastric or nasoduodenal tube. An intravenous form of Mucomyst is still considered experimental in the United States.

Activated charcoal adsorbs the antidote (n-acetylcysteine) to some degree. However, it is efficacious in binding most drugs, including acetaminophen. Therefore, give activated charcoal (1 g/kg), particularly when a mixed ingestion cannot be ruled out. After 20–30 minutes, lavage it out and instill the first dose of n-acetylcysteine through the lavage tube.

INDICATIONS FOR ADMISSION

- Possible acetaminophen toxicity, based upon amount ingested (>140 mg/kg) or serum levels
- Suicide gesture or attempt

REFERENCE

1. Lovejoy FH, Goldman P: PIR 1:117–121, 1979

Anticholinergics

INTRODUCTION

Anticholinergic poisoning in children is usually secondary to ingestion of a tricyclic antidepressant such as amitriptyline (Elavil), imipramine (Tofranil), or doxepin (Sinequan). Other etiologies include atropine, scopolamine, antihistamines, phenothiazines, antiparkinsonians, mydriatics, haloperidol, and jimson weed. For the tricyclics, the minimum toxic dose is about 10 mg/kg.

CLINICAL PRESENTATION

These agents cause an atropine-like syndrome (peripheral muscarinic blockade) manifested by dry mouth, flushed dry skin, confusion, mydriasis, blurred vision, constipation, urinary retention, tachycardia, and orthostatic hypotension or, less commonly, hypertension. Central anticholinergic blockade causes confusion, disorientation, hallucinations, seizures and coma. A severe poisoning can result in the triad of coma, grand mal seizures, and arrhythmias (sinus or supraventricular tachycardia, ventricular tachycardia or fibrillation, and A-V or intraventricular conduction disturbances).

DIAGNOSIS

Suspect an anticholinergic ingestion in any patient with an atropine-like presentation, coma, arrhythmia, or seizures.

On examination, the pupils are usually dilated and unreactive; reactive dilated pupils are found in *sympathomimetic ingestions*. The presence of tachycardia, dry mucous membranes, and dry flushed skin also suggests the diagnosis.

Obtain blood for a CBC, electrolytes and glucose, and dextrostix determination, as well as urine for ferric chloride testing (positive with phenothiazine ingestion) and an ECG. The hallmark of cardiotoxicity is QRS widening (>100 msec). Also obtain a KUB; the phenothiazines and tricyclic antidepressants are radioopaque.

ER MANAGEMENT

Institute basic measures of induced emesis/gastric lavage, activated charcoal (repeated q 2h), and a cathartic, and continuously monitor the ECG.

The treatment of coma is supportive. Treat seizures with diazepam (0.3 mg/kg IV), then give a loading dose of phenytoin (10–15 mg/kg slowly IV). Phenytoin is also effective for arrhythmias. If a life-threatening arrhythmia persists, give $NaHCO_3$ (1–2 mEq/kg over 30 minutes), which seems to facilitate the actions of phenytoin.

Continued seizures, ventricular arrhythmias unresponsive to standard therapy, supraventricular arrhythmias with hemodynamic compromise or severe agitation and hallucinations are indications for treatment with physostigmine. Do not use physostigmine merely to arouse a comatose patient. Give a test dose of 0.5 mg *slowly* over 2–3 minutes. This can be repeated up to four times q 5–10 minutes. Rapid administration may cause seizures, and an overdose can precipitate a cholinergic crisis (salivation, lacrimation, bradycardia, hypotension, or asystole). Always be prepared to give atropine (half the physostigmine dose) to a patient being treated with physostigmine.

INDICATIONS FOR ADMISSION

- Lethargy or signs of atropinism (tachycardia, postural hypotension, confusion, agitation)
- Coma, arrhythmia, A-V block or other conduction defect, or seizures

REFERENCE
1. Callahan M: JACEP 8: 413–425, 1979

Carbon Monoxide

INTRODUCTION

Carbon monoxide is in automobile exhaust, smoke from fires, and exhaust from a kerosene or gas heater. It avidly combines with hemoglobin, displacing oxygen, thus impairing the delivery of O_2 to the tissues.

CLINICAL PRESENTATION

Patients are asymptomatic until a carboxyhemoglobin (COHb) level of 10–20% is reached, when headache and dyspnea occur. At a COHb level of 30%, nausea, vomiting, and weakness are seen, followed by lethargy, tachycardia, and tachypnea at 40%. Coma and seizures occur at 50%, and 60% may be fatal.

DIAGNOSIS

Obtain a COHb level (0.5 cc of heparinized venous or arterial blood) if the patient is likely to have been exposed (fire victim, etc) to a source of CO. Ascertain the interval between the end of the exposure and when the level is obtained. If the interval is long or the patient was treated with oxygen prior to arrival in the ER, he may be more severely affected than the COHb level indicates.

ER MANAGEMENT

While waiting for the COHb level, institute treatment with 100% O_2 via a nonrebreathing mask. If the COHb level is over 20% or the patient is symptomatic, pregnant, or was unconscious at the scene of the fire (see pp 161–163), transport to a hyperbaric chamber (if available) or continue the 100% O_2 until the level is ≤ 5.

INDICATIONS FOR ADMISSION

- Initial COHb over 20%
- Any patient who required treatment for CO poisoning

REFERENCE

1. Binder JW, Roberts RJ: Clin Toxicol 16: 287, 1980

Caustics

INTRODUCTION

Corrosives burn the mucous membranes; alkalis frequently cause oropharygeal injury and serious esophageal ulcerations, while acids burn the stomach. Consequences include esophageal perforation with mediastinitis, gastrointestinal bleeding, gastric ulceration, and stricture.

Most caustic ingestions involve alkalis such as lye, ammonia, oven or drain cleaners, clinitest tablets, dishwasher detergents, and button batteries. Household bleach (5% sodium hypochlorite) is not a strong caustic and does not cause significant injury.

CLINICAL PRESENTATION

Oropharyngeal pain and drooling are common, and vomiting occasionally occurs. Although burns of the lips, tongue, and pharynx frequently occur, their presence or absence does not reliably predict the condition of the esophagus and stomach. Other findings may include perioral burns, stridor, or, rarely, dyspnea, retrosternal burning, or abdominal pain.

DIAGNOSIS

A serious esophageal injury (second- or third-degree burn) is unlikely in the absence of stridor, vomiting, drooling, or other serious sign. The presence or absence of oropharyngeal burns does not correlate with esophageal injury.

ER MANAGEMENT

If there is a history of possible caustic ingestion, give the patient milk to dilute the substance (if he or she is willing to drink) and obtain a CBC, type and cross-match, and a chest x-ray (looking for mediastinal widening indicative of mediastinitis). If the patient has vomiting, drooling, or stridor, he or she is at risk for serious esophageal injury. Make him or her NPO, begin maintenance IV hydration, and give IV ampicillin (100 mg/kg/day divided q 6h) and hydrocortisone (10 mg/kg/day divided q 6h). Do not insert an NG tube or try to neutralize the caustic. Consult with a skilled endoscopist and arrange endoscopy within 12–24 hours.

Patients with a history of possible caustic ingestion, with or without oropharyngeal burns, but without vomiting, drooling, or stridor are at low risk for serious esophageal injury. If the chest x-ray is normal and the patient is comfortable and can drink readily, he or she can be sent home with close telephone contact.

A chest x-ray usually locates an ingested button battery. Immediate endoscopy is indicated if the battery is lodged in the esophagus. If it has passed into the stomach, the patient may be sent home as long as close follow-up is possible. Repeat the x-ray in one week if the battery has not passed in the stool.

INDICATIONS FOR ADMISSION

- A history of caustic ingestion and vomiting, drooling, or stridor
- Button battery ingestion with signs of perforation or battery lodged in the esophagus

REFERENCES
1. Crain EF, Gershel JC, Mezey AP: Am J Dis Child 138:863–865,1984
2. Hawkins D, Demeter M, Barnett T: Laryngoscope 80:98–109,1980
3. Litovitz TL: Pediatrics 75:469–476 1985

Digitalis

INTRODUCTION
Digitalis ingestion is uncommon, as the drugs are available only where there is a patient with cardiac disease. The minimum toxic dose is about 0.07 mg/kg, which is roughly equivalent to 1.5 ml/kg of digoxin (Lanoxin) elixir. Twenty to 50 times the daily maintenance dose seems to be the lethal dose.

CLINICAL PRESENTATION
Anorexia, nausea, and vomiting occur early, followed by headache, somnolence, and bradycardia with A-V or S-A block. More serious poisonings cause visual disturbances, hyperkalemia, hypotension, and CNS depression. Cardiac findings include any arrhythmia, especially bradycardia associated with an increased P-R interval and ventricular premature contractions. Massive overdose leads to severe hyperkalemia with atrial or ventricular fibrillation, ventricular tachycardia, coma, and seizures. In up to 15% of patients (especially infants), ectopic rhythms are the first sign of intoxication.

Digitalis toxicity is increased by hypokalemia, hypercalcemia, hypomagnesemia, and concomitant quinidine use.

DIAGNOSIS
Suspect digitalis overdose when either a previously well patient who lives with someone taking digitalis presents with an arrhythmia, or a patient already taking digitalis presents with a new arrhthymia, hyperkalemia, hypotension, CNS depression, or visual disturbance.

Obtain a digitalis level (if available), electrolytes to check for hypo- or hyperkalemia, and an ECG.

ER MANAGEMENT

Institute basic measures, including emesis/gastric lavage, activated charcoal q 2h, and a cathartic. Obtain blood for electrolytes, calcium, magnesium, and a digitalis level (if available). Perform an ECG looking for arrhythmias and a prolonged P-R interval, and attach a cardiac monitor to follow changes in the rhythm.

Treat bradycardia with S-A or A-V block with atropine, 0.01 mg/kg IV (minimum dose 0.2 mg, maximum 0.5 mg). For ventricular arrhythmias and supraventricular tachycardias with A-V block give phenytoin (2 mg/kg IV slowly over 15 minutes) which decreases ventricular automaticity without slowing A-V conduction. Lidocaine is also effective for ventricular arrhythmias (1 mg/kg IV bolus, then 20–50 μg/kg/min continuous infusion). Propranolol is useful for supraventricular and ventricular tachycardias, but may be dangerous if there is A-V or S-A block. The dose is 0.01–0.1 mg/kg IV (1 mg maximum).

Hyperkalemia must be aggressively treated. For mild elevations (5–6 mEq/L) infuse D5 ⅓ NS with 15 mEq/L of $NaHCO_3$; moderate hyperkalemia (6–8 mEq/L) requires insulin (0.1 units/kg IV), 200–400 mg/kg of glucose IV (4–8 ml/kg of D5 ½ NS), and Kayexalate enemas (1 g/kg) q 4h. Hemodialysis or peritoneal dialysis is indicated for a potassium over 8 mEq/L.

Severe poisonings can be treated with antidigoxin Fab antibody fragments. Consult a Poison Control Center for information.

INDICATIONS FOR ADMISSION

- Possible serious digitalis overdose (≥0.07 mg/kg)
- New arrhythmia, visual disturbance, headache, CNS depression, hypotension

REFERENCE

1. Smith TW, Butler VP, Haber E, et al: N Engl J Med 307:1357–1362, 1982

Drug Abuse Reactions

INTRODUCTION

Many drugs, both prescribed and illicit, are abused by teenagers. In general, these are difficult patients who may not give accurate information, may be resistant to treatment, and may have ingested multiple substances. It must be remembered that an overdose may represent a suicide gesture or attempt, so that psychiatric intervention is usually necessary.

CLINICAL PRESENTATION

Narcotics. Morphine, heroin, codeine, meperidine, methadone, paregoric, Lomotil (diphenoxylate plus atropine), and propoxyphene cause toxicity via ingestion or injection. Presentation can include nausea and vomiting, euphoria, disorientation, drowsiness, seizures, orthostatic hypotension, hypothermia, and pulmonary edema. The classic triad of signs is coma, pinpoint pupils (except for demerol and early in Lomotil ingestions), and respiratory depression. Death can occur immediately after an injection or within hours of an ingestion.

Hallucinogens. LSD (''acid''), psilocybin, STP, or mescaline cause hallucinations, tachycardia, hyperthermia, hypertension, mydriasis, and increased deep tendon reflexes. *PCP* (''angel dust'') intoxication is similar, except that the pupils are usually small, and ataxia, nystagmus, rigidity, bizarre behavior, and agitation often occur. Seizures and coma are more common with PCP than with other hallucinogens, and intracranial hemorrhages have been reported.

Cannabis. Marijuana, hashish, and THC cause euphoria, time-space distortions, appetite stimulation, anxiety, orthostatic hypotension, conjunctival injection, and tachycardia. The pupils are unchanged and aggressive behavior is unusual.

CNS Stimulants. This group includes the amphetamines, cocaine, and some decongestants and antiobesity drugs such as phenylpropanolamine, ephedrine, and pseudoephedrine. Dilated (but reactive) pupils, tachycardia, palpitations, hypertension, hyperthermia, and increased DTR are seen along with paranoid ideation, diaphoresis. and dry mucous membranes. Arrhythmias, shock, seizures, and coma can also occur. Intracranial hemorrhage has rarely been reported.

CNS Depressants. These compounds can be classified as barbiturates and nonbarbiturates such as methaqualone (Quaalude), glutethimide (Doriden), mebrobamate (Miltown), and ethchlorvynol (Placidyl). Severe poisoning is rare in pure benzodiazepine (Valium, Librium, Dalmane) ingestions. Level of consciousness, respirations, and DTR are depressed, and ataxia, slurred speech, and nystagmus may be noted. Coma, hypotension, and shock can ensue. A barbiturate overdose causes small pupils and, after more than 12 hours, skin bullae.

Volatile Inhalants. Solvents, such as acetone and toluene, are found in glues, paints, and solvents. Inhalation initially causes euphoria, dizziness, and hallucinations, followed by headache, visual disturbances, and CNS depression. Nitrites (amyl, butyl, isobutyl) are used as incense and aphrodisiacs. Euphoria and confusion can be followed by convulsions, coma, and sudden death.

DIAGNOSIS

Without a reliable history from the patient or a concerned friend, the diagnosis may be very difficult to make. Remove all of the patient's clothes and check the pockets for pills, vials, "joints," etc. For comatose patients, note the response to a trial of glucose (1 cc/kg of D50) and Narcan (5 ampules IV). For comatose patients with dilated, unreactive pupils, a trial of physostigmine (0.5 mg *slow* IV over 2–5 minutes) may be diagnostic.

On examination (Table 13-7) look for "track" marks indicative of IV drug abuse (narcotics). Large reactive pupils suggest amphetamines and other sympathomimetics, cocaine, glutethamide, and LSD, but not PCP. Small pupils are seen with PCP, narcotics (not meperidine), and most sedative hypnotics (except glutethamide). Agitation suggests CNS stimulants and PCP; lethargy and respiratory depression occurs with the sedative hypnotics and narcotics.

ER MANAGEMENT

Treat *CNS depressant* and *volatile inhalant* overdose with cardiorespiratory supportive care. Maintain the airway and treat shock (p 11).

TABLE 13-7. CLINICAL FINDINGS OF DRUG ABUSE AND WITHDRAWAL

Drug	Intoxication/Overdose	Withdrawal
Narcotics Heroin Morphine Methadone Codeine Meperidine (Demerol) Hydromorphone (Dilaudid) Pentazocine (Talwin) Propoxyphene (Darvon)	*Pupils:* Constricted (dilated with meperidine) *BP:* Decreased *DTR:* Diminished to absent *Respirations:* Diminished to absent *Temperature:* Reduced Euphoria, somnolence, analgesia Stupor or coma Pulmonary edema Constipation Convulsions with propoxyphene or meperidine	Dilated pupils, increased pulse, gooseflesh, sweating, muscle jerks, tremulousness, vomiting, diarrhea, yawning, tearing
Hallucinogens LSD PCP (phenycyclidine) Mescaline Psilocybin STP	*Pupils:* Usually dilated (normal or constricted with PCP) *BP:* Elevated *Pulse:* Increased *DTR:* Brisk *Temperature:* Elevated Flushed face, blank stare, nystagmus, drooling Euphoria, anxiety, paranoia, inappropriate affect, time and visual distortions or hallucinations, depersonalization	No immediate withdrawal symptoms but patients can have flashbacks and abnormal behavior for a prolonged time afterwards

	Mutism, amnesia, analgesia Ataxia, muscle rigidity Impulsive/violent behavior (cyclic coma/hyperactivity with PCP) Convulsions	
Cannabis Marijuana Hashish THC	*Pupils:* Normal *BP:* Decreased while standing *Pulse:* Increased Injected conjunctivae Hunger Euphoria, fantasy-state Time–space distortions Impaired intellectual performance	No documented withdrawal syndrome
CNS Stimulants Amphetamines Cocaine Methylphenidate (Ritalin) Phenmetrazine (Preludin) Phenylpropanolamine (Dexatrim)	*Pupils:* Dilated, reactive *BP:* Elevated *Pulse:* Increased *DTR:* Brisk *Temperature:* Elevated *Respirations:* Shallow Cardiac arrhythmias, tremors Dry mouth, sweating Euphoria, confused or hyperacute sensorium, paranoia, hallucinations, hyperactivity, impulsivity Convulsions, coma, exhaustion	Muscle aches, abdominal pain Chills, tremors Hunger Sleep, lack of energy Profound depression

continued

TABLE 13-7. CONTINUED

Drug	Intoxication/Overdose	Withdrawal
CNS Sedatives Barbiturates Chlordiazepoxide (Librium) Diazepam (Valium) Flurazepam (Dalmane) Glutethimide (Doriden) Meprobamate (Miltown) Methaqualone	*Pupils:* Normal or constricted (dilated with glutethimide) *BP:* Decreased *DTR:* Depressed *Respirations:* Depressed Nystagmus, ataxia, slurred speech Drowsiness, coma, confusion, delirium Convulsions with methaqualone	Fever, sweat Tremulousness Insomnia Hypotension Agitation, delirium, hallucinations, disorientation Convulsions
Volatile Inhalants Nitrous oxide Amyl, butyl, and isobutyl nitrate Coolant Paint thinner Nail polish remover Gasoline Transmission fluid Glue	Euphoria Dizzyness, amnesia Confusion, inability to concentrate Convulsions Coma Sudden death	

(Adapted from The Medical Letter, 25: 88, 1983.)

In general, induction of emesis or gastric lavage is ineffective for the hallucinogens, cocaine, cannaboids, and inhalants. For the other chemicals, gastric decontamination may be helpful. Activated charcoal is of particular importance in the management of PCP and barbiturate overdoses, and can be used for other pill ingestions. Alkaline-forced diuresis is beneficial for the barbiturates. Although acid diuresis enhances excretion of the amphetamines and PCP, it is dangerous and not to be used.

Naloxone (Narcan) is the treatment of choice for *narcotic*-induced coma and respiratory depression, but comatose patients must be intubated first. The usual dose of 0.01 mg/kg (IV, IM, SQ) can be increased to 0.4 mg and repeated as often as necessary to keep the patient responsive. Larger doses may be required for propoxyphene but in nearly all cases, a response should be seen by the time 10 mg have been given. If the patient becomes comatose again after initially responding to a push of naloxone, use an IV drip (0.4 mg/hr). Observe patients for persistent respiratory depression for at least 24 hours after treatment (72 hours for methadone). Treat seizures with diazepam (0.3 mg/kg IV). Use Methadone (20 mg PO qd or bid) for narcotic withdrawal.

With the exception of *PCP* ingestions, the sedative of choice for *hallucinogens* is diazepam. Give patients on *PCP* haloperidol (5 mg IM) and place them in a quiet, darkened room. Treat seizures with diazepam (0.3 mg/kg IV). There is no specific therapy for *cannaboid* toxicity.

Patients severely toxic from *cocaine* and *CNS stimulants* may require lidocaine (1 mg/kg IV, then 20 to 50 μg/kg min) for ventricular arrhythmias, diazoxide (5 mg IV bolus) for hypertension, a cooling blanket for hyperthermia, and chlorpromazine (0.5 mg/kg IM) for sedation or acute paranoia.

Always obtain acetaminophin and ethanol levels, unless it is certain that the patient took only one drug.

The side effects of narcotic and CNS depressant withdrawl can be serious and, in some cases, life threatening (see Table 13-7). Admit all patients suspected of withdrawl from these substances for careful observation and treatment.

INDICATIONS FOR ADMISSION

- Any suicide gesture or attempt
- CNS or respiratory depression

- Hypertension, hypotension, hyperthermia
- Ventricular arrhythmia
- Narcotic overdose requiring naloxone treatment
- Suspected narcotic or CNS depressant withdrawl

REFERENCES

1. The Medical Letter 25:88, 1983
2. McGuigan MA: Emerg Clin North Am 2:87–101, 1984

Ethanol

INTRODUCTION

Ethanol is contained in alcoholic beverages (whiskey: 43–50%, beer: 3–5%, wine: 10–12%), colognes (up to 60%), mouthwashes (up to 50%), and liquid medications (acetaminophen: 7%; elixophylline: 20%). A patient is drunk at a blood level of 100 mg% and comatose at 300 mg%, while a level of 500 mg% may be fatal.

CLINICAL PRESENTATION

Mild intoxication presents with gross incoordination, ataxia, euphoria, and nausea and vomiting. With higher levels, drowsiness, slurred speech, and visual impairment occur. Finally, severe CNS depression results with stupor or coma. Young children are particularly at risk for hypoglycemia and seizures.

DIAGNOSIS

The diagnosis is usually evident, based upon the history, characteristic breath odor, incoordination, and sleepiness. *Sedative/hypnotic* (barbiturates, benzodiazepines, etc) and *narcotic ingestions* may present similarly, but without the odor of alcohol on the patient's breath. Adolescents may ingest a mixture of drugs, so the presence of alcoholic breath does not conclusively rule out other toxic substances (especially *acetaminophen*).

The diagnosis of ethanol intoxication is suggested by hyperosmolality and an increased anion gap metabolic acidosis. Obtain a serum alcohol level to confirm the diagnosis.

The volume of distribution (Vd) of ethanol is 0.6 L/kg. Therefore, the peak ethanol level (in mg/dl) can be estimated if the per cent of alcohol of the beverage (proof/2) and the approximate volume ingested are known:

$$[\text{Peak conc (mg/dl)}] = \frac{(\%\ \text{alcohol}) \times (\text{volume ingested in cc})}{0.6 \times (\text{patient's weight in kg})}$$

ER MANAGEMENT

Use ipecac with caution, as the patient may become stuporous prior to vomiting. Gastric lavage is the preferred route of gastrointestinal decontamination. Activated charcoal and cathartics do no harm and may be useful in the presence of a mixed ingestion.

If the patient is stuporous or comatose, give naloxone (4 ampules) and glucose (1 cc/kg of D50), after obtaining a dextrostix, electrolytes, glucose, CBC, and an ethanol level. Secure an IV and institute forced diuresis by giving D5 ½ NS at 2–3 times maintenance (a urine output of 3–6 cc/kg/hr is desired). Use a dextrose-containing solution to prevent alcohol-induced hypoglycemia. These patients may require respiratory support, so admit them to an intensive care setting.

If the patient is merely "drunk," close observation is all that is required. For an adolescent, this may be performed at home if the family is reliable.

Intoxicated patients are prone to falls, with resultant head trauma. A careful neurologic examination is mandatory, particularly if the history or clinical findings (bruises, scalp lacerations) are consistent with a fall. Focal findings on motor examination or asymmetric pupillary responses or extraocular movements suggest a structural component to the coma (see Head Trauma, p 393). Immediate neurologic consultation and CT scanning are indicated.

INDICATIONS FOR ADMISSION

- Intoxicated preadolescent
- Intoxicated adolescent with an unstable home environment or an alcohol level over 200 mg%
- Focal neurologic findings

REFERENCE

1. Becker CE: Emerg Clin North Am 2:47–61, 1984

Ethylene Glycol and Methanol

INTRODUCTION

Ethylene glycol is the primary ingredient in auto radiator antifreezes, and methanol is used as an antifreeze (windshield washer fluid), a solvent, and canned cooking fuel. Ethylene glycol is converted into oxalic acid, while methanol becomes formic acid and formaldehyde. The lethal dose of both is 1–2 cc/kg.

CLINICAL PRESENTATION AND DIAGNOSIS

Ethylene glycol initially causes an ethanol-like picture with nausea, vomiting, ataxia, incoordination, and euphoria. This is followed by tachypnea, cyanosis, pulmonary edema, seizures, shock, and coma. After a few days, oxalate crystals precipitate in the urine and cause acute tubular necrosis.

Methanol causes headache, nausea, and vomiting, followed by blurred vision and hyperemia of the optic discs. Respiratory failure, shock, and coma ensue.

Both chemicals cause an elevated serum osmolality and a severe increased anion gap acidosis with resultant tachypnea and stupor. A mnemonic for the poisonings and conditions which cause an anion gap acidosis is ''MUDPIES'': methanol, uremia, DKA, paraldehyde and phenformin, isoniazid and iron, ethanol and ethylene glycol, and salicylates. With ethylene glycol or methanol there is neither ketosis nor an acetone odor on the breath.

ER MANAGEMENT

Perform gastric lavage or induce emesis with ipecac. If available, obtain a methanol or ethylene glycol level, in addition to an ABG, CBC, glucose and electrolytes.

While waiting for *hemodialysis* to be arranged, treat with ethanol:

0.75 g/kg IV, followed by 0.5 g/kg IV q 4h. This must be diluted to a 5% ethanol solution in either normal saline or sodium bicarbonate. Sodium bicarbonate is also indicated for the acidosis: (16−measured HCO_3^-)×(0.3)×(weight in kg) is the dose (in cc) to be infused over 30–60 minutes.

Early hemodialysis is effective and prevents permanent vision loss in a methanol ingestion.

Admit the patient to an intensive care setting and support the respirations, if necessary.

INDICATION FOR ADMISSION

- Suspected ethylene glycol or methanol ingestion

REFERENCE

1. Becker CE: Emerg Clin North Am 2:47–61, 1984

Hydrocarbons

INTRODUCTION

Hydrocarbon ingestions cause either a chemical pneumonitis or CNS and liver toxicity. Aspiration of volatile aliphatic compounds (mineral seal oil, kerosene, gasoline, naphtha, charcoal lighter fluid) are responsible for the former, while ingestion of aromatics (benzene, nitrobenzene, toluene, xylene) and halogenated hydrocarbons (carbon tetrachloride) produce the latter. In some cases the hydrocarbon contains a toxic additive (camphor, insecticides, aniline dyes, heavy metals).

CLINICAL PRESENTATION

Most patients (especially toddlers) are asymptomatic, having only brought the bottle to their mouths, without swallowing any liquid. Often some of the material spills onto the patient's face or clothing, so that the child smells of the hydrocarbon. If an aliphatic is ingested, symptoms of tachypnea, dyspnea, coughing, gagging, and cyanosis may be seen as early as within 30 minutes of the ingestion. Conversely, the patient may remain asymptomatic for several hours.

With the ingestion of aromatic or halogenated hydrocarbons, insecticides, aniline dyes, and camphor, the patient may present with dizziness, headache, CNS depression (lethargy, coma), and seizures.

DIAGNOSIS

The nature of the compound must be determined. Therefore, have the family either call or return home in order to retrieve the bottle or read the contents label. If the ER staff is unfamiliar with a particular substance, consult a Poison Control Center, a reference text, the manufacturer, or a poisondex.

A chest x-ray is indicated for the pulmonary symptoms enumerated above, including the cases in which the patient is asymptomatic in the ER after being symptomatic at home. Otherwise, there is no need to routinely obtain radiographs in patients who may have ingested hydrocarbons.

ER MANAGEMENT

Once the substance is appropriately identified, the next issue is whether or not to induce emesis or perform gastric lavage. In general, almost all pediatric hydrocarbon ingestions are best managed by making no attempt to remove the poison. However, when the substance ingested has significant systemic toxicity and little pulmonary toxicity (benzene, nitrobenzene, heavy metals, insecticides, aniline dyes, camphor), remove any amount and admit the patient to an intensive care unit for observation.

With pine oil, halogenated hydrocarbons, xylene, toluene, and turpentine, the indication for removal is more than 1 cc/kg ingested (about four swallows). Two cc/kg (8–10 swallows) is the limit for kerosene, gasoline, naphtha, and charcoal lighter fluid. *Never* attempt to induce emesis or perform lavage if mineral seal oil (e.g., Old English furniture polish) has been ingested. Keep the patient sitting up and do not disturb him or her, as there is a serious risk of aspiration if vomiting occurs.

Immediately admit a symptomatic patient with an abnormal chest x-ray. If the patient is asymptomatic or has pulmonary symptoms but a normal x-ray, observe him or her for 6 hours. At the end of that period, discharge the patient if he or she is asymptomatic. Admit the symptomatic patient; repeat the chest x-ray and obtain an ABG and CBC, but prophylactic steroids and antibiotics are not warranted. If the patient worsens, positive end expiratory pressure (PEEP) is the treatment of choice.

INDICATIONS FOR ADMISSION

- Ingestion of hydrocarbons with significant systemic toxicity: benzene, nitrobenzene, heavy metals, insecticides, aniline dyes, camphor
- Pulmonary symptoms and an abnormal chest x-ray on arrival in the ER
- Pulmonary symptoms, with or without chest x-ray findings, after 6 hours of ER observation

REFERENCE

1. Anas N, Namasonthi V, Ginsburg CM: JAMA 246:840–843, 1981

Iron

INTRODUCTION

Iron toxicity occurs when the plasma level exceeds the iron-binding capacity (about 300 μg/dl), corresponding to an ingestion of at least 30 mg/kg of elemental iron. Ferrous gluconate is 12% elemental iron (32 mg Fe/325 mg tab), ferrous fumarate is 33% (100 mg Fe/325 mg tab), and ferrous sulfate is 20% (65 mg Fe/325 mg tab). Most multivitamins have only 10–15 mg of elemental iron per tablet.

CLINICAL PRESENTATION

Acute toxicity is triphasic. In the initial phase (first 6 hours), gastrointestinal symptoms predominate, with vomiting, hematemesis, upper abdominal pain, diarrhea, and melena. The following 6–24 hours is a latent period in which the symptoms abate. During the third phase, at 12–30 hours after ingestion, systemic toxicities are seen, with fever, hypotension, hepatic failure, shock, seizures, coma, metabolic acidosis, and hyperglycemia.

DIAGNOSIS

The diagnosis of iron overdose is easily overlooked if the history does not suggest the possibility of an ingestion. *Gastroenteritis,* especially *Salmonella* and *Shigella,* and acute *hepatitis* are likely misdiagnoses.

Clinically significant iron toxicity is possible if the history suggests that more than 30 mg/kg was ingested or the patient is symptomatic (abdominal pain, vomiting, or diarrhea).

ER MANAGEMENT

If an iron overdose cannot be ruled out, perform gastric decontamination. Use either ipecac-induced emesis or orogastric lavage with either 5% $NaHCO_3$ or Fleets Phosphosoda cathartic diluted 1:4 with water. Obtain a CBC, glucose, and KUB, to see if any radioopaque tablets remain in the gastrointestinal tract.

The following are risk factors for serious iron toxicity: (1) a white blood cell count (WBC) ≥ 15,000/mm³, (2) blood glucose ≥ 150 mg/dl, (3) vomiting before ipecac, (4) diarrhea, or (5) a positive KUB. For a patient with any of these, secure an IV and, if he or she is in shock, give 20 cc/kg of NS; otherwise, infuse a maintenance solution. Obtain an iron level and iron-binding capacity within 6 hours of ingestion (if readily available). A serum iron greater than the binding capacity (about 300 μg/dl) predicts toxicity; a level of 500 μg/dl is lethal. If an iron level is not readily available, give a test dose of 50 mg/kg of deferoxamine IM. A "vin rose" (salmon) color to the urine confirms that there is unbound iron and predicts a risk for systemic toxicity.

Positive Deferoxamine Challenge or Iron Level > 300 μg/dl. Obtain blood for electrolytes, calcium, phosphorous, liver function tests, prothrombin time (PT), and type and hold. Institute chelation therapy with deferoxamine (20 mg/kg IM q 4h) until the urine is clear. A continuous intravenous infusion (40 mg/kg over 4 hours) is reserved for patients in shock, but do not exceed an IV rate of 15 mg/kg/hr.

Negative Deferoxamine Challenge or Iron Level < 300 μg/dl. Observe the patient in the ER for 6 hours. Discharge home if he or she remains asymptomatic.

No Risk Factors. Discharge home; no observation is required (unless the patient has no phone for a follow-up check 2 hours after discharge).

INDICATION FOR ADMISSION

- Positive deferoxamine challenge or plasma iron ≥ 300 μg/dl

REFERENCES

1. Robotham JL, Lietman RS: Am J Dis Child 134:875–879, 1980
2. Lacoutre PG, Wason S, Temple AR, et al: J Pediatr 99: 89–92, 1981

Lead

INTRODUCTION

Lead toxicity usually results from chronic gastrointestinal absorption. Sources of lead include pre-World War II house paint, urban house dust, leaded gasoline, and improperly glazed pottery. A venous lead level over 56 μg/dl always requires chelation.

CLINICAL PRESENTATION

The majority of patients are asymptomatic, but are brought to the ER because they either have been observed eating paint chips or have an elevated free erythrocyte protoporphyrin (FEP) or lead on microsample screening. However, common symptoms with mild intoxications (Pb > 50 μg/dl) include restlessness, irritability, and poor appetite. With higher levels (Pb > 70 μg/dl) constipation, weakness, colicky abdominal pain, headache, and muscle soreness can occur. Acute lead encephalopathy, with persistent vomiting, focal or generalized seizures, ataxia, and increased intracranial pressure (IC), rarely occurs (Pb > 100 μg/dl).

DIAGNOSIS

Acute Encephalopathy. Always consider lead intoxication if a patient has seizures or signs of increased intracranial pressure (papilledema, VIth nerve palsy, bradycardia, hypertension). If the diagnosis is not evident, obtain a CTT scan. Once the scan is interpreted as normal, carefully perform a lumbar puncture, removing a few drops of spinal fluid. The usual findings are an elevated opening pressure, no pleocytosis, normal glucose, and an elevated protein.

Elevated Venous Lead Level. Always obtain a repeat venous specimen prior to provocation or treatment.

Elevated Micro Lead or FEP. Obtain a venous lead level, but the result is usually not rapidly available. If acute ingestion is suspected (history of eating paint chips in past 1–2 days), obtain a KUB as radioopaque lead particles may be seen in the colon (especially the sigmoid). Also obtain a CBC with peripheral blood smear and an FEP. A hypochromic, microcytic anemia with basophilic stippling of the erythrocytes is presumptive evidence of chronic lead toxicity, and an FEP over 160 μg/dl is highly suggestive of the diagnosis.

ER MANAGEMENT

Acute Encephalopathy. Prohibit oral fluid intake, establish urine output with a D10 IV solution, then limit fluids to insensible plus urinary losses. Institute chelation therapy with BAL (450 mg/M^2/day divided q 4h, deep IM). When the second dose of BAL is to be given, start a continuous IV infusion of $CaNa_2$-EDTA (1500 mg/M^2/day; no more than 500 mg/L of IV fluid). Continue therapy for 5 days. Obtain pretreatment, then daily urinalyses, electrolytes, creatinine, and calcium. Treat seizures with IV diazepam (0.3 mg/kg) and increased ICP with mannitol (0.5–1.0 g/kg IV).

Other Symptoms or Venous Lead > 70 μg/dl. Treat as for encephalopathy, using BAL (300 mg/M^2/day) and $CaNa_2$-EDTA either by continuous IV infusion (1000 mg/M^2/day) or q 4h doses of 175 mg/M^2 (IV or deep IM mixed with procaine). The BAL may be discontinued after 3 days if the Pb < 50 μg/dl. Once again, withhold oral intake and limit IV fluids to insensible plus urinary losses.

Venous Lead 56–69 µg/dl. Treat with $CaNa_2$-EDTA (1000 mg/M^2/day) via continuous IV infusion or IM (175 mg/M^2 q 4h) mixed with procaine for 5 days.

Venous Lead 25–55 µg/dl. If the FEP is >35 µg/dl, perform a $CaNa_2$-EDTA provocation test after obtaining a repeat venous lead. Give 500 mg/M^2 $CaNa_2$-EDTA IV in 250 cc/M^2 of D5 over 1 hour (or IM mixed with procaine). Collect all urine over the next 8 hours. If the ratio of urinary lead (in µg) to $CaNa_2$-EDTA given (in mg) is greater than 0.7, complete a 5-day course of 1000 mg/M^2/day of $CaNa_2$-EDTA. If the ratio is 0.60–0.69, treat children under 3 years of age, but repeat the test in 2–3 months for older patients.

INDICATIONS FOR ADMISSION

- Lead encephalopathy or other symptoms
- Venous lead level over 56 µg/dl (chelation)
- Venous lead level over 25 µg/dl with an FEP over 35 µg/dl, for $CaNa_2$-EDTA mobilization

REFERENCE

1. Piomelli S, Rosen JF, Chisolm J Jr, et al: J Pediatr 105:523–532, 1984

Mothballs

INTRODUCTION

Mothballs can be composed of two different chemicals, paradichlorobenzene, which is relatively nontoxic, and naphthalene, which can cause severe hemolysis in G-6-PD deficient patients.

CLINICAL PRESENTATION

In most cases the patient is asymptomatic. However, the onset of hemolysis in a G-6-PD-deficient patient may be delayed for up to 24–

48 hours. Weakness, pallor or jaundice, dark urine, and oliguria can occur.

DIAGNOSIS

When the chemical nature of the mothball is unknown, try dissolving a sliver in absolute ethanol—paradichlorobenzene (nontoxic) dissolves while naphthalene does not.

If the patient is symptomatic, a G-6-PD quantitative assay (not a qualitative screen) confirms that the child is at risk. The presence of hemolysis can be documented by serial hematocrit determinations, the peripheral smear (fragmented red cells), and a urinalysis (dipstix positive for blood and bilirubin, but no red blood cells [RBC] seen).

ER MANAGEMENT

Routine gastric decontamination procedures are indicated. Then, attempt to discern the nature of the mothballs and the patient's G-6-PD status. For asymptomatic patients no further work-up is necessary. Instruct the family to return at once if pallor, jaundice, lethargy, or dark urine is noticed.

If the patient is symptomatic, obtain a CBC, type and cross-match, urinalysis, electrolytes, BUN, and creatinine. If hemoglobinuria is present, institute aklaline diuresis with D5 ½ NS at three times maintenance and $NaHCO_3$ (1 mEq/kg q 4h, infused over 30 minutes). Maintain a urine output of 3–6 cc/kg/hr, using furosemide (1 mg/kg IV), if necessary. Give small transfusions (5 cc/kg) of packed red cells to maintain the hematocrit at about 80% of normal.

INDICATIONS FOR ADMISSION

- Suspected naphthalene ingestion in a patient known to be G-6-PD deficient
- Evidence of intravascular hemolysis

REFERENCE

1. Winkler JB, Kulig K, Rumack BH: Ann Emerg Med 14:30–32, 1985

Phenothiazines

INTRODUCTION

Phenothiazines such as chlorpromazine (Thorazine), thioridazine (Mellaril), and prochlorperazine (Compazine) are widely used as tranquilizers and antiemetics. The minimum toxic dose is about 15 mg/kg.

CLINICAL PRESENTATION

The most common toxic reaction is a syndrome of extrapyramidal effects, including torticollis, opisthotonus, difficulty speaking, facial grimacing, and oculogyric crisis. Onset can be delayed up to 24 hours after the ingestion. Other presentations include postural hypotension, seizures, and an anticholinergic picture (dry mouth, urinary retention, constipation, blurred vision, tachycardia).

DIAGNOSIS

The extrapyramidal syndrome can resemble *meningitis* (fever, meningeal signs) and *hysterical reactions* (previous history; strange affect, including indifference). When the diagnosis is in doubt, test the urine with either 10% ferric chloride (2 cc urine added to 0.5 cc of $FeCl_3$) or Phenistix. A purple color with either test confirms the ingestion.

ER MANAGEMENT

Since these compounds are antiemetics, ipecac may be ineffective. Gastric lavage with an orogastric hose may be required for successful gastrointestinal decontamination. Activated charcoal and cathartics are then effective.

Diphenhydramine (2 mg/kg, up to 50 mg, IV or IM) is both diagnostic and therapeutic for the extrapyramidal symptoms. Prescribe a 2-day course of diphenhydramine (5 mg/kg/day, maximum 300 mg/day, divided q 6h) to prevent a recurrence of the symptoms.

If the patient has seizures, give an IV loading dose of phenytoin (10 mg/kg) slowly over 15–20 minutes, with continuous ECG monitoring. Treat orthostatic hypotension with isotonic IV fluids (10–20 cc/kg of normal saline or lactated Ringer's). The management of an anticholinergic syndrome is detailed on p 341.

INDICATION FOR ADMISSION

- Seizures or persistent hypotension

REFERENCE

1. Lee AS: JACEP 8:351, 1977

Salicylates

INTRODUCTION

The most serious salicylate poisonings occur in patients taking aspirin chronically. In children, this often occurs as the result of therapeutic overdosage. Aspirin (acetylsalicylic acid) is in many nonprescription analgesics, and oil of wintergreen (methylsalicylate, 7.0 g/5 ml) is contained in skin liniments. The minimum acute toxic dose is 150 mg/kg; therefore the acute ingestion of an entire bottle of 36 80-mg children's aspirin tablets can poison a patient weighing up to 18 kg. A large number of salicylate tablets can retard gastric emptying or may coalesce in the stomach, resulting in prolonged absorption without a definite peak level. Chronic overdosage causes more serious toxicity at lower serum levels.

CLINICAL PRESENTATION

Mild poisoning causes tinnitus, abdominal pain, vomiting, and hyperpnea (respiratory alkalosis). With larger doses, marked hyperpnea, fever, lethargy, dehydration, metabolic acidosis, and hypo- or hyperglycemia (<300 mg%) occur. Severe poisoning leads to coma, seizures, severe metabolic acidosis, oliguria, pulmonary edema, and death. An unusual presentation is acute behavior change, including confusion, agitation, hallucinations, or a psychosis-like picture.

DIAGNOSIS

In an acute one-time overdose, a serum salicylate level at 6 hours postingestion predicts the severity of the poisoning and urgency of treatment. The minimum toxic level is 45 mg/dl; 65 mg/dl causes a moderate poisoning, 90 mg/dl is serious, and 120 mg/dl is often lethal (Fig. 13-2). Toxicity is more severe at any level in the presence of an uncorrected metabolic acidosis.

A urine $FeCl_3$ test provides qualitative proof of salicylate ingestion. To perform the test, add 0.5 ml of 10% $FeCl_3$ to 2 ml of urine—a purple color confirms the presence of salicylates. Acetone (in DKA) can also give a positive test, so heat the urine first to remove the acetone if the patient is diabetic.

A blood gas and serum electrolytes reveal a respiratory alkalosis early with a normal or elevated pO_2. An increased anion gap acidosis may develop at the same time or slightly later, and hypo- or hyperglycemia can occur.

Salicylate poisoning can be confused clinically with *diabetic ketoacidosis* (glucose usually > 300 mg/dl, polyuria), *influenza* (myalgias, upper respiratory infection [URI] symptoms), *pneumonia* (rales, infiltrate on chest x-ray), *gastroenteritis* (diarrhea more common, increased anion gap is uncommon), *ketotic hypoglycemia* (starvation, no acid-base disturbance unless postictal), *Reye syndrome* (elevated serum ammonia), or a *primary neuropsychiatric disturbance*. Other causes of an increased anion gap include (''MUDPIES''): methanol poisoning, uremia, DKA, paraldehyde, phenformin, iron, isoniazid, ethanol and ethylene glycol poisoning, and lactic acidosis (shock, idiopathic).

ER MANAGEMENT

Once the diagnosis is confirmed, institute basic measures (emesis/gastric lavage, activated charcoal, cathartic), secure an IV, and obtain blood for ABG, electrolytes, glucose, salicylate level, PT, and CBC.

If the patient has an altered mental status, give 0.5 g/kg of dextrose IV and maintain the serum glucose level at approximately 150 mg/dl. If the patient is dehydrated or in shock, give a bolus of 20 ml/kg of a solution made by adding one 50-cc ampule (44 mEq) of $NaHCO_3$ to 500 cc of D5 ½ NS. If adequate urine output (1 cc/kg/hr) is not established, give a second bolus of normal saline or lactated Ringer's.

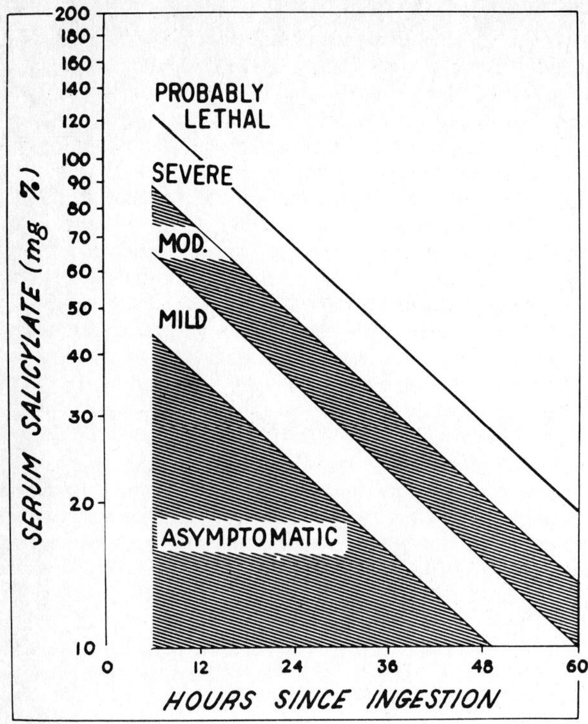

Figure 13-2. Nomogram relating serum salicylate level to severity of intoxication at varying intervals after acute ingestion of single doses of aspirin. Nomogram starts at 6 hours to ensure that levels will not be interpreted before they have reached their peak; it can be used earlier if more than one level is obtained to establish that level is on decline. *(Done AK: Aspirin overdosage: incidence, diagnosis, and management. Pediatrics 62 (5 Suppl): 895, 1978. Reproduced by Permission of Pediatrics.)*

Then, infuse a solution of D5W with 44 mEq/L of $NaHCO_3$ and 20–40 mEq/L of KCl at 2–4 times maintenance rate. The goal is a urine output of 3 cc/hr with a pH >7.5, since salicylate reabsorption in the kidney tubules is inhibited at an alkaline urine pH. Begin treatment before the 6-hour salicylate level is drawn.

Carefully monitor the serum K^+ since it is lowered by both $NaHCO_3$ administration and hyperventilation. A serum K^+ in the normal range is necessary for achieving an alkaline diuresis.

Dialysis is indicated for a salicylate level over 100 mg/dl, severe acidosis, oliguria or anuria, pulmonary edema, intractable seizures, or progressive deterioration despite appropriate therapy.

Treat fever with sponging or an ice mattress. Give vitamin K (2 mg IM), if the PT is more than 2 seconds longer than control.

INDICATIONS FOR ADMISSION

- Salicylate level >45 mg/dl 6 hours after an acute ingestion
- Signs and symptoms of salicylism in a patient taking salicylates chronically, regardless of the serum level

REFERENCE

1. Done AK: Pediatrics 62(5 Suppl):890–895, 1978

Theophylline

INTRODUCTION

Many bronchodilator medications contain either theophylline or aminophylline (80–85% theophylline) and are marketed under a multitude of brand names. While the therapeutic range of theophylline is 10–20 mg/L, there is little risk of serious toxicity until a serum level of 40 mg/L is reached. With a volume of distribution of about 0.5 L/kg, the minimum toxic dose of theophylline is about 20 mg/kg.

CLINICAL PRESENTATION

Vomiting, agitation, tremors, headache, and tachycardia are possible with a therapeutic serum level. Large doses can cause ventricular arrhythmias (premature ventricular contractions [PVC], ventricular tachycardia), hypertension, seizures, and coma. These more serious clinical findings may rarely occur without any preceding minor symptoms and the seizures may be particularly difficult to treat.

DIAGNOSIS

If a theophylline overdose is suspected, obtain a serum level. In general, the peak level occurs within 3 or 4 hours of ingestion. However, there are many sustained release preparations on the market. If one of these is ingested, the serum level may continue to rise for up to 12–16 hours or more. Always obtain a second specimen 4–6 hours after the first.

ER MANAGEMENT

Gastric decontamination is effective, including emesis/lavage, activated charcoal, and cathartics. Repeating the instillation of activated charcoal every 2 hours is beneficial.

Charcoal hemoperfusion, performed in an intensive care setting, is the treatment of choice for patients with dangerously high levels (≥60 mg/L), coma, seizures, and severe arrhythmias (ventricular tachycardia).

INDICATIONS FOR ADMISSION

- Coma, seizures, ventricular tachycardia
- Initial theophylline level ≥30 mg/L
- Any theophylline ingestion that is a suicide gesture or attempt

REFERENCE

1. Gaudreault P, Wason J, Lovejoy FH: J Pediatr 102: 474–476, 1983

14

Neurologic Emergencies

Acute Ataxia

INTRODUCTION

Disorders affecting the cerebellum or its major pathways cause ataxia, manifested as an unsteady, reeling, wide-based gait or truncal instability (titubation). Dysmetria, intention tremor, slow, dysrhythmic "scanning" speech, and lateral gaze nystagmus may also be present. Although intoxications (especially alcohol, phenytoin) and viral infections are the most likely causes (Table 14-1), always consider an intracranial (posterior fossa) mass lesion and hydrocephalus.

CLINICAL PRESENTATION

Acute Cerebellar Ataxia Typically, a 1- to 3-year old presents with a short history (hours to days) of uncoordination, unsteady gait, or tremor. The mental status and the remainder of the examination are normal. Most often, the syndrome occurs several days to weeks following a viral respiratory infection. The ataxia may precede or follow the appearance of an exanthem. The cerebrospinal fluid (CSF) may be normal, or there may be a mild pleocytosis or elevation of the protein. The prognosis is excellent; recovery is rapid (usually within 4–6 weeks), but as many as 10–20% of patients have sequelae of variable severity.

Other Causes of Ataxia In most of the disorders noted in Table 14-1, the lethargy associated with the ataxia helps to distinguish them from acute cerebellar ataxia. Posterior fossa tumors are associated with headaches, vomiting, and an insidious onset. In the Miller-Fisher variant of Guillain-Barré syndrome, ataxia is accompanied by ophthalmoplegia and areflexia. This may be followed by an ascending

TABLE 14-1. CAUSES OF ACUTE ATAXIA

Acute cerebellar ataxia
- Viral infections
  - Infectious mononucleosis
  - Mumps, measles, varicella, CMV, enteroviruses

Intoxications
- Ethanol
- Phenytoin
- Antihistamines

Posterior fossa tumor

Otitis media (labyrinthitis)

Guillain-Barré syndrome

Bacterial meningitis

Disorders of lactate and pyruvate metabolism

Hydrocephalus

weakness and autonomic symptoms (flushing, pulse and blood pressure changes, gastrointestinal symptoms).

DIAGNOSIS

Attempt to ascertain the time of onset of the symptoms (chronic ataxia usually results from tumors or metabolic disorders), and whether there was any antecedent *trauma, viral illness,* rash, or *toxin* exposure. Inquire about the possibility of ingestion or overuse of an anticonvulsant, sedative, or antihistamine preparation.

Pertinent physical examination findings include a typical exanthem (*varicella, measles*); cervical adenopathy, nasal congestion, and splenomegaly (*infectious mononucleosis*); the odor of *alcohol* on the breath (intoxication); or fever and nuchal rigidity (meningitis).

A careful neurologic examination is necessary to confirm the presence of ataxia, search for associated findings, and rule out a posterior fossa mass lesion. Note the head circumference and carefully examine the fundi (disc margins, presence of spontaneous venous pulsations) for evidence of intracranial hypertension (p 397). Remember that in toddlers, the sutures may split before eye ground changes appear. Other evidence of a posterior fossa tumor may include neck stiffness, head tilt, cranial nerve palsies (facial weakness, ophthalmoplegia), or long tract findings (hemiparesis, extensor plantar responses). Tone and reflexes may be diminished in the ataxic patient, but consider Guillain-Barré syndrome if the patient is areflexic.

In acute cerebellar ataxia the sensory examination is normal, and although tone may be somewhat diminished, there is no focal weakness.

ER MANAGEMENT

A CTT scan must be obtained prior to preforming a lumbar puncture if the patient is lethargic in order to rule out an expanding posterior fossa lesion. Other indications for an immediate CTT scan include papilledema or focal neurologic findings. The management of increased intracranial pressure is discussed on p 398.

Perform a lumbar puncture, including a measurement of the opening pressure. Obtain serum electrolytes for comparison of the glucose with the CSF glucose, and, if intoxication is suspected, a serum osmolality (increased with ethanol).

In cases of suspected ingestion (see pp 334–338), obtain a blood level of the drug (eg, ethanol, phenytoin, phenobarbital). If infectious mononucleosis (p 302) is suspected, a complete blood count (CBC), heterophile, and slide agglutination test are indicated.

INDICATIONS FOR ADMISSION

- All patients with ataxia until the diagnosis is established and the course stabilized

REFERENCE

1. Weiss S, Carter S: Neurology 9:711, 1959

Acute Hemiparesis

INTRODUCTION

Acute hemiparesis is a rare event during childhood. The numerous causes can be grouped into a few etiologic categories including thrombotic and embolic events, hemorrhage, trauma, mass lesions, and the idiopathic syndrome of acute infantile hemiplegia (Table 14-2).

TABLE 14-2. CAUSES OF ACUTE HEMIPARESIS IN CHILDHOOD

Intracranial hemorrhage
- Arteriovenous malformation rupture
- Aneurysm
- Blood dyscrasia
- Hemorrhage into a tumor

Head trauma

Mass lesion
- Abscess (trauma, cyanotic heart disease)
- Neoplasm

Thrombotic events
- Posttraumatic carotid occlusion
  - Penetrating oral trauma
  - Tonsillectomy
- Venous thrombosis
  - Dehydration
  - Cyanotic heart disease with polycythemia
  - Infection (meningitis, mastoiditis, encephalitis, sinusitis)
  - Sickle cell anemia
  - Collagen vascular disease (lupus, polyarteritis nodosa, mucocutaneous lymph node syndrome)
- Idiopathic occlusion of the intracranial carotid artery

Embolic event
- Subacute bacterial endocarditis
- Prosthetic valve
- Atrial myxoma

Hemiplegic migraine[a]

Acute infantile hemiplegia[a]

[a]Diagnosis of exclusion.

CLINICAL PRESENTATION

In the mildest form, acute hemiparesis presents as a tendency to adopt the decorticate posture. This involves shoulder adduction, flexion of the elbow, wrist, and fingers, pronation of the hand, extension of the knee, and plantar flexion of the foot. More severe or acutely evolving lesions can produce flaccidity and hemiplegia. Usually, hemiparesis is accompanied by hyperreflexia, spasticity, and extensor plantar reflexes (corticospinal tract signs).

An intracranial hemorrhage typically has a sudden onset and rapid evolution. Headache, vomiting, and obtundation are common, and there may be other signs of increased intracranial pressure, such as hypertension, bradycardia, and papilledema (p 397).

Acute infantile hemiplegia presents with sudden weakness, accompanied by fever, altered mental status, and prolonged or repetitive seizure activity. The motor deficit persists for more than 1 week and is often followed by intractable seizures and slowed mentation. The typical patient is under 3 years of age and previously well.

DIAGNOSIS

In general, determining the etiology of the hemiparesis can be deferred to the inpatient setting. However, inquire about the rate of onset of the weakness, and the occurrence of seizures, fever, *intraoral* or *head trauma, infections* (upper respiratory, sinusitis, mastoiditis), or change in mental status. Ask about past medical illnesses (*sickle cell disease, cardiac malformations, lupus, coagulopathies, seizure disorder*).

On physical examination, check for nuchal rigidity. If present, suspect an infectious process (*meningitis, encephalitis*) or a *subarachnoid hemorrhage*. Look for cyanosis or signs of head or neck trauma and auscultate the head and neck for a bruit and the chest for a cardiac murmur.

Perform a thorough neurologic examination. Assess the mental status. A limited unilateral, nonexpanding structural hemispheric lesion does not in itself cause a change in mental status. If the patient is lethargic, consider a hemorrhage, stroke, bilateral disease, accompanying metabolic defect, infectious disease, or postictal state.

ER MANAGEMENT

Management is the priority over etiologic diagnosis. Perform a quick survey to assess the adequacy of the airway, breathing, and cardiovascular function, and obtain a complete set of vital signs. Check the pupils, extraocular movements, fundi (for papilledema) and level of consciousness. Secure an IV with D5 ½ NS after obtaining blood for a CBC, platelet count, erythrocyte sedimentation rate (ESR), sickle prep (if patient's status is unknown), electrolytes, glucose and dextrostix, PT and PTT, liver function tests, arterial blood gas, and blood culture (if febrile).

Immediately summon a pediatric neurologist and neurosurgeon and arrange for a CTT scan. If there is no evidence of increased intracranial (ICP) pressure on the scan, perform a lumbar puncture (including opening pressure) and obtain specimens for cell count, protein and glucose, culture, and Gram stain.

The management of increased intracranial pressure (p 398), meningitis (p 286), sickle cell disease (p 273), headache (p 391), and enecephalitis (p 296) is discussed elsewhere.

INDICATION FOR ADMISSION

- Acute hemiparesis or hemiplegia

REFERENCES

1. Gold AP, Carter S: Pediatr Clin North Am 23:413–433, 1976
2. Gold AP, Challenor YB, Gilles FH, et al: Stroke 4:835, 1007, 1973

Acute Weakness

INTRODUCTION

Although acute weakness is uncommon in childhood, it usually heralds a significant neurologic disorder.

CLINICAL PRESENTATION AND DIAGNOSIS

The history is vital in defining the underlying process. Determine the time of onset, progression, pattern of weakness (unilateral, bilateral, hemi-, di-, or quadriparetic, flaccid versus spastic) and associated systemic features.

Guillain-Barré Syndrome. Guillain-Barré syndrome is usually a post infectious or postinfluenza vaccination phenomenon, characterized by premonitory vague sensory symptoms, ascending motor weakness, and depressed or absent reflexes. About 10% of patients have significant respiratory and/or autonomic dysfunction.

Botulism. Botulism-induced weakness (see p 292), resulting from release of endotoxin, is characterized by a fairly rapid progression of cranial nerve dysfunction (diplopia, ptosis, dysarthria, dysphagia), and weakness.

Polio and Diptheria. Polio and diptheria, now rare, can also cause acute weakness.

Spinal Cord. Spinal cord pathology can produce acute weakness with either paraplegia or quadriplegia. *Trauma* is the most likely cause. Patients with *Down syndrome* are particularly susceptible to C_1-C_2 subluxations that can result in quadriparesis. The presence of fever and vertebral tenderness strongly suggests a *spinal epidural abscess*—a neurosurgical emergency. *Myelitis,* an inflammatory process of the spinal cord, may result in para- or quadraparesis.

Metabolic Causes. Metabolic causes (hypokalemia, hypo- and hypercalcemia, hypo- and hyperthyroidism) are quite rare in childhood and usually have associated systemic manifestations.

Acute or subacute weakness with a rash, fever, and myalgias, suggests an inflammatory process such as *dermatomyositis, polymyositis,* or *systemic lupus erythematosus.*

When weakness is more episodic, consider the *periodic paralyses* and *myasthenia gravis.* The latter is characterized by fatigue which is provoked by repetitive or prolonged activity. Associated symptoms may include horizontal and vertical diplopia, ptosis, dysphonia, dysarthria, and respiratory symptoms.

Certain *toxins,* especially the anticholinesterase-inhibiting insecticides (organophosphates, carbamates) cause acute weakness.

Psychogenic Causes. Consider psychogenic causes when the history and physical examination fail to suggest an organic etiology, and the neurologic examination shows neurophysiologic inconsistencies.

ER MANAGEMENT

Perform a careful neurologic examination to define the extent and pattern of weakness. Ask about bladder fullness, and percuss the lower abdomen for a distended bladder, and check the rectal tone. Obtain a CBC, electrolytes, and glucose, and, if the patient is febrile, a blood culture and ESR. A lumbar puncture is indicated, particularly if Guillain-Barré is suspected, but it can be delayed until after consultation with a pediatric neurologist.

Observe the patient's respiratory efforts, and obtain an arterial blood gas (ABG) to document the adequacy of ventilation.

The management of the *trauma* victim is detailed on p 488. If there is any history of trauma, the patient must not be manipulated. Obtain the appropriate spine films (cervical, areas of tenderness) and consult with a neurosurgeon and a pediatric neurologist.

INDICATION FOR ADMISSION

- Acute weakness of any etiology except psychogenic

REFERENCE

1. Spiro AJ: Pediatr Ann 6:149–161, 1977

Bell Palsy

INTRODUCTION

Bell palsy is idiopathic facial weakness arising from a peripheral VII nerve lesion.

CLINICAL PRESENTATION

The typical presentation is a sudden, nonprogressive unilateral weakness involving the upper and lower halves of the face, often preceded by ipsilateral periauricular pain. Other complaints may include hyperacusis, excessive tearing from the ipsilateral eye, or difficulty with eating or drinking. Occasionally there is an associated ipsilateral otitis media or mastoiditis.

DIAGNOSIS

Other etiologies of acute facial nerve palsy include *trauma* to the face or fractures of the petrous bone or styloid process, *infections* (Lyme disease, varicella, parotitis, infectious mononucleosis), *tumors* (neurofibromatosis, cerebellopontine angle brainstem tumors), *hypertension,* and the *Guillain-Barré syndrome* (usually bilateral facial palsy and ascending symmetric flaccid weakness with areflexia). Chronic causes such as *birth trauma, hypothroidism, infantile hypercalcemia,* and congenital absence of the VII nerve nuclei (*Möbius syndrome*) can almost always be excluded by the history.

Ascertain that the weakness is isolated to the peripheral or intranuclear facial nerve. Peripheral facial lesions are manifested by weakness of *all* the ipsilateral muscles of facial expression, while central or supranuclear lesions cause weakness of the lower facial muscles with sparing of the frontalis muscle (the patient can wrinkle his entire forehead).

A careful neurologic examination, including testing of cranial nerves II–XII (especially V, VI, and VIII), is essential to rule out other neurologic etiologies (Guillain-Barré). Evaluate gait, coordination, reflexes, and plantar responses; abnormalities suggest a *posterior fossa lesion.*

On physical examination, note the blood pressure and look for rashes (Lyme disease, varicella, herpes), café-au-lait spots (neurofibromatosis), otitis media, a displaced pinna (mastoiditis), and generalized adenopathy and splenomegaly (infectious mononucleosis).

ER MANAGEMENT

Bell Palsy. Perform a fluorescein test (p 410) to rule out a corneal abrasion. Give artificial tears to be instilled in the affected eye (1–2 gtt q 2h) and an eye patch to be worn at night to prevent drying of the cornea. Contact lenses should not be worn. If the patient is seen on the first or second day of the illness, start a 10-day course of prednisone (2 mg/kg/day to a maximum of 60 mg divided qid) if there is no evidence of infection.

Advise the patient to report any eye pain or discomfort (possible corneal abrasion) immediately. See all patients again within 10 days to check for improvement. If none is noted, refer the patient to a neurologist for electromyography.

The prognosis varies with the severity of the initial palsy. Approximately 80% of patients recover completely, generally within 2 months, and improvement usually begins within 1 to 2 weeks of diagnosis.

Other Etiologies. The presence of facial nerve weakness does not usually alter the treatment of the associated problem. The management of mastoiditis (pp 101–110), Guillain-Barré syndrome (p 376), infectious mononucleosis (p 302), head trauma (p 393), and increased intracranial pressure (p 397) are discussed elsewhere. If otitis media associated with a facial nerve palsy does not improve after two days of oral antibiotics, perform tympanocentesis, culture the middle-ear fluid, and admit the patient for IV antibiotics (ampicillin and chloramphenicol). If the diagnosis is in doubt, consult a pediatric neurologist.

INDICATIONS FOR ADMISSION

- Acute facial nerve palsy associated with progressive weakness, evidence of a mass lesion, hypertension, central nervous system (CNS) infection, mastoiditis, acute trauma, or other serious signs
- Acute facial nerve palsy associated with otitis media unresponsive to oral antibiotics

REFERENCE

1. Adour KK: N Engl J Med 307:348, 1982

Breathholding Spells

INTRODUCTION

Breathholding spells typically begin between 6 and 18 months of age and usually disappear by 6 years. Most patients have no more than one attack per month, although 10% have two or more each day. In 25% there is a positive family history of breathholding.

CLINICAL PRESENTATION

Breathholding spells are brief, lasting about 30 seconds. There are two distinct types, cyanotic and pallid. A *cyanotic* spell follows a frustrating event in which the child cries briefly, then develops apnea, cyanosis, and loss of consciousness. Rigid limbs and opisthotonus may be seen. A *pallid* spell has a more rapid onset following a frightening event or occipital trauma, after which the child starts crying, stops breathing, loses consciousness, and becomes pale and limp.

DIAGNOSIS

The diagnosis is made by history, as these children generally appear well by the time they arrive in the ER. Breathholding spells are most often confused with *seizures*. However, before a convulsion there is rarely an external precipitating factor, sustained crying, or cyanosis. Infrequently, a *syncopal episode* may be misdiagnosed. Fainting is very unusual in young children and is usually not associated with rigidity or opisthotonus.

ER MANAGEMENT

If the history of the event is typical and a thorough neurologic examination is normal, reassure the family as to the benign nature of the episode (no risk of epilepsy). Instruct the parents to be consistent when disciplining the child and not allow him or her to derive some secondary gain from the episodes (do not pick up the child). Refer patients with frequent (one/day) breathholding spells to a pediatric neurologist.

If the history is unusual or unclear, obtain a CBC, dextrostix, electrolytes, glucose, and calcium, and perform an electrocardiogram (ECG) with rhythm strip (see syncope, p 44, and cyanosis, p 37). If a seizure cannot be ruled out from the history, ask about a family history of seizures or a possible ingestion, look for ash-leaf or café-au-lait spots on the skin, and schedule an electroencephalogram (EEG).

INDICATION FOR ADMISSION

- Cyanotic episode that cannot be confidently diagnosed as a breathholding spell

REFERENCE
1. Lombroso CT, Lerman P: Pediatrics 39:563, 1967

Coma

INTRODUCTION

Coma results from dysfunction of either the brainstem or both cerebral hemispheres. Structural lesions compress or destroy the brainstem. In children the etiology is usually intracranial bleeding and swelling secondary to head trauma, while tumors, spontaneous hemorrhages, and ischemic strokes are rare. Toxic-metabolic (TM) states depress function in both cerebral hemispheres and may affect the brainstem as well. TM coma results from either endogenous (uremia, liver failure, respiratory failure, DKA) or exogenous (salicylate, tricyclic, sedative, carbon monoxide, narcotic poisonings) toxins, cerebral hypoxia or hypoperfusion, or hypoglycemia. Distinguishing between structural and TM coma is critical since structural coma represents a potential surgical emergency while TM coma can usually be managed medically.

CLINICAL PRESENTATION AND DIAGNOSIS

> Three elements of the physical examination allow differentiation of structural from TM coma: the pupillary response, the extraocular movements (EOM), and the motor response to pain.

Fixed or asymmetrical pupils strongly suggest structural coma. A minimal but symmetrical response usually indicates a functioning brainstem, implying TM coma. However, the earliest stage of central herniation can produce small, sluggish pupils indistinguishable from those seen in many TM states. Therefore, clinical evidence of a structural etiology (signs of trauma) or neurologic signs of asymmetry or progression (Table 14-3) must never be ignored. The few TM states that can truly fix the pupils must be considered (Table 14-4) whenever nonreactive pupils are encountered.

The EOM can be tested with the doll's eyes maneuver or, when

TABLE 14-3. CLINICAL PROGRESSION OF HERNIATION SYNDROMES

Stage	Consciousness	Pupils	EOM	Motor
CENTRAL HERNIATION				
Diencephalic	+/−	Small Reactive	Normal	Normal Decorticate
Midbrain	−	Fixed Midposition	Normal Asymmetrical	Decorticate Decerebrate
Pons	−	Fixed Midposition	Absent	Decerebrate Flaccid
Medulla	−	Fixed/dilated	Absent	Flaccid
UNCAL HERNIATION				
Early	+/−	One eye dilated	Normal Asymmetrical	Normal Asymmetrical
Late	−	Fixed/dilated	Asymmetrical Absent	Decorticate Decerebrate

head or neck injury is suspected, cold water vestibular stimulation. Intact doll's eyes are manifested by transient conjugate deviation away from the direction of rapid head rotation, and intact cold caloric responses involve conjugate deviation toward the stimulated ear. These responses usually indicate a functioning brainstem (TM coma), asymmetrical responses are seen with structural coma, and absent EOM imply brainstem depression from either structural lesions or profound TM states.

An asymmetrical motor response to painful stimuli (pin prick, pinch) is seen with structural coma. Absent motor responses or symmetrical posturing can result from either structural lesions or profound TM states. Progression from meaningful responses to posturing and then to flaccidity suggests one of the herniation syndromes listed in Table 14-3.

ER MANAGEMENT

The priority is stabilization of the vital signs (see pp 1–5). Initial blood tests include a CBC, electrolytes, BUN, dextrostix and glucose, and

TABLE 14-4. TOXIC-METABOLIC CAUSES OF FIXED PUPILS

	Pupils	Characteristics	Diagnosis/ Laboratory
Anoxia	Fixed, dilated	Antecedent history of shock, cardiac or respiratory arrest, etc	None
Anticholinergic agents, eg, tricyclics, atropine	Fixed, dilated	Tachycardia; warm, dry skin QRS >.12 sec	Physostigmine[a]
Cholinergic agents, eg, organophosphates	May be small with barely perceptible reflex	Diaphoresis, vomiting, incontinence	Atropine
Opiates, eg, heroin	Very small with barely perceptive reflex	Needle marks, history of overdose	Naloxone
Hypothermia	May be fixed	History of exposure	T < 90°F
Barbiturates, glutethimide	May be midsized or dilated and fixed	History of overdose	Serum levels

[a]Do not use routinely.

an ABG. If the etiology is unknown, a serum osmolality, prothrombin time (PT), liver function tests, and various toxicologic levels (barbiturates, alcohol, aspirin) may be useful. Save an additional red top tube for future analysis. Establish an intravenous line and give all patients IV glucose (1 cc/kg of D50) and naloxone (0.01 mg/kg) for diagnostic and therapeutic purposes.

The management of head trauma is directed at decreasing intracranial pressure and identifying neurosurgically treatable lesions, although the vital signs remain the first priority. When head trauma is suspected, the neck must be immobilized until cervical fractures are ruled out (p 481). The Glasgow Coma Scale (p 395) provides a rapid means of assessing progression and prognosis in these patients. Intubate all comatose head trauma victims and give 100% O_2 to minimize brain hypoxia and edema. Other initial measures for managing these patients are described on pp 397–399, including hyperventilation to a pCO_2 of 25 torr, IV mannitol (0.5–1 g/kg), IV dexamethasone (0.4 mg/kg to maximum 16 mg), and placement of an orogastric tube and Foley catheter. Once the C-spine is cleared radiographically, an emergency CT scan is indicated to assess the need for surgery.

When the etiology of the coma is unknown and the vital signs are stable, treatment can be directed by the results of the coma examination, as outlined above. If structural coma is suspected, management is as described for head trauma, including an emergency CT scan to identify the lesion. If TM coma is suspected, the situation is generally less urgent. A key exception is the patient with suspected meningitis who requires an immediate lumbar puncture followed by appropriate antibiotics (pp 285–288). The general approach to TM coma involves supporting the vital signs and correcting abnormalities in acid-base and electrolyte status. A toxic ingestion may require gastric lavage, activated charcoal, cathartics, and supportive therapy (see pp 334–338).

INDICATION FOR ADMISSION

- All comatose patients

REFERENCES

1. Plum F, Posner JB: The Diagnosis of Stupor and Coma, 3rd ed. Philadelphia, Davis, 1980
2. Cardonna J, Simon R: Int Anesthesiol Clin 17:3–18, 1979

Febrile Seizures

INTRODUCTION

Febrile seizures occur in 3–4% of children from 3 months to 6 years of age during a febrile illness which does not involve the central nervous system. The risk of a seizure is greatest on the first day of the illness, and the convulsion often occurs before the parents detect the child's fever.

CLINICAL PRESENTATION

Typically, the seizure is generalized and brief (usually <10 minutes), and it almost always has stopped prior to arrival in the ER. "Complex" febrile seizures, on the other hand, have one or more of the following features: focality (before, during, or after the seizure), prolonged duration (>15 minutes), and multiple occurrences within 24 hours. Seizures occurring with fever in a patient with prior central nervous system dysfunction or developmental problems are also considered "complex."

DIAGNOSIS

Approximately 10% of patients with CNS infections, particularly *bacterial meningitis,* present with a seizure. Older patients often have meningeal signs, but younger children may lack the typical clinical manifestations and simply be irritable or lethargic. Other, less common, causes of seizures with fever include *Shigella gastroenteritis* (seizure may occur prior to the diarrhea), a diptheria, pertussis, tetanus *(DPT) reaction, subdural hematoma,* certain *ingestions* such as anticholinergics or salicylates, and *electrolyte abnormalities,* particularly hypoglycemia, severe hyponatremia (<120 mEq/L), and hypocalcemia (<7.0 mEq/L).

ER MANAGEMENT

The primary objectives are (1) prevention of further convulsions, (2) diagnosis of central nervous system infection, (3) determination of other etiologies for the seizure, and (4) control of fever. Treat a prolonged febrile seizure, continuing at the time of arrival in the ER, as status epilepticus (see p 401).

Determine whether the seizure was indeed typical (brief, generalized, and solitary in a patient without prior CNS dysfunction or infection). Ask about oral intake (hypoglycemia and electrolyte disturbances), diarrhea in the patient or family members, recent immunizations (pertussis), or medication use. Physical examination usually reveals a source for the fever that should be appropriately treated.

Because young children can have meningitis without the typical manifestations (stiff neck, headache), perform a lumbar puncture in every patient under 18 months of age unless he or she is able to walk and act in what seems to be his or her normal fashion.

If there is no identifiable fever source and the patient is under the age of 2 years, evaluate for occult bacteremia. Obtain a CBC, dextrostix, urinalysis, cultures of the blood, urine and stool, and a chest x-ray. Obtain serum electrolytes and glucose if the destrostix is borderline or low (<45–90 mg%), there is any suspicion of other electrolyte disturbances, or a lumbar puncture is to be performed. A calcium determination is unnecessary unless hypocalcemia seems likely (carpopedal spasm, stridor, or laryngospasm).

There is no evidence that EEG findings influence prognosis or guide treatment, even for patients with risk factors for epilepsy; an EEG is certainly not indicated for patients with simple febrile seizures.

Routine measures for the treatment of the fever (acetaminophen, encouraging fluid intake) are the mainstay of therapy. Anticonvulsant therapy is not necessary in patients with simple febrile seizures, and is typically not instituted until there have been multiple febrile seizures (>3). Some children have 2 (or more) febrile seizures within the same illness. In general, only vigorous antipyresis is required. However, suspect a CNS infection, and carefully reevaluate the child's behavior and mental status to decide whether a lumbar puncture is indicated.

Anticonvulsant therapy is usually reserved for patients with two or more risk factors for epilepsy (see below) or three or more febrile seizures. Once instituted, treatment is usually continued for 2 years or 1 year after the last seizure, whichever is longer. Phenobarbital is the drug of choice. Give a loading dose of 10–15 mg/kg, preferably orally, to a maximum of 500 mg, followed in 18–24 hours by maintenance therapy of 5 mg/kg/day in one or two doses. Warn parents about transient (7–14 days) sedation and unsteadiness. "Hyperactivity," however, is usually not transient and is often so bothersome that it is an indication for stopping therapy. Do not use phenytoin or carbamazepine. Although valproate has been shown to be as efficacious as phenobarbital, the risk of hepatotoxicity outweighs the benefits of preventing future febrile seizures.

One-third of the children who have a febrile seizure have at least one recurrence, and one-half of these have a third convulsion. Nearly one-half of the recurrences happen within 6 months and 75% within a year of the initial seizure. The likelihood of recurrences varies inversely with the age of onset (> 50% in those <1 yr). However, recurrence of febrile seizures does not increase the risk of epilepsy. The risk factors for epilepsy include (1) a family history of epilepsy (not febrile seizures), (2) a complicated initial seizure (prolonged, focal, multiple), and (3) a preexisting neurologic or developmental abnormality. Patients with one risk factor have a 2% chance of developing epilepsy by age 7 years, while children with two risk factors have a 10% risk. Although it is controversial, treat the latter group with phenobarbital (see above). Reassure the parents that febrile seizures do not cause brain damage or mental retardation. Inform them that most children never have a second febrile seizure and that few develop epilepsy.

See patients with a first febrile seizure within a week. This is especially important for patients who have started anticonvulsant medication. Repeated seizures, lethargy, or irritability and fever are indications for immediate return to the ER.

INDICATIONS FOR ADMISSION

- Suspicion of a serious underlying disease (meningitis)
- Parents too anxious to cope with the situation

REFERENCES

1. Nelson KB, Ellenberg JH: Pediatrics 61:720–726, 1978
2. Consensus Statement: Pediatrics 66:1009–1012, 1980
3. Gerber MA, Berliner BC: Am J Dis Child 135:431–433, 1981

Headache

INTRODUCTION

Although most headaches in children are psychogenic (emotional or functional headaches) or due to muscle contraction (tension headaches), there are a number of serious intracranial and extracranial etiologies (Table 14-5) that must always be eliminated from consideration before the patient is discharged from the ER.

TABLE 14-5. COMMON CAUSES OF HEADACHE

Psychogenic (emotional, functional)	Muscle contraction (tension)
Intracranial Etiologies	Extracranial etiologies
Meningitis	Sinusitis
Brain abscess	Dental infection
Brain tumor	Visual abnormality
Pseudotumor cerebri	Migraines (vascular)
Head trauma	Common
Systemic Infections	Classic
Group A *Streptococcus*	Hemiplegic
Influenza	Ophthalmoplegic
Mycoplasma pneumoniae	Basilar artery

CLINICAL PRESENTATION

Psychogenic Headaches

These usually occur between 6 years of age and adolescence. They may be triggered by a recent emotional or traumatic event and tend to be dull, occipital, and prolonged, sometimes lasting for a week or more. The headaches typically occur in the late afternoon or evening, are relieved by analgesics, and are not accompanied by other neurologic signs and symptoms. The severity and frequency are not progressive. Often there are associated personality changes such as poor school performance, sleep disturbances, aggression, lack of energy, and self-deprecatory behavior.

Muscle Contraction Headaches

Tension headaches are of prolonged duration, without prodromal symptoms. The pain is symmetrical, dull or achy, and usually starts in the neck or muscles of the shoulder or upper back and moves anteriorly to the forehead or top of the head.

Intracranial Etiologies

Meningitis. The headache of bacterial meningitis is generalized, constant, often described as "throbbing all over," and associated with fever, toxicity, nuchal rigidity, and other meningeal signs. Viral meningitis causes a similar presentation, usually during summertime epidemics, but with a variable degree of nuchal rigidity.

Brain Abscess. A child with a brain abscess may present with a nonspecific headache, usually accompanied by fever, vomiting, and sometimes diplopia, convulsions, or altered mental status. Predisposing factors are congenital heart disease with right-to-left shunting and ethmoid or frontal sinusitis that has been unresponsive to therapy.

Brain Tumor. The headache of a brain tumor is intermittent initially, but very quickly increases in frequency and severity. It is often present in the very early morning hours, may awaken the child from sleep, and can be associated with projectile vomiting. Localization is uncommon, but severe occipital pain may indicate an occipital tumor and frontal headache may reflect a supertentorial mass.

Pseudotumor Cerebri. Patients with pseudotumor cerebri can present with intermittent headaches, vomiting, blurred vision, papilledema, and occasionally diplopia. However, there is no alteration in the level of consciousness or intellectual functioning.

Head Trauma. A headache is quite common after minor head trauma. It usually is localized to the area of impact and may be associated with vomiting and sleepiness. There are no focal neurologic deficits or signs of increased intracranial pressure. Headache, minutes to days after significant head trauma, may be caused by an epidural or subdural hematoma. Worrisome signs are a decreasing level of consciousness, projectile vomiting, and signs of increased intracranial pressure (bulging fontanelle, split sutures, unequal pupils, VI nerve palsy, hypertension with bradycardia). Head trauma (p 393) and increased ICP (p 397) are discussed elsewhere.

Extracranial Etiologies

Sinusitis. The headache of sinusitis (p 121) may be referred to the teeth or cheek in young children, and the frontal or retrorbital area in older patients. There may be cough, mucopurulent unilateral nasal discharge, fever, and facial pain and tenderness. Often the pain occurs in the early morning and is accentuated by leaning forward.

Dental Infection. Dental infections (p 48) cause pain in the cheek or mandibular area as well as temporal headaches. The involved tooth or gum is extremely sensitive upon percussion or manipulation.

Visual Abnormality. Headaches secondary to visual abnormalities usually occur in the late afternoon or evening, after much visual activity. If there has been late-night, poorly lighted reading, the headache may occur in the morning.

Systemic Infection. Systemic infections, such as group A *Streptococcus,* influenza, and *Mycoplasma* pneumonia can cause a headache in addition to the other symptoms (fever, sore throat, cough, coryza, conjunctivitis, or myalgias).

Vascular Headaches

Migraine headaches, uncommon in children less than 5 years, are paroxysmal, throbbing or pulsating, unilateral, accompanied by nausea (or vomiting), and frequently associated with a positive family history. The frequency varies from several times a year to 1–2 weeks. Children often experience common migraines, which last ½–2 hours and are followed by 1–3 hours of sleep. These can be bilateral and without an aura or accompanying nausea.

Vascular headaches may present with a variety of other symptoms, determined by the distribution of the blood vessels involved. There may be a visual or olfactory aura (classic migraine), recurrent episodes of paralysis (hemiplegic migraine), transient ptosis or III nerve paralysis (ophthalmoplegic migraine), or an acute confusional state (basilar artery migraine).

DIAGNOSIS

Despite the wide spectrum of etiologies, the most common childhood headaches are psychogenic, followed by tension, These patients are afebrile, awake and alert, nontoxic, and have normal physical and more importantly, neurologic examinations. A small minority of headaches in children are secondary to some serious intracranial process, but these must always be considered.

Describe the headache(s) fully, including onset, duration, location, quality, usual time of day they occur, what (if anything) makes the pain better or worse, and whether the severity and frequency are increasing. Ask about recent emotional stress, personality changes, head trauma, warning signs (aura), family history of migraines, and associated symptoms, including fever, nausea or vomiting, nasal discharge, visual disturbances, cough, and photophobia.

Perform a complete physical examination, looking for fever, hypertension, split sutures and bulging fontanelle, facial tenderness, gingival swelling, dental caries and tooth percussion sensitivity, otitis media, nuchal rigidity and meningeal signs, and signs of a systemic infection. A thorough neurologic examination is necessary, including fundoscopy. Asymmetry of the pupils, EOM, or motor response suggest a structural abnormality such as a brain tumor or an abscess, or a subdural or epidural hematoma (see coma, p 382). Finally, check the visual acuity and visual fields and measure the blood pressure.

ER MANAGEMENT

The priority is expeditious diagnosis and treatment of *increased intracranial pressure*. The management of a suspected mass lesion, meningitis, head trauma, pseudotumor cerebri, sinusitis, systemic infections, and dental infections is discussed elsewhere in the appropriate sections.

The treatment of *psychogenic* and *tension* headaches in the ER is limited to oral analgesics (aspirin, acetaminophen) and reassurance that a serious disease process is not underway. Refer these patients to a primary care setting, where the stresses causing the headaches can be addressed.

Migraines can be a chronic, debilitating disease. For that reason, give mild analgesics only, and refer to either a primary care setting or a child neurologist. The ER is not the appropriate site for instituting prophylactic therapy with ergotamines or propranolol.

INDICATIONS FOR ADMISSION

- Focal neurologic findings, suspected intracranial hypertension
- Meningitis
- Acute confusional state
- Frontal sinusitis
- Severe headache after head trauma

REFERENCES

1. Shinnar S, D'Souza BJ: Pediatr Clin North Am 29: 79–94, 1982
2. Rothner AD: Headache 19: 156–162, 1979
3. Honig PS, et al: Am J Dis Child 136:121, 1982

Head Trauma

INTRODUCTION

Head trauma can result from falls from windows (toddlers) and bicycle, motorcycle, and automobile accidents (children and adolescents). Consider child abuse (shaking, whiplash injuries) in infants and young children.

CLINICAL PRESENTATION

Most pediatric head trauma victims do not suffer serious injury, although soft tissue swelling or laceration is common. Occasionally the patient is sleepy or lethargic (but fully arousable); however, the neurologic examination is otherwise normal.

Serious signs and symptoms include persistent headache or vomiting, ataxia, blurred vision, altered level of consciousness, focal neurologic signs, seizures, a compound skull fracture, retinal hemorrhage and evidence of increased intracranial pressure.

A less obvious presentation is the young afebrile infant with a full fontanelle who is lethargic or vomits food. He or she may be a "shaken baby," with or without other physical evidence of abuse (see p 430).

DIAGNOSIS

Determine the nature of the trauma, including whether the patient lost consciousness or cried immediately. Ask about vomiting, seizures, recollection of the event and the activities both prior to and after it, and past medical problems (seizure disorder, neurologic handicap). Once the patient is medically stabilized, obtain a developmental history. Many severe head trauma victims have a prior history of behavioral or developmental problems.

Perform a complete physical examination, including vital signs. Look for scalp lacerations and hematomas, a depressed skull fracture, and evidence of a basilar skull fracture (retroauricular or periorbital ecchymoses, hemotympanum, serous or serosanguinous rhinorrhea or otorrhea). Palpate for neck tenderness (pp 481–483) and check for sources of bleeding and other major injuries (see multiple trauma, p 488).

Head trauma per se does not cause hypotension, except in very young infants or patients with serious scalp lacerations. Hypotension demands an immediate, thorough evaluation of the rest of the body (particularly chest, abdomen, pelvis, and thighs) for sources of blood loss. Tachycardia, particularly in association with a narrowed pulse pressure, suggests impending shock (p 11).

Hypertension and bradycardia associated with slow or irregular respirations (Cushing triad) indicates increased intracranial pressure. Treatment must be instituted at once (see below).

Perform a careful neurologic examination, paying particular attention to the signs of structural coma (p 382): asymmetry of pupillary responses, extraocular movements, or motor response. Examine the cranial nerves, perform fundoscopy (for papilledema), and test the reflexes, strength, sensation, and coordination, comparing one side to the other.

The Glasgow Coma Scale (GCS) indicates the initial severity of the head injury and facilitates monitoring changes in the patient's status (Table 14-6).

The neurologic examination, the nature of the injury, and the age of the patient determine the need for skull x-rays. Indications for radiographs are summarized in Table 14-7. If a depressed skull fracture is suspected (trauma caused by a sharp, high velocity object; large scalp hematoma preventing palpation of the skull below), obtain an x-ray tangential to the area in question. Skull x-rays are usually not needed to rule out a linear compound fracture in a patient with a scalp laceration, since these wounds will be explored under local anesthesia.

Contact seizures occur at the moment of or within several seconds of the head trauma. Although frightening to the parents, contact seizures are of no clinical significance. Early posttraumatic seizures, occurring 1 minute to 1 week after the head trauma, carry some risk for future epilepsy.

ER MANAGEMENT

The priorities are securing the airway, maintaining vital signs, and treating increased intracranial pressure.

First, assess the airway and adequacy of ventilation. Since a patient with a depressed level of consciousness may have inadequate ventilation despite respiratory movements, obtain an ABG and give 100% O_2 if he or she is not fully awake and alert. Intubate any patient with a

TABLE 14-6. GLASGOW COMA SCALE[a]

Best Verbal Response:	
None	1
Incomprehensible sound	2
Inappropriate words	3
Confused	4
Oriented	5
Eyes Open:	
None	1
To pain	2
To speech	3
Spontaneously	4
Best Motor Response:	
None	1
Abnormal extensor	2
Abnormal flexion	3
Withdraws	4
Localizes	5
Obeys	6

[a]Total GCS is the sum of the scores of the three parts.

GCS $\leq$ 9, regardless of whether cervical spine x-rays have been obtained or interpreted. Use a jaw thrust or chin lift maneuver (pp 3–4). Evaluate the chest for the presence of bilateral breath sounds and signs of respiratory distress.

Next, measure the vital signs at least every 15 minutes, but more frequently in patients with severe head trauma or an abnormal pulse or

TABLE 14-7. INDICATIONS FOR SKULL X-RAYS IN PATIENTS WITH HEAD TRAUMA

1. Suspected basilar skull fracture
2. Vomiting or sleepy afebrile infant <1 year of age
3. Suspected depressed skull fracture (tangential views)
4. Penetrating head trauma

blood pressure. Secure a large bore IV in patients with hypotension or a GCS < 15. The treatment of hypotension with 20 cc/kg boluses of isotonic crystalloid and packed red cell transfusions takes precedence over concerns about increased intracranial pressure (p 11). Once a normal blood pressure is maintained, infuse D5 ½ NS at a ⅔ maintenance rate.

Patients with a depressed skull fracture, focal neurologic findings, or an early posttraumatic seizure are at risk for the development of epilepsy. Give a loading dose of phenytoin (10–15 mg/kg) IV slowly over 30 minutes. Give oxacillin (25 mg/kg up to 1 gm) to patients with a compound skull fracture prior to debridement. Do not give antibiotics routinely to patients with basilar skull fractures.

GCS < 9 or GCS > 9 But Worsening. Immediately intubate the patient and call for neurologic and neurosurgical consultations. Hyperventilate the patient to a pCO_2 of 25–30 torr, keep the head in the midline and the bed elevated to 40 degrees , and restrict fluid (⅔ maintenance). Give dexamethasone (0.4 mg/kg, to maximum 16 mg) and mannitol (0.5–1 g/kg). To be effective, mannitol must be given rapidly, preferably as an IV push. Arrange for an immediate CTT (see increased intracranial pressure, p 397).

GCS 9–14. Insert a large bore IV for access and repeat the GCS every 15 minutes. Admit the patient, unless his or her mental status returns rapidly to his or her usual baseline (GCS=15).

GCS=15. If the parents can follow instructions and return immediately, the patient may be sent home, unless there is persistent vomiting or dizziness. Allow the child to sleep, but have the parents awaken him every 2 hours. The patient must *immediately* return to the ER if he cannot be aroused or, has diplopia, unsteady gait, several episodes of vomiting, or a headache unresponsive to aspirin or acetaminophen.

INDICATIONS FOR ADMISSION

- GCS < 15
- Early posttraumatic seizure
- Compound or depressed skull fracture
- Persistent vomiting, dizziness, or abnormal neurologic findings in the ER

REFERENCES
1. Dershewitz RA, Kaye BA, Swisher CN: Pediatrics 72: 602–605 1983
2. Leonidas JC, Tinge M, Binkiewicz A, et al: Pediatrics 69: 139–143, 1982

Increased Intracranial Pressure

INTRODUCTION

An increase in the volume of any intracranial compartment (blood, CSF, or parenchyma) can cause an elevation in ICP, a true neurosurgical emergency. Head trauma is the most common cause of increased ICP in children. Although the onset is usually acute, symptoms of a subdural or epidural hematoma may have a delayed onset. Other etiologies include brain tumor, meningitis, rupture of an aneurysm, intracerebral abscess, pseudotumor cerebri, or an obstructed shunt in a patient with hydrocephalus. Intracranial hypertension is also the major life-threatening complication of Reye syndrome.

CLINICAL PRESENTATION

Lethargy is an important finding in the patient with increased ICP. A patient with a GCS <9 or a falling GCS following head trauma requires an immediate evaluation for intracranial hypertension.

Patients with either a history of head injury or increased ICP on a nontraumatic basis may complain of early morning headache and vomiting or headaches of recent onset that have become more frequent and severe. Altered mental status, a change in personality (constant crying or irritability in an infant), or a head tilt are also suggestive of increased ICP. Papilledema is a highly reliable finding but may not be present for 24 or more hours.

In infants, increased ICP causes irritability, vomiting, widening of the sutures, an increasing head circumference, and a full or bulging fontanelle.

Clinical signs of imminent cerebral herniation include a deteriorating level of consciousness, unequal pupils (the dilated pupil is usually on the same side as the herniation), asymmetrical EOM, and decerebrate (extensor) posturing. Abnormal respirations, bradycardia, and hypertension (Cushing triad) occur with severely increased ICP.

DIAGNOSIS

Assume that any patient who has suffered significant head trauma is at risk for increased ICP. Always check the pupillary responses, EOM, and level of consciousness. Perform a careful fundoscopic examination and a sensory and motor exam, comparing one side of the body to the other. Coma can be due to *toxic-metabolic* causes (see p 382) but typically the pupils are reactive and miotic, and there are no focal findings.

Congenital anisocoria, the use of *mydriatic drops,* or *direct trauma* to the eye can cause pupillary inequality. These are always diagnoses of exclusion in a patient with lethargy or any other signs suggesting increased ICP.

Vomiting is a common symptom in pediatric patients. In the absence of other neurologic signs, vomiting in an alert child nearly always reflects a different diagnosis, including *infection* (abdominal pain, diarrhea, posttussive emesis, fever), *intestinal obstruction* (bilious vomiting, distended abdomen above the obstructed site), *pregnancy* (adolescent female with amenorrhea), etc.

The evaluation of headaches is discussed on p 388. Morning headaches, or headaches that are increasing in frequency and intensity are worrisome. However, headaches in an alert patient with no other abnormal neurologic findings are most likely to be *psychogenic, tension,* or *migrane headaches.*

ER MANAGEMENT

If increased ICP is suspected, immediately arrange for a CTT scan and notify a neurosurgeon and a neurologist to assist in further management. See p 393 for the treatment of head trauma.

If the patient has an altered level of consciousness, but does not have unequal pupils, bradycardia, hypertension, or decerebrate posturing, continuously monitor the heart rate and blood pressure and assess the adequacy of ventilation with an ABG. Secure an IV with D5 ½ NS for vascular access. If the patient is hypotensive, restoration of a normal blood pressure takes priority over treatment of the increased intracranial pressure (see p 11). Always keep the patients head in the midline and, unless the patient is in shock or has a cervical spine injury, the head of the bed at 40° of elevation. Provide 100% oxygen, and intubate any patient who is hypoxic, hypercarbic (pCO_2 > 40 torr), comatose, has a depressed level of consciousness, or is leaving the ER for diagnostic procedures (where he or she cannot be easily monitored).

If the patient has signs of markedly increased ICP (unequal pupils, bradycardia and hypertension, or abnormal posturing), employ all available modalities to lower the ICP while a neurologist and neurosurgeon are summoned. These include immediate intubation and hyperventilation to a pCO_2 of 25–30 torr (if the patient is intubated, increase the rate of ventilation), and the administration of IV dexamethasone (0.4 mg/kg to maximum 16 mg), and mannitol (0.5–1 g/kg). Insert a Foley catheter prior to giving the mannitol. Limit the IV fluid rate to KVO unless the patient is in shock.

If required, perform intubation under controlled circumstances to avoid further increasing the intracranial pressure. Hyperventilate the patient with a bag-valve-mask with 100% O_2. Measure the blood pressure to be sure that the patient is not hypotensive, then give thiopental, 3–5 mg/kg IV. Follow this with pancuronium, 0.2 mg/kg IV to prevent any movement by the patient during the intubation. The onset of paralysis is in 30 seconds, the peak effect is at 3–4 minutes, and the duration is less than an hour. As soon as intubation has been accomplished, insert a nasogastric tube, aspirate the stomach contents, and connect the tube to suction. Pass a Foley catheter using sterile technique to monitor urine output.

Order a shunt survey if there is a suspected shunt obstruction. Consult with a neurosurgeon who should tap the reservoir, and send the CSF for culture, cell count, and chemistries.

INDICATION FOR ADMISSION

- Intracranial hypertension

REFERENCE

1. Griffith JF, Brasfield JC: PIR 2:269–276, 1981

Night Phenomena

INTRODUCTION AND CLINICAL PRESENTATION

Nightmares. Nightmares are frightening dreams that occur commonly in childhood. The patient reawakens fully, is anxious, and typically has good recall of the dream. Diaphoresis and tachypnea may occur, but there is no vocalization.

Night Terrors. With night terrors, the child (usually preschool age) suddenly sits up, emits a loud scream or cry, and appears truly terrified. The child is confused and not awake, and, in fact, appears to be hallucinating. Tachycardia, dilated pupils, diaphoresis, and tachypnea occur. The patient returns to sleep after several minutes and there is no recollection of the event in the morning. Night terrors is a transient disorder that usually resolves spontaneously.

Somnambulism. Somnambulism, or sleepwalking, occurs at least once in up to 15% of children and as often as four times a week in 1–6%. The child sits up, leaves the bed, performs some clumsy movements, and may even respond somewhat to verbal commands. There is generally no recall of the event when the child awakens. Most children outgrow sleep-walking.

DIAGNOSIS

The diagnosis is usually evident from the history of the event. Nightmares are differentiated from night terrors by the full arousal, good recall, and the absence of vocalizations and tachycardia in the former. If the two cannot be distinguished, instruct the parents to measure the child's pulse rate during the next episode (tachycardia occurs with night terrors only). Somnambulism can be confused with psychomotor epilepsy, but there are no sleep-walking episodes during the daytime.

ER MANAGEMENT

Take a careful history, including the nature and frequency of the events and recent stresses in the child's life. In general, the only treatment is reassurance. If the child is sleep-walking, have the parents secure an area so he or she cannot be injured (lock doors and windows, remove dangerous objects). Refer patients with recurrent episodes to a primary care provider who can assess the family situation in depth.

REFERENCES
1. Keith PR: J Am Acad Child Psych 14:447, 1975
2. Pesikoff RB, Davies PC: Am J Psychiatry 128:779, 1971

Status Epilepticus

INTRODUCTION

Status epilepticus is defined as 30 minutes or more of either continuous seizure activity or serial convulsions without recovery of consciousness between seizures. The immediate consequences of status epilepticus include hypoxia and hypercarbia, metabolic and respiratory acidosis, and increased cerebral oxygen consumption with increased cerebral blood flow (possibly causing intracranial hypertension). In time, hypoglycemia may develop. Physical injury and vomiting with aspiration are additional hazards.

CLINICAL PRESENTATION

Convulsive status epilepticus is easily recognized. Typically, the child has rhythmic jerking of one or more extremities with unresponsiveness. Less commonly, the child presents with tonic eye deviation, complex automatic motor behavior, or dilated unresponsive pupils, without overt tonic or clonic activity. In neonates, seizures are often more subtle, consisting of apnea, nystagmus, vasomotor changes, and lipsmacking or sucking. Motor activity may include bicycling or swimming movements.

DIAGNOSIS

The most common cause of status epilepticus is *noncompliance with the anticonvulsant medication regimen* in a child with documented epilepsy. Other provocative factors in known epileptics, especially those with poorly controlled seizures, include fever, vomiting, and intercurrent infections (*breakthrough seizures*). A *prolonged febrile seizure* (lasting > 30 min and continuing past the child's arrival in the ER) is a frequent cause of status epilepticus . Less commonly, status epilepticus is symptomatic of an acute encephalopathic process such as a *CNS infection* (meningitis, encephalitis), *metabolic disturbance* (hypoxia, hypoglycemia, hyponatremia, hypocalcemia), *intoxication* (theophylline, tricyclic antidepressants, amphetamines, and camphor), or *head trauma.*

ER MANAGEMENT

The goals of ER management are to stop the seizures as quickly as possible, prevent recurrence, and avoid any complications (aspiration, self-induced injuries). Suction the oral cavity and apply a face mask with 100% O_2. Next, secure an intravenous line with D5 ½ NS and obtain blood for anticonvulsant levels, CBC, electrolytes, glucose, and calcium, as well as a rapid dextrostix determination of the serum glucose. Always obtain an additional red top tube. The vital signs must be carefully measured and the ECG continuously monitored.

Diazepam (0.3–0.5 mg/kg to maximum 10 mg) by slow IV push usually terminates the seizures rapidly. Three doses may be given at 10-minute intervals.

As soon as the seizure has stopped, flush the line with normal saline and administer a loading dose of a long-acting anticonvulsant. The first choice is *phenytoin* (15 mg/kg IV to maximum 1 g) given no faster than 50 mg/min. Monitor the blood pressure and the ECG for P-R prolongation.

If the seizures persist, *phenobarbital* can be given (10–15 mg/kg IV to maximum 350 mg). Electively intubate the patient if phenobarbital is required (if it has not already been done), since respiratory depression is a distinct possibility in patients given a loading dose of phenobarbital after receiving diazepam.

If the patient is known to recently have had a therapeutic anticonvulsant level, give an extra dose of that medication rather than a full loading dose. For example, give 5 mg/kg of phenobarbital IV or 5 mg/kg of phenytoin IV slowly over 15–20 minutes (*never IM*). If there are subsequent seizures, give a loading dose of a second drug (as described above).

If the seizures persist, give paraldehyde IV (10 cc of a 4% solution in 90 cc of saline), and titrate the dose against the seizures. Paraldehyde cannot be exposed to light or used in plastic IV bags.

Within 2 hours of the patient's arrival in the ER, he or she can be treated with diazepam, given a loading dose of phenytoin and phenobarbital, and treated with paraldehyde, if needed. If the seizures persist, intubate and mechanically ventilate the patient. Then give general anesthesia with a neuromuscular blockade, after correction of any existing metabolic abnormalities.

In the unusual situation when an IV cannot be secured, diazepam can be given per rectum (0.5 mg/kg of the parenteral form). Paraldehyde can also be given rectally (0.15–0.4 mg/kg mixed with an equal volume of mineral oil).

For the rare patient who does not have a history of epilepsy and does not respond to diazepam, check the electrolytes and obtain an ABG. A patient with a metabolic or hypoxic basis for the status epilepticus needs correction of the underlying problem and usually does not require treatment with anticonvulsants. Treat hyponatremic seizures with hypertonic saline (4 mEq/cc). The dose (in mEq) is:

$$(125 - \text{measured serum sodium}) \times (0.6) \times (\text{weight in kg})$$

Treat hypertensive seizures with a rapid IV push of 5 mg/kg of diazoxide (300 mg maximum). Fever and irritability are indications for a blood culture and a lumbar puncture once the status has been terminated (see febrile seizures, p 385). If the dextrostix is low (<45–90), give an IV push of 0.5 g/kg of glucose (1 cc/kg of D50).

Once the seizures have stopped, obtain a careful history from the parents or a witness regarding how the seizure activity started (focal versus generalized at the outset). Does the child have a known seizure disorder, what medications does he or she take, and are there any recent anticonvulsant levels? Did the patient stop taking medication (noncompliance, supplies exhausted), or is this a patient on substantial doses of several medications whose seizures are difficult to control? Perform a careful physical and neurologic examination to assess the patient's level of consciousness, (see Glasgow Coma Scale, p 395), pupillary reflexes, eye movements, and to look for asymmetries of movement, muscle tone, and reflexes, or upgoing toes (see coma, p 382).

Admit all patients with status epilepticus for further evaluation and/or observation. Patients with evidence of increased intracranial pressure or persistent focal findings on neurologic examination must undergo CTT scanning immediately (see management of increased ICP, p 397).

INDICATIONS FOR ADMISSION

- Status epilepticus
- Patients with increasing numbers of breakthrough seizures
- Focality or evidence of increased ICP

REFERENCES

1. Delgado-Escueta AV, Wasterlain C, Treiman CM, et al: N Engl J Med 306:1337, 1982
2. Rothner AD, Erenberg G: Pediatr Clin North Am 27:592–602, 1980
3. Knudsen FU: Arch Dis Child 54:855–857, 1979

15

Ophthalmologic Emergencies

Excessive Tearing in Infancy

INTRODUCTION

Excessive tearing in infancy can be caused by obstruction to lacrimal drainage (most common) or an increase in tear formation secondary to serious ocular disease (glaucoma, iritis, chronic lid irritation).

CLINICAL PRESENTATION

Nasolacrimal duct obstruction causes persistent excessive tearing punctuated by recurrent episodes of conjunctivitis or dacryocystitis. There should not be any associated photophobia, corneal enlargement, or decreased corneal clarity (loss of crisp red reflex) as occur with glaucoma. Iritis is painful, with decreased visual acuity, photophobia, diminished pupillary response, and a ciliary flush.

DIAGNOSIS

Check for the signs of *glaucoma* or an *iritis* (enumerated above) as well as for *chronic irritation* of the lids. Recurrent infections are seen with *flow obstruction.* Ocular symptomology suggests tearing secondary to ocular pathology.

ER MANAGEMENT

Treat nasolacrimal obstruction by digital massage of the nasolacrimal sac (qid), with finger pressure at the medial canthus directed toward the nose. Treat acute infections with antibiotic drops (10% sulfacetamide) qid. Eighty percent of obstructions will resolve by 8 months, so that ophthalmologic referral can be deferred until that time, unless there have been recurrent infections which may compromise the success of future probing.

Tearing suspected to be secondary to ocular pathology (glaucoma, iritis) requires immediate ophthalmologic evaluation.

REFERENCE

1. Peterson RA, Robb RM: J Pediatr Ophthalmol Strabismus 15:246, 1978

Eyelid Inflammation

INTRODUCTION

Infection of the eyelid margin, or *blepharitis,* is most commonly secondary to *Staphylococcus aureus*. Other etiologies include molluscum contagiosum, herpes simplex, seborrhea, and lice. Inflammation of the glands of the lid is termed a *hordeolum* (stye). It is usually caused by *S. aureus* and may be acute or subacute. A *chalazion* is a granulomatous, noninfectious inflammation of the tarsal Meibomian gland. This occurs secondary to blockage of the gland orifice at the lid margin, frequently as a result of a blepharitis.

CLINICAL PRESENTATION AND DIAGNOSIS

Staphylococcal blepharitis presents as lid margin inflammation with accumulation of crusting material at the bases of the eye lashes (collarettes). A concomitant conjunctivitis, occasionally with phlyctenules (white conjunctival nodules near the limbus) may be present. *Molluscum* appear as 1–5 mm, umbilicated, flesh-colored papules usually associated with similar lesions on the periorbital skin. Patients are usually asymptomatic, although involvement of the lid margins can produce a concomitant conjunctivitis. The vesicles of *herpes simplex* may involve the lid margin as well as the surrounding skin and are associated with preauricular adenopathy. *Seborrhea* causes a greasy scaling of the lid margins in association with scaling of the scalp and retroauricular areas. A pruritic infestation, with visible moving *lice* can occasionally occur in the eye lashes.

A *hordeolum* presents as an erythematous, tender swelling of the lid margin. Often the abscess is pointing. A *chalazion,* on the other hand, is an asymptomatic or mildly tender, often recurrent, well-circumscribed swelling within the lid itself.

ER MANAGEMENT

Treat staphylococcal blepharitis with regular washing and shampooing. The base of the eyelashes may be scrubbed with a moistened applicator, tid. A sulfonamide ointment (10% sulfacetamide) qid for 2 weeks is also helpful. Molluscum is usually a self-limited disease, but if cosmetic concerns are an issue, refer the patient to a dermatologist for curettage. If herpex simplex infection involves the lid margin, refer the patient to an ophthalmologist for antiviral prophylaxis of the cornea. Treat seborrheic blepharitis with removal of the scales with a moistened applicator followed by a keratolytic shampoo (Selsun, Sebulex). Treat pediculosis with either petrolatum tid or 0.5% physostigmine ointment applied once to the lash base.

Therapy for a hordeolum includes warm compresses (for 15 minutes q 4–6h) followed by a sulfonamide ointment (10% sulfacetamide) qid. Any associated blepharitis should be appropriately treated. If there is no response in 2–3 days, refer the patient to an ophthalmologist for incision and drainage.

Warm compresses are also effective for a chalazion, although therapy may be necessary for several weeks. Once again, an underlying blepharitis should be appropriately treated and ophthalmologic referral (for incision and drainage) considered if there is no response.

REFERENCE

1. Harley RD: Pediatr Clin North Am 30:1156–1158, 1983

Eye Trauma

INTRODUCTION

Any patient with ocular (and facial) trauma requires a thorough eye evaluation. Concomitant damage to other ocular structures may be overlooked when focusing solely on an obvious injury.

CLINICAL PRESENTATION

Burns. Chemical and thermal burns are true emergencies. Acids coagulate proteins, which limit further penetration, while alkalis penetrate deeply and continue to damage the eye for a period of several days. The patient may present with burns of the face or periorbital skin, ocular pain, lacrimation, decreased corneal clarity, or decreased visual acuity.

Corneal Abrasion. Disruption of the corneal epithelium produces moderate to severe ocular pain. There is often a foreign body sensation, especially with lid movement. Conjunctival injection, photophobia, and lacrimation occur, while visual acuity and extraocular movements (EOM) are normal. Although many abrasions can be seen with a penlight, fluorescein staining is necessary to determine the extent of the injury.

Hyphema. A significant blow to the globe can cause a hyphema, bleeding into the anterior chamber. Frequently, there is associated damage to intraocular structures (iris, lens, retina, and filtration angle). The patient presents with decreased visual acuity and a blood layer in the anterior chamber, which is best seen in the upright position. A dangerous rise in intraocular pressure may result, especially in patients with sickle cell disease or trait. Rebleeding may occur, usually 3–5 days after the injury, and damage to the filtration angle may produce future glaucoma.

Lid Laceration. Although a laceration is obvious, the eye must be carefully examined. The wound may go through the lid and involve the globe.

Orbital Floor Fracture. Blunt trauma to the globe may result in a "blow-out" fracture of the floor of the orbit. Entrapment of ocular muscles (or surrounding tissues) can occur, restricting ocular movements (especially upward gaze) and causing diplopia.

Palpate the orbital rim in all cases of blunt trauma—point tenderness suggests a fracture. Injury to the trigeminal nerve branch in the orbital floor can cause hypesthesia in its distribution (lower orbital rim and upper lip). Incarceration of orbital tissues in the maxillary sinus may cause enophthalmus. A Water's view x-ray may reveal the bony fracture, clouding of the maxillary sinus, or incarcerated tissue appearing as a "tear drop" in the superior maxillary sinus.

Ruptured Globe. Hallmarks of ocular perforation include decreased visual acuity (can be severe), a distorted pupil (peaked, pointed, pulled to one side or with a flat side), a shallow or absent anterior chamber, and protrusion of iris or other intraocular contents. Perforation is obvious if the globe is collapsed, but more often, brownish iris tissue plugs the perforation and distorts the pupil.

Subconjunctival Hemorrhage. Blood beneath the conjunctiva appears bright red. It is generally a benign, asymptomatic finding, only rarely associated with a bleeding diathesis.

Superficial Foreign Bodies. Retained superficial conjunctival and corneal foreign bodies present like corneal abrasions, with injection, pain, photophobia, tearing, and normal visual acuity. Fluorescein staining may help locate the object.

DIAGNOSIS

A thorough evaluation includes a history of the trauma, including the nature and velocity of any traumatizing material.

Note symptoms of diplopia, visual disturbance, and ocular pain. Inspect the periorbital skin, lids, and globe and assess anterior chamber clarity, pupillary reactions, and extraocular movements. Ophthalmoscopy allows evaluation of optic nerve and retinal dysfunction, while the presence of the red reflex assures clarity of the optical media. The examination must always include an assessment of visual acuity.

Perform fluorescein staining if there is any pain or foreign body sensation, lacrimation, conjunctival injection, or decreased visual acuity. The only exception is if the globe might be ruptured. Fluorescein dye stains the corneal stroma green if there is a loss of corneal epithelial integrity (corneal abrasion, burn, or foreign body). Touch a wetted fluorescein strip to the inferior conjunctiva, wait a few minutes, then examine with a blue or black light.

ER MANAGEMENT

Burns. Immediately (preferably at the site of the accident) begin irrigating the eye with water or saline, using 1–2 liters. Apply two drops of a topical opthalmic anesthetic and use a lid speculum or retractor to elevate the lids off the globe. After irrigation, search for foreign bodies, stain the cornea with fluorescein, and call an ophthalmologist.

Corneal Abrasion. Instill one drop of both an ophthalmic anesthetic and an antibiotic (10% sulfacetamide). Then apply a pressure patch by putting two eye pads over the closed lid, securing one end of a piece of tape on the central forehead, and placing the other end over the pads onto a raised cheek. Releasing the cheek tightens the tape. Apply three or four more pieces of tape in the same manner.

Reassess the abrasion after 24 hours. Symptomatic improvement, improved or stable visual acuity, and continued corneal clarity indicate satisfactory progress. If the abrasion persists, refer the patient to an ophthalmologist. Use aspirin or acetaminophen; do not use anesthetic drops, except at the time of the initial patching.

Hyphema. Place the patient at bedrest and sedate as necessary (chloral hydrate 20 mg/kg q 6h). Close ophthalmologic follow-up is imperative. If the family cannot comply with the instructions, admit the patient.

Lid Laceration. Give tetanus toxoid and antibiotic prophylaxis (cat or dog bites), if indicated. If suturing is required, consult an ophthalmologist.

Orbital Floor Fracture. If a patient with blunt ocular trauma has point tenderness of the orbital rim or limitation of extraocular movements (especially upward gaze), obtain x-rays of the orbit, including a Water's view. Ophthalmologic referral is indicated for close follow-up and possible surgical repair if the patient has diplopia that does not resolve. Instruct the patient to refrain from blowing his nose.

Ruptured Globe. Any suspicion of a penetrating injury is an indication for immediate ophthalmologic consultation to arrange surgical repair. Do not instill any drops, cover the eye with a plastic shield, and have the patient lie supine.

Subconjunctival Hemorrhage. No therapy is required. Clearing gradually occurs over 1–2 weeks.

Superficial Foreign Body. If the patient is cooperative, attempt removal by irrigation or gentle wiping with a moist cotton applicator. Instillation of an anesthetic drop and the use of a lid retractor may facilitate the procedure. If the object is metallic, deeply imbedded, or not easily removed, refer to an ophthalmologist after instillation of an antibiotic drug. Once the foreign body is removed, treat any associated corneal abrasion.

INDICATIONS FOR ADMISSION

- Chemical or thermal burn
- Hyphema, if bedrest and ophthalmologic follow-up is not guaranteed
- Ruptured globe

REFERENCES

1. Ervin-Mulvey LD, Nelson LB, Freeley DA: Pediatr Clin North Am 30: 1167–1183, 1983
2. Frey T: Pediatr Ann 12:487–497, 1983

The Red Eye

INTRODUCTION

Conjunctival hyperemia, or the "red eye," may be a consequence of simple conjunctival inflammation or may be a sign of corneal or intraocular disease.

Etiologies of conjunctivitis include viruses (adenovirus, herpes simplex 1, measles, varicella), *Chlamydia* (especially in neonates), bacteria (*Pneumococcus, Haemophilus influenzae, Staphylococcus,* group A *Streptococcus*), allergy, and irritants (pollutants, $AgNO_3$ drops in newborns). Gonococcal infection is always a concern in the first few weeks of life.

Keratitis, a superficial corneal inflammation, may be caused by ocular trauma, infection (adenovirus, herpes, *Chlamydia),* or an immunologic process initiated by a staphylococcal blepharitis or conjunctivitis.

Iritis is an inflammation of the anterior uveal tract, usually caused by trauma. Alternatively, it may be associated with immune diseases (juvenile rheumatoid arthritis), infections (adenovirus, herpes, syphilis), sarcoidosis, keratitis, or a primary posterior uveitis (ciliary body or choroidal inflammation).

CLINICAL PRESENTATION AND DIAGNOSIS

Conjunctivitis. Inflammation of the bulbar and tarsal conjunctival mucous membranes produces vascular engorgement, appearing as diffusely distributed, discrete, red vessels. Although itching or a "sandy" sensation is frequently noted, there is no ocular pain and photophobia is mild, at most. Visual acuity is normal. On examination, a discharge ranging from mucus and crusting to frank pus may be present, along with lid edema.

A viral etiology is suggested by a mucoid discharge, preauricular lymphadenopathy, and, occasionally, an associated pharyngitis (adenovirus pharyngoconjunctival fever). A purulent discharge, often associated with otitis media, suggests a bacterial cause, while a seasonal watery or mucoid discharge with itching and inflamed conjunctival papilla (conjunctival cobblestoning) is seen with an allergic etiology.

The most common cause of neonatal conjunctivitis is a chemical irritation from $AgNO_3$, which presents in the first 24 hours of life. Gonococcal ophthalmia typically causes a hyperacute purulent or bloody discharge at 24–72 hours of age. Perform a Gram stain of the pus. Gram-negative intracellular diplococci and polys are seen with gonorrhea. Other bacteria and *Chlamydia* cause a purulent discharge but are generally not implicated until the fourth day of life.

Keratitis. Corneal inflammation usually occurs with a concomitant conjunctivitis. Viral keratitis may be epithelial (painful) or subepithelial (painless), visual acuity may be normal or decreased, and photophobia may be moderately intense. Herpes is initially epithelial and may cause pain, but decreased corneal sensation frequently coexists. If the corneal epithelium is disrupted, green fluorescein staining of the underlying stroma may be noted (normally it does not stain).

Iritis. Exudation of protein and cells into the anterior chamber causes decreased visual acuity, ocular pain, and photophobia, all of which may be severe. Conjunctival inflammation is also present, but with an iritis there is hyperemia of the deeper scleral vessels at the corneal margin. These vessels are not seen discretely through the conjunctiva, but rather appear as a pink band (''ciliary flush''). The pupil is frequently affected, appearing smaller with a diminished response to light, and the ocular dischage is clear.

ER MANAGEMENT

The *determination of visual acuity* is of paramount importance; any decrement is an indication for immediate ophthalmologic referral. Other evidence of intraocular involvement includes severe photophobia or ocular pain, vascular engorgement at the limbus (corneoscleral junction), and pupillary abnormalities. Always inquire about a history of ocular trauma (p 408).

Conjunctivitis. In general, bacterial cultures are not needed. An ocular antibiotic (10% sulfacetamide) 1–2 drops q 3–4 h, rapidly treats most uncomplicated bacterial cases and prevents secondary bacterial infection if the etiology is viral. Instruct the mother to gently wipe away any crust with a damp washcloth prior to instilling the drops, to be meticulous about hygiene, washing hands, and sharing towels, and to keep the child from community settings (school, day care). Do not prescribe neosporin or steroid preparations without ophthalmologic consultation. Continue treatment for 7 days or for 3 days after clinical resolution. If there is no response after 72 hours, obtain a bacterial culture by swabbing the conjunctiva and change antibiotics (polymixin drops, bacitracin ointment). Refer a patient with persistant conjunctivitis to an ophthalmologist.

Neonatal Conjunctivitis. No treatment is required for $AgNO_3$ chemical inflammation. If there is any discharge, obtain a Gram stain and conjunctival cultures for routine bacteria, gonococci (Thayer-Martin medium), and *Chlamydia* (if available) and begin a topical sulfonamide preparation. If the Gram stain reveals gram-negative intracellular diplococci or gonococci are cultured, treat with intravenous penicillin G (50,000 units/kg/day divided q 12h for 7 days) and frequent saline irrigations. Isolate the patient for at least 24 hours.

If the Gram stain in an infant 1–12 weeks of age reveals polys but few organisms, and culture or serologic testing for *Chlamydia* is not available, treat for presumed *Chlamydia* conjunctivitis: give topical 1% tetracycline or 0.5% erythromycin ointment and oral erythromycin (40 mg/kg/day divided qid) for at least 3 weeks.

Keratitis and Iritis. Patients with ocular pain, photophobia, decreased visual acuity, pupillary changes, or ciliary flush must be immediately referred to an ophthalmologist.

INDICATION FOR ADMISSION

- Gonococcal ophthalmia

REFERENCES

1. Pernoud FG: Pediatr Ann 12: 517–526, 1983
2. Gigliotti F, Williams WT, Hayden FG, et al: J Pediatr 98:531–536, 1981

16

Orthopedic Emergencies

Arthritis

INTRODUCTION AND ETIOLOGIES

Arthritis is defined as joint swelling, pain, and limitation of motion. It results from synovial inflammation due to infectious and noninfectious causes (Table 16-1). Arthritis must be differentiated from arthralgia, which is joint pain only.

CLINICAL PRESENTATION

By definition, the arthritic joint presents with a combination of swelling, erythema, warmth, pain, and decreased range of motion. The patient may limp or refuse to use the affected extremity.

Septic Arthritis. The onset of septic arthritis (see p 316) is usually abrupt, associated with fever, erythrocyte sedimentation rate (ESR) > 50 mm/hr, and systemic toxicity. Typically, the patient resists any attempts to move the affected joint. In nearly all cases, it is monoarticular. However, gonococcal (GC) arthritis can be migratory initially, then monoarticular or pauciarticular. Adolescents with GC infection may have tenosynovitis and a rash (erythematous, hemorrhagic, papular, or vesicopustular) rather than a vaginal discharge or urethritis.

Arthritis may occur during the course of *rubella, Kawasaki disease,* and occasionally in the prodromal phase of *hepatitis B* infection.

Lyme Disease. Lyme disease is caused by a spirochete transmitted by a tick bite. The arthritis is monoarticular or pauciarticular (large joints, especially knees) and it occurs weeks to months after a dis-

TABLE 16-1. CAUSES OF ARTHRITIS

- Infectious
  - Group B *Streptococcus*—infants
  - *H. influenzae, Pneumococcus, Staphylococcus*—toddlers and older children
  - *Pseudomonas aeruginosa*—puncture wounds
  - Lyme disease
  - Viruses (rubella, hepatitis B, Epstein-Barr)
  - Mycoplasma
  - Tuberculosis
  - Kawasaki disease?
- Rheumatic diseases
  - Acute rheumatic fever
  - Juvenile rheumatoid arthritis
  - Systemic lupus erythematosis
  - Inflammatory bowel disease
- Vasculitis
  - Henoch-Schönlein purpura
  - Serum sickness
- Trauma
- Malignancies
  - Leukemia
  - Neuroblastoma

tinctive eruption, erythema chronicum migrans (expanding erythematous lesions with central clearing).

Acute Rheumatic Fever. Typically, acute rheumatic fever (ARF) (p 288) presents with a migratory polyarthritis and fever, occasionally associated with carditis.

Systemic Lupus Erythematosus. Systemic lupus erythematosus (SLE) may present with symmetrical arthritis of both large and small joints. A butterfly rash, polyserositis, fever, and nephritis (hematuria, proteinuria) may be present.

Inflammatory Bowel Disease. Patients with arthritis associated with inflammatory bowel disease may also have weight loss, failure to thrive, bloody diarrhea, and erythema nodosum.

Juvenile Rheumatoid Arthritis. There are three major types of juvenile rheumatoid arthritis: pauciarticular (four or fewer large asymmetrical joints, iridocyclitis), polyarticular (five or more small or large symmetrical joints), and systemic onset (arthritis similar to polyarticular type, spiking fevers, evanescent salmon-pink macular rash, lymphadenopathy, hepatosplenomegaly). The arthritis persists for at least 6 weeks.

Henoch-Schönlein Purpura. Henoch-Schönlein purpura presents with some combination of arthritis, purpuric rash of the buttocks and lower extremities, abdominal pain, hematuria, and hematochezia.

Serum Sickness. Serum sickness causes arthritis, fever, urticaria, and lymphadenopathy 1–3 weeks after exposure to foreign proteins, including drugs (sulfonamides, penicillins, diphenylhydantoin) and infectious agents (hepatitis B virus, Epstein-Barr virus).

Malignancies. Malignancies cause arthritis by cellular infiltration of the synovium. Weakness, weight loss, bleeding, fever, and pallor are usually present as well.

DIAGNOSIS

Monoarticular Arthritis. Consider monoarticular arthritis to be *infectious* in etiology. Ask about antecedent trauma, upper respiratory infection (URI) symptoms, and the time of onset of the symptoms. Obtain a complete blood count (CBC) with differential, ESR, blood culture, and two additional red top tubes in the event septic arthritis is ruled out. Obtain an x-ray of the involved joint, and have an orthopedist perform arthrocentesis as soon as possible. Culture of the joint fluid is most important; inoculate it into a blood culture bottle. If there is enough fluid, prepare a Gram stain and do a cell count as well. Save the remainder to send for complement levels if septic arthritis seems unlikely. Interpretation of the results of joint fluid analysis is summarized in Table 12-8 p 319.

Polyarticular Arthritis. In patients with involvement of more than one joint, a history of migration of the arthritis suggests ARF or, in adolescents, gonococcal arthritis. Inquire about *hepatitis* exposure, fevers, weight loss, aspirin and drug use, change in bowel habits, rash, recent sore throat, or previous episodes of joint swelling or pain. Perform a complete physical examination looking for lymphadenopathy, petechiae, rash, pharyngitis, hepatosplenomegaly, and in the adolescent, vaginal or urethral discharge. Consider Lyme arthritis if there is a history of a tick bite or a rash consistent with erythema chronicum migrans.

Obtain a CBC with differential, ESR, ASLO, FANA, complement (C3, C4, CH50), rheumatoid factor, HBsAg, heterophile antibody, urinalysis, and stool guiac. If petechiae or pustules are present, unroof a lesion with a scalpel blade and Gram stain the contents looking for organisms. Leukocytosis with a shift to the left suggests an infectious process. Hematuria (*HSP, serum sickness, lupus*) and hematochezia (*inflammatory bowel disease,* HSP) may be helpful findings.

Suspect that an adolescent with mono- or pauciarticular arthiritis associated with tenosynovitis, pustules, or necrotic lesions has *gonococcal arthritis.* Obtain genital, rectal, and pharyngeal cultures for GC in addition to cultures of the joint fluid and blood.

True migratory polyarthritis (especially knees, ankles, elbows, wrists) is highly suspicious for *ARF.* Obtain a chest x-ray and an ECG to look for evidence of carditis (cardiomegaly, tachycardia out of proportion to the fever, prolonged P-R interval).

ER MANAGEMENT

Septic arthritis is an emergency since significant joint destruction may occur in a short period of time. As soon as joint fluid and blood cultures have been obtained, secure an IV and admit the patient for IV antibiotics.

After the appropriate blood tests have been obtained, if the parents are reliable, afebrile, well-appearing patients with multiple (but not migratory) joint involvement may be evaluated as outpatients. Refer them to an office setting within a week, at which time the serologic tests can be checked and the patient reevaluated.

Treat suspected Lyme arthritis (erythema chronium migrans) with tetracycline (250 mg qid) unless the patient is less than 8 years old or possibly pregnant. Treat these patients with penicillin (50 mg/kg/day, 1–2 g/day). Treat for at least 10 days with tetracycline, 20 days with penicillin. For penicillin-allergic patients, use erythromycin (30 mg/kg/day) for 15–30 days. Admit patients with frank arthritis for IV penicillin.

INDICATIONS FOR ADMISSION

- Suspected septic arthritis, rheumatic fever, malignancy
- Arthritis associated with weight loss, systemic toxicity, or severe pain

- Migratory polyarthritis
- Follow-up not guaranteed

REFERENCES
1. Schaller SG: Pediatr Clin North Am 24: 775–790, 1977
2. Mandell GL, Douglas RG, Bennett JE: Principles and Practice of Infectious Diseases 2 ed, New York: John Wiley and Son, pp. 1343–1349, 1985.

Fractures, Dislocations, and Sprains

INTRODUCTION

Although the definitive treatment of a serious orthopedic injury requires an orthopedist, the primary care physician must be able to diagnose these conditions so that appropriate orthopedic consultation can be obtained.

Fracture. A fracture is a break or crush injury involving bone. When the growth plate or epiphyseal ossification center is affected, acute or chronic growth disturbances may result. The *Salter classification* scheme of epiphyseal injuries (Fig. 16-1) is useful for describing the fracture and predicting the likelihood of growth disturbance. *Pathologic fractures* can occur in areas of bone weakness. Etiologies in-

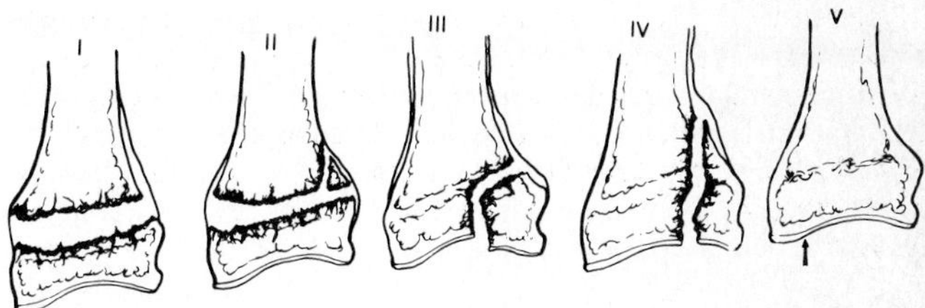

Figure 16-1. Salter-Harris classification of fractures. As the number of the fracture increases from 1 to 5, the likelihood that bone growth will be impaired increases. *(Rund: Essentials of Emergency Medicine, New York: Appleton-Century-Crofts, 1982, p 265.)*

clude rickets, bone cysts, osteogenesis imperfecta, and malignancies. *Open* or *compound* fractures communicate with the outside environment via a puncture wound or laceration.

Sprain. A sprain is disruption of a ligament. Grade I is minor, without any tear. A grade II sprain is an incomplete tear of the ligament, while a grade III injury results in a complete disruption. Sprains of the knees and ankles are most common.

Dislocation. A dislocation is a complete disruption of the normal articular relationships of a joint. The most common sites are the shoulder (anterior), MCP and IP finger joints (p 483), and patella (pp 422–424). A *subluxation* is an incomplete dislocation, most commonly involving the radial head of a toddler (''nursemaid's elbow'').

CLINICAL PRESENTATION

Fractures. Fractures usually present with point tenderness, ecchymosis, and swelling after an episode of trauma. There may be an obvious deformity. Infants and toddlers, however, may merely refuse to use the involved limb which is neither swollen nor markedly tender (''toddler's fracture''). Significant blood loss, leading to shock, can occur with fractures of the femur or pelvis. With a compound fracture, bone may be seen protruding through the skin.

Sprains. Sprains present as joint swelling, with ecchymosis and tenderness over the involved ligament, after an episode of trauma. There may be pain on palpation over the ligament without any instability (grade I), increased joint laxity upon stress (grade II), or total joint instability (grade III).

Dislocations. A dislocated or subluxed joint appears deformed, with a limited, painful range of motion. A *nursemaid's elbow* is caused by axial traction on the arm. The toddler is comfortable, but refuses to actively flex his or her elbow, preferring an extended, internally rotated position. There is no swelling and minimal tenderness, unless passive flexion of the elbow is attempted.

DIAGNOSIS

A complete history includes the mechanism of the injury, location of maximal pain, chronic medical problems (rickets, renal failure, liver disease, malignancy), and drug use (diphenylhydantoin can produce a rickets-like picture). For open fractures, ascertain the patient's tetanus status and whether the trauma occured in a dirty environment. Unfortunately, an accurate history is not always possible with infants and toddlers.

The priority on physical examination is assessment of the neurovascular status of the injured extremity. Palpate the pulses, check the warmth, capillary filling, and active motion of the fingers or toes, and evaluate sensation, using the uninjured limb for comparison. The presence of any of the "six P's" suggests neurovascular compromise: *pain, pulselessness, pallor, paralysis, paresthesias, and painful passive motion.*

Next, examine the injured site, looking for deformity, swelling, ecchymoses, point tenderness, and range of motion, again using the other side for comparison.

Perform a complete examination of the ligaments of all injured knees and ankles. For knees, check for valgus (medial collateral) and varus (lateral collateral) laxity. Perform a Lachman test (anterior draw at 15 degrees of flexion) to check the anterior cruciate, and a posterior draw test (at 30 degrees of flexion) for the posterior cruciate. For ankles, check inversion (tibulocalcaneal) and anterior draw (talofibular). If the patient cannot cooperate, immediately consult an orthopedist who may perform the examination under anesthesia. Complete the physical examination, looking for associated injuries.

AP and lateral x-rays are indicated if there is an obvious deformity, point tenderness, or marked swelling or ecchymosis, suggestive of a fracture or dislocation. Splint the extremity first and obtain views that include the joints above and below the site of injury. No radiographs are necessary if a nursemaid's elbow can be confidently diagnosed clinically. If the radiologist or orthopedist is experienced at interpreting pediatric films, comparison views of the uninjured extremity are not routinely indicated (with the exception of elbow fracture).

The differentiation between sprains and Salter I epiphyseal injuries can be difficult, as routine x-rays are normal in both. With a sprain the ligament is tender and the joint may be lax, while Salter I injuries cause tenderness over the growth plate. Obtain stress films that may show joint line opening with a sprain. However, do not stress the ankle when there is tenderness over the lateral malleolus; a nondisplaced Salter I fracture may be converted into a more serious injury.

ER MANAGEMENT

Immediate orthopedic consultation is necessary for suspected *neurovascular compromise.*

Prior to radiographic examination, cover *open fractures* with sterile dressings, obtain a culture of the bone or exposed soft tissue, start an IV, and give antibiotics (oxacillin or cephalothin 100 mg/kg/day; clindamycin 40 mg/kg/day if allergic to penicillin). Splint deformities in a physiologic position prior to obtaining x-rays.

Refer all *fractures, grade II* and *III sprains,* and *shoulder* and *patella dislocations* to an orthopedist. The management of MCP and IP dislocations is discussed on p 487.

If orthopedic consultation is not immediately available, elevate and apply ice and a compression bandage to the extremity. If the patient must travel to see an orthopedist, apply a Jones dressing. Wrap the extremity in 2–3 layers of cotton, followed by an ace bandage. Repeat the process 3–4 times.

A *nursemaid's elbow* can be reduced by flexing the elbow to 90 degrees, then supinating fully while palpating the radial head. Usually a click is felt, and within 10–15 minutes (sometimes longer) the child actively flexes the elbow.

INDICATIONS FOR ADMISSION

- Open fracture
- Neurovascular compromise
- Serious injury (supracondylar, tibia-fibula, radius-ulna, cervical spine, or femur fracture; grade III knee sprain; shoulder dislocation)

REFERENCES

1. Rang NC, Willis RB: Pediatr Clin North Am 24: 749–773, 1977
2. Harvey J: PIR 217–222, 1981

Knee Injuries

INTRODUCTION

The knee is a common site for sports injuries, especially in football players and skiers. The ligaments or menisci may be torn or the patella dislocated.

CLINICAL PRESENTATION AND DIAGNOSIS

The patient may complain of pain or swelling, or he or she may be limping or unable to bear weight. The evaluation of an injured extremity is discussed on pp 420–421, but with knees in particular compare with the uninjured side.

The mechanism of injury is particularly important: a blow to the lateral knee surface can cause a *medial collateral* or *anterior cruciate* injury. *Meniscal injuries* occur while weight bearing with the foot externally rotated, pushing off. *Patellar dislocations* are noncontact injuries that occur while alighting with the foot externally rotated and the knee flexed.

With *anterior cruciate* tears, the patient or bystanders may report hearing a "pop" or "snap," the patient refuses to bear weight, and swelling begins almost immediately. Locking occurs with a *meniscal injury,* but these patients want to continue the activity. A ripping sound suggests a *patellar dislocation,* and a sensation of "tightness" behind the knee suggests a small effusion.

After the initial evaluation of the injured extremity, as described on p 421, the integrity of the ligaments must be checked. With the patient supine, hip extended, and knee at 0 degrees, place one hand above the ankle and the other on the lateral knee. Abducting the lower leg then causes valgus knee stress, testing the medial collateral ligament. Place the upper hand on the medial knee and adduct the lower leg (varus stress, lateral collateral). If instability is present, stop the examination; if the knee is not unstable, repeat the examination at 30 degrees flexion. Now, test the cruciate ligaments by flexing the hip to 45 degrees and the knee to 90 degrees with the foot flat on the table. Sit on the patient's toes, place both hands on either side of the patient's calf, and gently pull the tibia forward (anterior draw, anterior cruciate) and push it backward (posterior draw, posterior cruciate). Repeat the anterior draw at 15 degrees of knee flexion, which relaxes the quadriceps (secondary anterior stabilizers of the knee). For each ligament, assess the range of motion and whether there is a definite endpoint, using the other side as a reference.

To evaluate the menisci, perform the McMurray test. With the knee flexed and the foot turned laterally, slowly extend the knee while applying valgus (medial meniscus) and varus (lateral meniscus) force. A palpable click reflects a positive test.

Patellar dislocation is obvious when the patella is lateral to the joint and the anterior aspect of the knee appears concave and empty. Since knee extension causes patellar relocation, the patient often arrives in the ER complaining of knee pain with no obvious deformity. The patellar apprehension test is useful if relocation has occurred. Slightly flex the knee and prepare to push the patella laterally. The patient will become anxious and stop the procedure.

ER MANAGEMENT

After the clinical evaluation is complete, obtain anteroposterior (AP) and lateral radiographs of the knee. Obtain stress films to rule out a Salter I fracture if a ligamentous injury is diagnosed (see p 421). Patients with grade II or III collateral or cruciate sprains, meniscal injuries, and dislocated patellas must be evaluated immediately by an orthopedist. While awaiting consultation, elevate the leg and apply ice and a compressive bandage to the knee.

REFERENCES

1. Smith JB: Pediatr Clin North Am 24: 841–855, 1977
2. Garrick JG: PIR 4: 235–243, 1983

Limp

INTRODUCTION

Limp in children is most often secondary to trauma. Other etiologies include infections, connective tissue disorders, and sickle cell disease. In addition, if the pain can be localized to either the hip or knee joint, there are specific, age-dependent disorders to consider (Table 16-2).

CLINICAL PRESENTATION

Trauma

The most common cause of limp and pain is trauma. The insult may be minor, such as a sore from an ill-fitting shoe or a foreign body in the sole of the foot. Alternatively, there may be a more serious injury (fracture, sprain, dislocation; p 419) with ecchymosis, swelling, localized tenderness, or obvious deformity.

TABLE 16-2. COMMON ETIOLOGIES OF LIMP

Trauma	Knee Disease
Soft tissue injury (bruise)	Osgood-Schlatter disease
Fracture	Chrondromalacia patella
Dislocation	Osteochondritis dissecans
Sprain	Other Etiologies
Foreign body	Viral infection
Hip Disease	Henoch-Schönlein purpura
Transient synovitis	Inflammatory bowel disease
Legg-Perthes disease	Serum sickness
Slipped capital femoral epiphysis	Acute rheumatic fever
Infection	Juvenile rheumatoid arthritis
Osteomyelitis	Systemic lupus erythematosus
Septic arthritis	Sickle cell disease
Intervertebral discitis	

Infections

Osteomyelitis. Osteomyelitis (p 307) causes fever, toxicity, and limp or unwillingness to use the extremity. Point tenderness is typical, with or without overlying cellulitis.

Septic Arthritis. Septic arthritis (p 316) causes the sudden onset of fever and toxicity, limp or complete unwillingness to move the leg, and erythema, warmth, and tenderness over a joint. The patient resists passive joint movement. The hip is most commonly involved and it is held in flexion, external rotation, and abduction.

Intervertebral Discitis. Intervertebral discitis is an infectious or inflammatory disease occurring primarily in 2 to 7-year olds. The patient may present with limp, back pain, refusal to sit or walk, irritability, and low grade fever. On examination, there is localized tenderness directly over the spine, paravertebral muscle spasm, and limited straight leg raising.

Other Etiologies

Arthritis. Arthritis (nonseptic) presents with swelling, erythema, tenderness, and warmth of single or multiple joints (p 415). Both passive and active movements are limited. Associated findings may include fever, rash, heart murmur, generalized adenopathy, and hepatosplenomegaly.

Sickle Cell Disease. In sickle cell disease (p 273) the patient may have diffuse bone pain secondary to infarcts, leading to tenderness and limp. Associated findings may include fever, jaundice, abdominal pain, and swelling of the dorsums of the hands and feet.

Hip Diseases. With hip diseases, the pain may be in the hip or anterior thigh, or referred to the anteromedial aspect of the knee.

Transient synovitis is a benign, self-limited, inflammatory hip disease seen predominantly in males 3–12 years old. Acute or gradual onset of limp and either hip or knee pain may follow a mild URI with or without low grade fever. The child does not appear toxic. The hip is held in mild flexion, external rotation, and abduction, but there is no erythema or increased warmth. Abduction and internal rotation are limited by pain at the extremes of motion.

Legg-Perthes disease, or aseptic necrosis of the femoral head, usually occurs in males 4–9 years of age. There is a gradual onset of limp and pain in the hip, groin, or medial knee. Hip abduction and internal rotation are limited.

Slipped capital femoral epiphysis (SCFE) causes a displacement of the normal relationship between the femoral head and neck. Most patients are obese adolescent males who present with a limp and subacute or chronic groin pain, which can be referred to the anterior thigh or knee. The hip is held in flexion and external rotation. Flexion of the hip may accentuate the external rotation deformity, while internal rotation and abduction may be limited.

Knee Diseases. Although there are a number of specific conditions which affect the knee, remember that hip diseases can also present with knee pain. Therefore examine the hips carefully in all patients with knee pain.

Osgood-Schlatter disease, or apophysitis of the tibial tuberosity, is a self-limited disease that usually occurs in active adolescents. Patients present with a gradual onset of limp, especially after exercise. On examination, there is tenderness and swelling over the tibial tuberosity.

Chondromalacia patellae is a softening of the patellar cartilage that also occurs in active patients. Patellar pain after activity, episodes of buckling (but not locking), and crepitance and tenderness upon palpation of the patellar articular surface are typical.

In *osteochondritis dissecans,* an area of bone, usually on the lateral aspect of the medial femoral condyle, develops ischemic necrosis and subsequent fracture (a piece of bone and cartilage may break loose). This causes intermittent painful limp after exercise, buckling, locking, and a tender medial femoral condyle. It is most common in adolescent males.

DIAGNOSIS

The priority is the prompt diagnosis of a septic arthritis, osteomyelitis, or SCFE.

Inquire about trauma, rate of onset (acute versus chronic), similar previous episodes, fever, and location and radiation of the pain. On examination, check the neurovascular status of the extremities, look for erythema, warmth, and tenderness and put the joints through complete active and passive ranges of motion.

Unless it is clear that the etiology of the limp is minor trauma, obtain standard AP and lateral x-rays of the suspicious areas. If the limp is associated with decreased hip range of motion, obtain AP and frog leg lateral radiographs. Possible findings include fractures, SCFE, joint space widening (septic arthritis, Legg-Perthes disease), increased density of the femoral epiphysis (Legg-Perthes disease), or subchondral bone fragmentation (osteochondritis dissecans). X-rays of the knee are not needed when Osgood-Schlatter disease is suspected and the films are normal in chondromalacia patella.

Obtain a CBC (with differential) and ESR when there is no definite history of trauma. Leukocytosis, a shift to the left, and a markedly increased ESR (>60mm/hr) may occur in inflammatory conditions such as septic arthritis, osteomyelitis, and discitis. With synovitis, the ESR is elevated, but usually less than 60mm/hr.

Occasionally, synovitis may resemble septic arthritis (high fever and ESR; markedly decreased range of motion). An AP pelvic x-ray, obtained while bilateral axial traction is applied to both legs, causes a curvilinear lucency to be seen within the normal hip joint space. If a lucency is also seen in the affected hip joint space, there is no joint effusion (no septic arthritis).

ER MANAGEMENT

If a *septic arthritis* or *osteomyelitis* is suspected, refer the patient immediately to an orthopedist for aspiration of joint fluid or subperiosteal pus. Intravenous antibiotics are then indicated (see pp 316–319 and 307–308).

Some patients with transient *synovitis* have a good hip range of motion with maximal tenderness away from the joint line (over one of the flexor tendons). If the patient is afebrile, with an ESR <40mm/hr, he or she may be treated at home with bedrest and aspirin (10–15 mg/kg q 4h) until the symptoms have resolved completely (less than 10–14 days). For patients with more severe symptoms, consult with an orthopedist and admit for bedrest and skin traction, until the range of motion is normal.

Immediately obtain orthopedic consultation for patients with *SCFE*, as minor trauma can cause complete displacement of the femoral epiphysis. Weight bearing must be discontinued and the patient placed at rest with the affected leg in traction. Ultimate treatment is operative. SCFE is associated with hypothyroidism; draw thyroid function tests in addition to a CBC.

Although no emergency treatment is required for *Legg-Perthes disease*, refer these patients to an orthopedist so that a comprehensive plan of treatment can be arranged.

The treatment of *Osgood-Schlatter disease* is salicylates and limitation of activity until the acute symptoms resolve (2–6 weeks), then titration of activity level to tolerance. Similar therapy is useful for *chondromalacia*, in addition to quadriceps exercises (straight leg lifting, hip flexion while sitting). Refer patients with suspected *osteochondritis dissecans* to an orthopedist, since treatment usually requires nonweight bearing and casting.

Since *discitis* is difficult to distinguish from osteomyelitis, treat with bedrest, IV oxacillin (100 mg/kg/day), and observation in the hospital.

INDICATIONS FOR ADMISSION

- Slipped capital femoral epiphysis
- Septic arthritis, osteomyelitis, discitis
- Transient synovitis with fever or markedly decreased range of motion

REFERENCES

1. Hensinger RN: Pediatr Clin North Am 24: 723, 1977
2. Chung S: Pediatr Clin North Am 24: 857, 1977

17

Psychologic and Social Emergencies

Abandonment

INTRODUCTION

Abandonment of infants and small children is an extreme form of parental neglect. Abandoned children are very likely to suffer physical harm unless there is immediate intervention.

CLINICAL PRESENTATION AND DIAGNOSIS

Every abandoned child must have a thorough physical examination, with particular attention to a general assessment of the state of nutrition and hygiene. Undress and examine the child thoroughly for physical stigmata of abuse (p 431).

ER MANAGEMENT

Immediately file a telephone report of abandonment with the local Child Protection Services (CPS), even if complete information about the family is lacking. A written report must be filed within 48 hours in most states.

There are several options available in the management of an abandoned child. He or she may be transferred into the custody of a relative who is judged suitable by the CPS worker, or he may be placed in temporary shelter or foster care. However, if medical care is necessary or temporary placement is not available, admit the child to the hospital. In most states, abandoned children who are referred to the local CPS may be legally placed in another home without a court order. The biologic parents may contest the placement in a court of law.

INDICATIONS FOR ADMISSION

- Abandoned child who requires medical care
- Temporary placement unavailable

REFERENCE

1. Fontana VJ: Pediatr Ann 13: 736–744, 1984

Child Abuse

INTRODUCTION

Physical abuse can be defined as nonaccidental physical injury to a child, while neglect is a parent's or caretaker's failure to meet a child's needs for food, clothing, shelter, hygiene, medical care, education, or supervision. There has been an alarming increase in the incidence of both child abuse and neglect throughout the United States during the past 2 decades. Health professionals are required to report all such cases to their state CPS.

CLINICAL PRESENTATION AND DIAGNOSIS

When evaluating a child with an injury, be suspicious of abuse or neglect if the history reveals an unusual delay in seeking medical care, the parents' explanation of the injury is not compatible with the physical findings, the cause of the injury is unknown, or there is a previous history of similar episodes. Parents may be reluctant to give information or their reaction may be inappropriate to the seriousness of the injuries. Other worrisome signs are a lack of primary care (no immunizations) and a history of parental psychosis, substance abuse, or alcoholism.

While examining the child, maintain a high index of suspicion for abuse or neglect if his or her weight is below the third percentile for age, there is poor personal hygiene, lack of adequate clothing, behavioral disturbance (especially undue compliance with the examiner), or an abnormal interaction between the parent and child (unwarranted roughness or extreme aloofness).

Remove all the child's clothing and examine the skin carefully for bruises, abrasions, burns, and lacerations in various stages of resolution. Certain skin lesions are typical for specific types of abuse, such as circular cigarette burns, human bite marks, J-shaped curvilinear marks from a wire cord or belt, circumferential rope burns, "grid" marks from an electric heater, and symmetrical scald burns of the buttocks or extremities. Other dermatologic manifestations may include cutaneous signs of malnutrition (decreased subcutaneous fat, increased creases), scalp hematomas, and signs of trauma to the genital area.

Fractures are suggested by refusal to bear weight or move an extremity, gross deformity, or soft tissue swelling and point tenderness over an extremity. Neurologic manifestations may include retinal hemorrhages (whiplash injury) and unexplainable irritability, coma, or convulsions. Finally, an acute abdomen, poisoning, or drug withdrawal which cannot be explained may in fact represent forms of child abuse.

The differential diagnosis of the abused child includes diseases with skeletal involvement (*osteogenesis imperfecta*, *Caffey disease*, *scurvy*, *rickets*, *birth trauma*, *TORCHS infection*, and *accidental trauma*). Diseases with dermatologic manifestations include *bleeding disorders* idiopathic thrombocytopenic purpura (ITP), leukemia, hemophilia, von Willebrand disease, *recurrent pyodermas*, *scalded skin syndrome*, and *accidental trauma*. Finally, the *sudden infant death syndrome* and *accidental poisonings* may be mistaken for child abuse.

ER MANAGEMENT

If child abuse is suspected, obtain a complete skeletal survey for all children under 5 years of age and for older patients if the physical examination suggests a fracture. Order other radiologic studies, such as a CTT scan or liver-spleen scan when indicated by the nature of the injuries. If the parents deny any knowledge of the etiology of skin bruises, obtain a complete blood count (CBC) with differential, platelet count, prothrombin time (PT) and partial thromboplastin time (PTT), and a bleeding time.

Immediately notify (telephone) the CPS if abuse or neglect is suspected. The CPS is required to initiate action in all cases reported and may not refuse to accept a referral made in good faith by a competent reporter. A written report must be filed by a physician, nurse, or social worker within 48 hours.

A protected environment for these children must be guaranteed. The CPS worker must evaluate the case and decide whether the child can safely return home or must go to a temporary shelter or foster placement. Hospitalize the child if adequate placement is not available or medical care is needed. In all cases appropriate follow-up must be arranged. If the parents refuse to allow hospitalization, it may be necessary to have law enforcement officials intervene. In most states, hospital personnel may place a child under temporary protective custody without either parental consent or a family court order. However, it is the responsibility of the CPS worker to decide whether the child can be placed in the custody of a relative or guardian.

Working with the families of abused children can be a difficult experience. Avoid an accusatory attitude, as the majority of these parents love their children and deserve a supportive approach. Keep the parents informed and involved, emphasize that the goal of all concerned is to keep the family together, explain the role of the social worker and supportive services, and assure confidentiality. Avoid police involvement unless absolutely necessary. Finally, arrange to examine the siblings within 24 hours as up to 20% have also been abused.

INDICATIONS FOR ADMISSION

- Medical care required
- Safe placement not available

REFERENCE

1. Fontana VJ: Pediatr Ann 13: 736–744, 1984

Death in the ER

INTRODUCTION

The loss of a child has a devastating effect on a family, particularly if unexpected or without any readily identifiable cause. These families do not have the opportunity for "preparatory grief."

CLINICAL PRESENTATION AND MANAGEMENT

An initial period of denial and disbelief occurs, often without any visible signs of grieving. The diagnosis may be questioned at this time.

There usually follows a period of guilt, at which time the family questions whether they may have somehow contributed to the child's death. The parents may blame themselves for the death or they may direct their anger to another family member or the medical staff, especially if medical care was sought prior to the patient's demise. Grieving follows, during which the family may repeatedly review the events leading to the death. Grieving may last for months or even years, and anniversary reactions are common.

ER MANAGEMENT

The parents must be informed promptly and privately of the child's death, assuring them that everything possible was done. The exact words used are not nearly as important as the sentiment and concern expressed by the physician.

Have a staff member remain with the family at all times, preferably in a private area, and have a trained clergyman present, if possible. If the family is denying the death, do not argue with them or reinforce their denial. Allow the parents to be angry, but try to relieve their guilt, if possible. Listen to the parents, as they desperately need to express their thoughts and feelings.

See to the personal needs of the family (coffee, telephone) and offer to help them with funeral arrangements. If an autopsy is necessary, make sure the parents comprehend that the child is dead before requesting it. A clear explanation of the reasons for performing the postmortem (determine cause of death, possibility of familial or infectious diseases, medical knowledge) facilitates obtaining consent. In most cases (sudden infant death syndrome [SIDS], possible homicide, unexpected death), however, an autopsy is required by law.

Arrange a follow-up appointment to ascertain that a normal grieving process is underway. At that time the events leading up to the death and autopsy results can be reviewed.

REFERENCE

1. Soreff SM: Crit Care Medicine 7: 321–323, 1979

Emergency Care of the Chronically Ill Child

INTRODUCTION

Children with congenital malformations and chronic illnesses pose special problems for the emergency physician. In many instances the problem is uncommon and the physician is unsure of the ramifications and implications. It may therefore be helpful to employ a set of general questions that is applicable to the assessment of a great many different conditions. Answers to these questions provide a framework for making appropriate management decisions.

CLINICAL PRESENTATION AND ER MANAGEMENT

Is the Situation a Life-Threatening Emergency? If yes, the general principles of ventilation and support of cardiac function are critical, regardless of the baseline health status of the patient. Maintain vital functions in the usual manner. If time allows, consider important specific issues of fluid and electrolyte management and modification of drug doses in light of special metabolic needs (eg, renal failure, liver, endocrine or cardiac disease), but the first priority is to resuscitate the patient.

What is the Usual Baseline Status of This Child? When treating healthy children, the physician can generally assume that the baseline status of the child is within normal limits. However, such assumptions can be misleading in the case of children with special health conditions. The parents frequently can give detailed information including diagnosis, medications, laboratory results, and usual physical findings. Sometimes they have documentary evidence including medical summaries, names and numbers of the child's physicians, and photographs. Pictures can be extremely useful in verifying the presence of "old" rather than acute findings, such as a facial nerve paresis revealed in an asymmetrical smile.

Is the Illness or Accident in Any Way Related to the Child's Ongoing Health Problem? The acute complaint may be comparable to that of a normal child or it can be secondary to the underlying disease. Inaccurate assumptions can be made about the nature of the causes of the current problem. For example, the physician must consider the possibility of a pathologic fracture in the demineralized bones of a patient with malignancy, osteogenesis imperfecta, or vitamin D deficiency secondary to liver or renal disease. Similarly a shunt obstruction or urinary tract infection must be ruled out in a child with myelodysplasia who presents with fever and vomiting, before a viral etiology is assumed.

Does the Underlying Chronic Condition Place the Child at Risk for Having an Unusual Medical Problem? The risk may result directly from the underlying condition, such as sepsis in a febrile child with an immune deficiency or sickle cell anemia. Alternatively, it may be due to previous or ongoing treatment of the underlying health problem, as in the case of a child who is unable to mount a stress response because of suppression of the adrenal pituitary axis following recent high dose steroid treatment. If the disease or its treatment places the child at special risk, it is important to identify the risk and so that the evaluation and treatment are appropriate.

Does the Child's Condition Require Any Special Management in View of the ER Diagnosis? Do the patient's usual medicines need to be adjusted? For example, it may be necessary to alter insulin dosage for a diabetic who presents with an illness or accident. Similarly, the child who takes anticonvulsants may require an alternate route of administration of the medication if he or she is vomiting. Such preventive measures are extremely important and often avoid unnecessary hospitalizations.

Why Did the Parent Bring the Child for Care? Were the parents advised to seek medical attention or alerted to respond urgently to a particular symptom? What changes do they see in the child? Alternatively, are they coming primarily for reassurance or to check out a concern because they view the child as especially vulnerable and therefore are unsure whether to treat a minor symptom in the usual way. Parents often view children with ongoing health problems as being at special risk. Failure to address the specific basis for their concerns may lead to oversight of important special considerations or to parental dissatisfaction with the care, even when it is medically sound.

Attention to these questions will enable the ER physician to provide better care to children with chronic illnesses.

REFERENCE

1. Stein REK, in Shelov SP, et al: *Primary Care Pediatrics*. Norwalk, Conn: Appleton–Century–Crofts, 1984, pp. 14–24

Psychiatric Emergencies

INTRODUCTION

Although behavioral problems are common in pediatrics, true psychiatric emergencies are not. The priorities in the ER are assessment of whether the patient's condition is dangerous to him- or herself or others and whether or not the family can adequately care for the child at home.

CLINICAL PRESENTATION

Suicide Attempt. The most common adolescent psychiatric emergency is the *suicide gesture* or *attempt* (see p 444). A polydrug ingestion by an adolescent female is a typical example. However, some accidents, particularly those that occur when the patient is alone, may be suicide attempts.

Depression. The depressed patient may present with recurrent somatic complaints (stomachaches, headaches, myalgias) for which no organic cause can be found. Rarely, depression can present with acting out behavior, running away, stealing, or fire setting. Occasionally the parent is concerned about a loss of appetite, poor school performance, or a change in the sleep pattern.

Psychosis. The psychotic patient, who cannot distinguish reality from fantasy, may present with a history of hallucinations, extreme variations in mood and, occasionally, violent behavior. The adolescent with *schizophrenia* has delusions, auditory hallucinations, inappropriate affect, and abnormal speech, although recent memory is relatively intact.

DIAGNOSIS AND ER MANAGEMENT

Suicide Attempt. The diagnosis and management are discussed on p 444. Once the patient is medically stabilized, admit him or her to the hospital. Suicide precautions are needed for the patient who has made a serious attempt. The goals of hospitalization are to facilitate early psychiatric intervention and to remove the patient from the situation that led to the attempt.

Depression. Somatic complaints with no identifiable organic basis or changes in the patient's normal behavior or mood suggest depression. Ask the patient how he is sleeping, whether or not he enjoys school, and what he does for fun. Ask about a family history of depression and suicide. Have the patient name his best friend and tell you when he last saw that person. If the patient appears to be depressed (loss of interest in school, friends, usual hobbies, or sports), ask whether he has ever thought of committing suicide. Far from putting thoughts in the patient's mind, these kinds of questions may actually help him feel better, since he can now discuss something that is troubling him. Patients who have considered suicide must be seen immediately by a psychiatrist or psychologist. If the suicidal ideation has reached the point of actual planning, hospitalization is indicated.

Psychosis. The first step is to rule out an organic cause for the psychosis. The most common organic etiology is *drug ingestion* (LSD,

PCP, amphetamines, anticholinergics). Other causes include *hypoglycemia, increased intracranial pressure* (tumor, brain abscess, Reye syndrome), *temporal lobe seizures, encephalitis, porphyria,* and *Wilson disease.*

Ask about possible drug ingestion (p 348) and have the family bring in all medications in the home (and from the homes of friends or relatives that the patient has visited recently). Inquire about a family history of schizophrenia, and try to determine when the symptoms were first noticed. With an *organic psychosis,* the onset is acute and the hallucinations are often visual, olfactory, tactile, or gustatory, rather than auditory. With *schizophrenia* and other *functional psychoses,* the hallucinations are typically auditory and the onset is more insidious.

On physical examination, there may be fever (brain abscess, encephalitis, anticholinergic or amphetamine ingestion), tachycardia (anticholinergic, hallucinogen or amphetamine ingestion, sepsis), and hypertension (anticholinergics, amphetamines, LSD, PCP). The vital signs are usually normal in patients with a functional etiology. Note the pupil size and reactivity; there may be inequality (mass lesion, brain abscess), mydriasis (hypoglycemia, LSD, amphetamines, cocaine, anticholinergics), or miosis (PCP).

Immediately order a CTT scan in patients with any neurologic abnormalities, signs of increased intracranial pressure, or fever. Febrile patients require a lumbar puncture after the CTT (if it is normal). Also obtain a CBC, electrolytes, serum glucose and dextrostix, liver function tests, and urinalysis.

Unless an organic cause for the psychosis can be definitely ruled out in the ER, admit the patient to a pediatric service to continue the evaluation after consultation with a psychiatrist. Do not initiate antipsychotic medications in the ER unless a psychiatrist, who can provide the necessary close follow-up, has examined the patient. If sedation is required for agitation use diazapem (0.1–0.3 mg/kg/dose).

INDICATIONS FOR ADMISSION

- Suicide attempt or gesture
- Depression with concrete suicidal plans (relative)
- Psychotic episode

REFERENCES

1. Rothenberg MB: Pediatr Digest 21: 33, 1979
2. Pearce J: J Child Psychol Psychiatry 18: 79 1977

Sexual Abuse

INTRODUCTION

Sexual abuse is the exposure of a child to sexual stimulation inappropriate for his or her age, cognitive development, or position in the relationship. The legal definition is nonconsensual sexual contact. Incest is legally defined as a marriage or intercourse (oral, anal, genital) with a person known to be related as an ancestor, descendent, brother, sister, uncle, aunt, nephew, or niece. Rape is legally defined as nonconsensual sexual intercourse. For all offenses, a child under 17 years is legally incapable of consent. Specific laws vary from state to state.

CLINICAL PRESENTATION

A number of behavioral findings may signal the possibility of sexual abuse, including difficulties in school, unwillingness to change for or participate in gym class, enuresis and encopresis, sleep disturbances, running away, and attempted suicide. Incest victims may exhibit seductive or regressive behavior. More specific complaints include difficulty walking or sitting, and genital trauma, pain, or itching. Venereal disease or pregnancy in a child under the age of 12 years is sexual abuse or rape until proven otherwise.

DIAGNOSIS

Insure privacy for the patient and whomever accompanied him or her, and keep the number of staff members involved to a minimum. Because sexual abuse usually evokes intense feelings, maintaining objectivity requires effort. Use language that is appropriate for the child's age, and ask specifically about all types of sexual contact. It may be useful to use anatomically correct dolls or pictures. Try to ascertain when the last sexual activity occurred and what the child has done since the assault (changed clothes, bathed, urinated, defecated). Assure the child that he or she was right to reveal information about the sexual abuse.

Consent for the physical examination is often an issue. However, consent from the minor (regardless of age) is all that is required since the examination also serves to rule out venereal disease.

If the child has not changed clothes since the sexual activity, have him or her undress on a sheet and save all clothing for legal evidence. If the child has changed, but not bathed, collect only the underwear. If the child has pubic hair, comb it onto a paper towel and seal the paper towel, combings, one plucked pubic hair, and the comb in a labeled envelope. Perform a complete and careful physical examination looking for marks, bruises, or other signs of physical injury or illness, and note the child's Tanner stage of pubertal development.

Perform a perineal-genital examination in young children in the frogleg position or as described on p 247. If the examination is performed less than 48 hours after the sexual activity, examine the potential areas of contact with a Wood light. Areas of fluorescence may be seminal fluid and should be swabbed with a saline-moistened cotton swab, and placed on a labeled slide to air day. In girls, spread the labia with two fingers to examine the hymenal ring, the introitus, and the area between the labia majora and minora. In the prepubertal female, if there are no acute signs of pelvic injury, a speculum exam is not necessary. If there are obvious signs of physical injury (bleeding, lacerations), consult a pediatric gynecologist regarding the need for a pelvic examination under anesthesia.

In boys, examine the penis and scrotum for bruises, swelling, teethmarks, erythema, or other signs of trauma. In both boys and girls, spread the buttocks with both hands to examine the anus and perineal area. If there are obvious signs of physical injury or severe pain, anoscopy or sigmoidoscopy is indicated, under anesthesia if necessary.

Obtain gonorrhea and chlamydial cultures from the cervix (postmenarchal), vagina (premenarchal), urethra, rectum, and pharynx, regardless of the nature of the sexual contact. Examine vaginal specimens for the presence of *Trichomonas*. Obtain wet preps from all involved areas to look for sperm: mouth up to 6 hours postassault, rectum up to 24 hours, vagina up to 24 hours. If a speculum exam is performed, obtain a PAP smear and ask the hospital laboratory to specifically note the presence of sperm. Immotile sperm are present up to 2½ weeks after intercourse. Obtain a VDRL on all patients and a pregnancy test on all pubertal females.

ER MANAGEMENT

Report all cases of suspected sexual abuse to the Child Protective Services, although it is not your responsibility to determine whether or not the abuse actually occurred. Make careful documentation, in writing, of all findings on the physical examination; diagrams and drawings are very useful. Take photographs of any bruises or other evidence of physical injury. Label all specimens taken for evidence and place them in evidence envelopes to be logged and secured by the security department of the hospital or given directly to the police. Give prophylaxis against gonorrhea and and *Chlamydia* as outlined in Table 17-1.

Offer a postcoital contraceptive to the postmenarchal adolescent female who is seen within 72 hours. Lo-Ovral (0.3 mg norgestrel, 0.03 mg ethinyl estradiol), 4 tablets at once, and 3 tablets 12 hours later is one regimen that has few side effects (nausea and vomiting).

TABLE 17-1. ANTIBIOTIC PROPHYLAXIS OF SEXUAL ABUSE VICTIMS

Gonorrhea, *Chlamydia*	Amoxicillin 3.0 g (50 mg/kg) or Ampicillin 3.5 g (100 mg/kg) PLUS probinecid 1 g (25 mg/kg) in a single dose[a] followed by Tetracycline 500 mg (10 mg/kg) qid for 7 days (doxycycline 100 mg bid for 7 days) or Erythromycin 500 mg (50 mg/kg/day) qid for 7 days for patients under 8 years of age or possibly pregnant

[a]Use spectinomycin 2 g (40 mg/kg) IM once for penicillin-allergic patients; use penicillin G procaine 4.8 million U (100,000 U/kg) IM plus probenecid if prophylaxis against syphilis is a concern.

Reassure the patient that his or her body is not harmed, that he or she was not responsible for the sexual assault, and that you believe him or her, and will do everything to protect the patient from further assault.

Schedule a visit within the next several days with a skilled psychotherapist. A follow-up physician visit in 2 weeks is necessary for repeat cultures (repeat the VDRL in 6 weeks).

INDICATIONS FOR ADMISSION

- Incest unless alternative arrangements can be made to ensure that the abuse cannot take place again
- Sexual abuse that occurred very near the home or when the patient's family is unable to provide the necessary support

REFERENCES

1. Selman YM, Nekitas JA: NY State J Med 83(3):341–343, 1983
2. Sgori SM. Management of the Physically and Emotionally Abused: Emergency Assessment, Intervention, and Counselling. Norwalk, Conn: Capistrano Press Ltd, 263–279, 1982

Sudden Infant Death Syndrome

INTRODUCTION

The sudden infant death syndrome (SIDS) is defined as "the sudden death of an infant or young child, unexpected by history, in which a thorough postmortem examination fails to demonstrate an adequate cause." SIDS is the leading cause of death during infancy, after the first week of life.

CLINICAL PRESENTATION

The peak incidence is at 2–4 months, although there have been autopsy-proven occurrences at up to 12 months of age. The incidence is higher in males and prematures, and when the mother smokes, is a drug addict, or is of lower socioeconomic status. Most cases occur between midnight and 9 AM during the cold weather months. Typically, a previously healthy baby either does not awaken for a morning feed or is found cold and lifeless in his or her crib.

On occasion, the infant is found pale or cyanotic, apneic, or limp and resuscitation is initiated at home or enroute to the ER. It is not clear if these "near miss" episodes are one end of the spectrum of SIDS.

DIAGNOSIS

The diagnosis of SIDS cannot be confirmed until an autopsy and other postmortem studies exclude other possible causes of sudden death in infancy. These include *adrenal insufficiency, overwhelming pneumonitis, bacterial sepsis* (especially in sickle cell disease), *child abuse,* and *poisoning.*

Near miss episodes may result from prolonged *sleep apnea, gastroesophageal-reflux-induced apnea,* and *seizures,* in addition to the diseases listed above.

ER MANAGEMENT

The management of the SIDS victim involves obtaining a detailed history of the circumstances surrounding the child's death and notifying the medical examiner that an autopsy must be performed. The management of a bereaved family is discussed on p 433.

If the resuscitation of a near miss victim is successful, admit the infant to an intensive care setting for continual cardiopulmonary monitoring and further evaluation. Obtain an electrocardiogram (ECG) with rhythm strip, chest x-ray, and blood for a CBC with differential, electrolytes, glucose, and culture. Perform a lumbar puncture for cytology, chemistries, and culture and obtain a urinalysis and urine culture. Treat with IV ampicillin and chloramphenicol if there are any findings suggestive of bacterial sepsis (pp 281–282) or meningitis (p 285).

INDICATION FOR ADMISSION

- Near miss episode

REFERENCE
1. Shannon DC, Kelly DH: N Engl J Med 306: 16, 1982

Suicide

INTRODUCTION

Suicide is the third leading cause of death among teenagers, although it also occurs in younger children. Suicide gestures, which are seen most frequently in females, are perhaps 100 times more common than successful suicides, which occur more often in males. Females are more likely to employ nonviolent methods (ingestion), whereas males more frequently use violence (firearms, blades).

CLINICAL PRESENTATION AND DIAGNOSIS

A suicide attempt is usually triggered by a crisis situation, such as the death or departure of a loved one, a fight with a boyfriend or girlfriend, or an argument with a parent. There are a number of danger signals that may signify that a patient is potentially suicidal (Table 17-2).

TABLE 17-2. DANGER SIGNALS OF POTENTIAL SUICIDE

Behavioral	Physical
Change in eating or sleeping pattern	Somnolence
History of many recent "accidents"	Anorexia
Increased tension or anxiety	Weight loss
Temper outbursts	Constipation
Episode of running away from home	Pregnancy
Drop in school performance	
Onset of truancy	
Preoccupation with bodily symptoms	
Start of drug or alcohol use	
Depression or frank psychosis	

In the ER, these patients may present as *trauma* (p 488) or *overdose* (p 320) victims, or in a *coma of unknown etiology* (p 382). Every adolescent who takes a medication overdose or ingests a household product (caustics, hydrocarbons, insecticides) is making a suicide gesture or attempt, until proven otherwise. Also, consider any developmentally normal child over 5 years of age who ingests a poison to be potentially suicidal.

ER MANAGEMENT

The patient's clinical condition and the method of attempted suicide determine the priorities of ER management. However, the majority of patients are well enough to be interviewed when first seen. Assess the seriousness of the attempt; a "suicidal" patient needs one-to-one nursing on admission. Greater "lethality" of intent is suggested by a previous suicide attempt, a plan to commit suicide, no communication of intent to others, no request for help after the attempt (discovered accidentally), and taking action that is clearly lethal (jumping from a rooftop). Once the patient is medically stable, obtain psychiatric evaluation.

Admit all patients making a suicide gesture or attempt. Removing the patient from his or her usual social/family milieu is in itself therapeutically beneficial. In general, a pediatric or adolescent unit, where the patient can be among peers, is preferable to a psychiatric service.

INDICATION FOR ADMISSION

• Suicide gesture or attempt

REFERENCE

1. Curran BE: Pediatr Clin North Am 26: 737–746, 1979

18

Pulmonary Emergencies

Asthma

INTRODUCTION AND CLINICAL PRESENTATION

Asthma, the most common chronic disease of childhood, is defined as episodic reversible lower airway obstruction. The airway lumen is narrowed by a combination of mucous plugs, smooth muscle constriction, and airway wall edema. Air flow through the narrowed passage then causes the typical expiratory wheezing sound.

The asthmatic airway has heightened responsiveness to external stimuli. Common triggers of attacks are upper respiratory infections (URI), exercise, aspirin, and allergens. Other precipitants of wheezing include irritants (pollutants, odors, smoke), weather changes, cold air, and emotional stress. Quite often there is a family history of asthma, allergies, or eczema, or the patient is known to have allergies.

Clinical presentation varies from nighttime coughing to acute wheezing with a prolonged expiratory phase, to the absence of air movement and severe dyspnea. Status asthmaticus is defined as failure to respond to appropriate ER treatment, and therefore can be life threatening.

DIAGNOSIS

The diagnosis of asthma is suggested by the acute onset of expiratory wheezing, especially if the patient has had previous similar episodes or a history of bronchopulmonary dysplasia (BPD). Occasionally the patient has subcostal and intercostal retractions, tachycardia, and a prolonged expiratory phase with few audible wheezes. The absence of wheezing in a patient with other clinical findings compatible with asthma is suggestive of a more severe attack.

Upper Airway Obstruction. Lack of air movement can be caused by either upper or lower airway obstruction. In general, upper airway obstruction (croup, epiglottitis, extrathoracic tracheal foreign body) causes inspiratory stridor instead of expiratory wheezing. Also, suprasternal retractions are prominent. Although croup and asthma can occur simultaneously, in most instances the clinical picture of upper airway obstruction is sufficiently different from asthma that there is no confusion over the diagnosis.

Bronchiolitis. Expiratory wheezing in children under 2 years of age is frequently due to bronchiolitis, most commonly secondary to respiratory syncitial virus infection. The clinical and radiographic picture is often indistinguishable from asthma and the treatment of patients over 1 year of age is generally the same as for asthma.

Mycoplasma pneumoniae. Mycoplasma pneumoniae is the most common cause of wheezing-associated respiratory illness in school age children. Cold agglutinins, which are positive in about 50% of patients over 8 years of age, or a chest x-ray with bilateral diffuse interstitial infiltrates can help make the diagnosis.

Foreign Body. Aspiration of a foreign body can produce local or diffuse wheezing. A history of coughing or choking while eating or playing with small toys is suggestive, especially in the toddler with a first wheezing episode and no family history of atopy. The chest x-ray, if one is obtained, may show only hyperaeration, and the wheezing may clear with treatment, only to recur hours, days, or weeks later. If the diagnosis is suspected, obtain bilateral decubitus chest x-rays (see pp 107–109). A lung that is obstructed by the foreign body will not decrease in size when it is in the dependent position.

Congestive Heart Failure. Congestive heart failure can cause wheezing (cardiac asthma). Usually the patient has a history of heart disease, and there are other signs of failure, including hepatomegaly, tachycardia, and distended neck veins.

Cystic Fibrosis. Suspect cystic fibrosis in any child with recurrent pneumonias and wheezing episodes. A sweat chloride determination confirms the diagnosis.

ER MANAGEMENT

Diagnosis and assessment of the severity of the attack are performed simultaneously. A peak flow measurement compared to known standards based on height allows a quick assessment of the clinical status of cooperative patients. To determine the severity of the wheezing in patients who cannot perform spirometry, evaluate the degree of intercostal and suprasternal retractions, air movement, heart and respiratory rates, and ratio of inspiration to expiration, and note the presence or absence of cyanosis.

X-rays are not usually indicated for children over 1 year of age during their *first wheezing episode*. Exceptions include patients in respiratory distress after treatment (respirations >60/min, pulse >160/min), those with localized posttreatment auscultatory findings, and children requiring admission. However, during subsequent attacks, x-rays are unnecessary for admitted patients unless there is suspicion of an alternative diagnosis (pneumonia, heart failure, etc) or complication (pneumothorax) that requires a change in therapy.

Acute Therapy

The goal of ER therapy is to rapidly reverse the bronchospasm.

Epinephrine. Epinephrine (1:1,000 aqueous solution) has been the mainstay of emergency asthma treatment for decades. The dose is 0.01 cc/kg (up to 0.3 cc) given subcutaneously every 20 minutes, up to a maximum of three doses. Common side effects include palpitations and tachycardia, agitation, tremor, and, less frequently, hypertension and ventricular arrhythmias. Epinephrine (given *prior* to obtaining a blood gas) is the initial therapy of choice in the patient whose peak flow is less than 10–15% of expected or who has a silent chest with evidence of marked respiratory distress.

B_2 Agonists. B_2 agonists, such as metaproterenol (Alupent) and albuterol (Salbutamol), nebulized in oxygen, are frequently used as the first-line emergency treatment. The efficacy is comparable to epinephrine, with fewer side effects and without the need for painful injections. Exact doses have not been determined as yet, but 0.01 cc/kg up to 0.3 cc of metaproterenol or 0.01 cc/kg up to 1 cc of albuterol in 5 cc of saline are appropriate. These must be delivered by face mask—the parent cannot hold the nebulizer in front of the child's face. The onset of action is within 10 minutes, and the dose may be repeated once an hour later. A B_2 agonist may be useful for a patient who has not responded to epinephrine. Tachycardia and tremors are possible side effects but occur less commonly than with injected epinephrine.

Oxygen. Oxygen at 6 liters/min of flow is helpful in moderate or severe attacks. Epinephrine can cause pulmonary vasodilation prior to bronchodilation, thus worsening the ventilation–perfusion mismatch. Oxygen helps to alleviate the resultant hypoxemia.

Postural Drainage. Postural drainage loosens mucous plugs and decreases airway obstruction and atelectasis.

Hydration. Hydration is an important adjunct to medical management. Encourage patients who can drink to take juice or other palatable liquids. Give maintenance IV hydration to seriously ill patients.

Aminophylline. Aminophylline (80% theophylline) by intravenous bolus in the ER is controversial, but do not withhold it if the patient is in extremis. When the patient clearly has not taken any theophylline preparation in the past 24–48 hours, give a 5 mg/kg bolus of theophylline. Otherwise, use an initial bolus of 3 mg/kg. A smaller bolus can be given to patients with a known theophylline level who have recently taken their medication if it is remembered that the volume of distribution of theophylline is about 0.5 L/kg (a 1 mg/kg theophylline dose raises the serum level approximately 2 mg/L). If a patient who usually has a level of 10 mg/L presents with severe wheezing, he or she can be given a 3–4 mg/kg bolus of theophylline to raise his or her serum level to 16–18 mg/L. Ideally, for the severe asthmatic with acidosis or hypercapnia, follow the bolus with a continuous infusion of 0.9–1.3 mg/kg/hour, depending on age. Use bolus aminophylline in the ER only for the seriously ill patient, and ensure that there are personnel to observe the patient carefully for hypotension and arrhythmias.

Sedatives. Sedatives are contraindicated in the ER during an acute attack. Agitation most probably represents hypoxia. Obtain an arterial blood gas (ABG) and give 40% FIO_2 to agitated patients.

Complications

If the patient presents in extreme respiratory distress or suddenly worsens, suspect a complication such as pneumothorax (see p 493), atelectasis, or pneumonia (p 458). Other complications include mediastinal and subcutaneous emphysema, as well as profound respiratory acidosis and hypoxemia. Patients who continue to worsen after subcutaneous epinephrine and an inhaled B_2 agonist should have an IV placed and be given a bolus of aminophylline (as above) and steroids

(Decadron, 0.1 mg/kg, or hydrocortisone, 10 mg/kg). If there is no improvement in the blood gas and clinical status, obtain a chest x-ray and start an isoproterenol infusion at 0.1 μg/kg/min (see p 8). Titrate the infusion rate to changes in the blood gas, blood pressure, and electrocardiogram (ECG). Prepare for intubation and ventilation with positive pressure and admit the patient to an intensive care setting for further management.

Discharge Management

The asthmatic is ready to go home when the peak flow is above 60% of the expected value, there are minimal or no wheezes heard, and there are no other signs of respiratory distress (retractions, flaring, tachypnea). Susphrine (0.005 cc/kg up to 0.15 cc) subcutaneously is useful for patients who have not been treated with a nebulized beta agonist to prevent relapse before outpatient medications can take effect. As a general rule intensify (number of drugs or doses) outpatient medication regimen after acute ER therapy.

Theophylline. Theophyllines are used in a dose to achieve a therapeutic level of 10–20 mg/L. Convenient total daily starting doses are 24 mg/kg for children 1–9 years, 20 mg/kg for 9–12 years, 18 mg/kg for 12–15 years, and 16 mg/kg (1200 mg maximum) for patients over 15 years. For infants between 6 months and 1 year, estimate the total daily dose by:

$$\text{Mg theophylline/kg} = 8 + 0.3 \times \text{age (in weeks)}$$

Theophylline is not recommended on an outpatient basis for infants less than 6 months of age.

Give short-acting preparations every 6 hours for occasional episodes of wheezing, but use long-acting formulations every 8 or 12 hours for patients taking theophylline chronically. Regardless of the interval, the total daily dose remains the same. Gastrointestinal side effects (nausea, vomiting) are common and may occur below the accepted toxic serum level of 20 mg/L. Palpitations, tachycardia, headaches, hypo- and hypertension, and seizures can be other signs of theophylline toxicity.

Serum theophylline levels are *increased* by heart failure, liver disease, erythromycin, propranolol, cimetidine, upper respiratory infections, and influenza infection. Levels are *decreased* by concomitant phenobarbital or phenytoin use and by smoking. Obtain serum levels when there is a change in the dose, any suspicion of toxicity, or persistent wheezing despite continuous theophylline therapy. In young children, long-acting theophylline "sprinkle" preparations (given before meals) are useful and often better tolerated than liquid theophylline preparations.

B_2 Agonists. B_2 agonists can be inhaled or administered orally as an adjunct to theophylline or as first-line drugs. They are most effective when delivered by a metered dose inhaler. Albuterol is a highly selective B_2 agonist with less B_1 side effects than metaproterenol. The dose for either is 2 puffs 5 minutes apart, every 6 hours. Onset of action is rapid (5 minutes) with a prolonged duration (4–6 hours) and fewer side effects than the theophyllines. Children who are unable to use an inhaler may benefit from adding a plastic device (Inhal-aid, Inspirease) which does not require a coordinated inhalation. B_2 agonists can also be administered orally (metaproterenol 1.3–2.6 mg/kg/day divided q 6–8 h). Since serum levels are not available, clinical evaluation for signs of toxicity is necessary. These include nervousness, tremor, and tachycardia, while palpitations, vomiting, and hypertension occur less commonly.

Prednisone. Prednisone may be helpful for outpatient management of asthmatics on maximal doses of theophylline and B_2 agonists who have been to the ER several times in a week or more than once in 24 hours but have cleared at each visit. Give 2 mg/kg/day (60 mg maximum) divided tid or qid for 5 days (dose tapering unnecessary).

Follow-up

Arrange a follow-up visit within a week for all patients with a first wheezing attack, patients with new or altered medications or doses, and all patients given steroids. Obtain a serum theophylline level within 72 hours for all patients under one year of age who have started taking theophylline preparations.

INDICATIONS FOR ADMISSION

- Continued wheezing in association with any other sign of respiratory distress 1 hour after nebulized B_2 agonist or immediately after three doses of subcutaneous epinephrine

- Repeated emergency visits in a short period of time, especially if the patient is already receiving maximum bronchodilator therapy and taking steroids
- Hypercapnea ($pCO_2 > 40$ mm/Hg)
- Altered level of consciousness
- $PaO_2 < 70$ mm Hg in room air
- Pneumothorax or pneumomediastinum
- Persistent tachypnea

REFERENCES

1. Hendeles L, Weinberger M: Pharmacotherapy 3: 2–43, 1983
2. Easton S, Hilman B, Shapiro G, et al: Pediatrics 68: 874–879, 1981
3. Leffert F: J Pediatr 96: 1–12, 1980
4. Gershel JC, Goldman H, Stein REK, et al: N Engl J Med 309: 336–339, 1983

Bronchiolitis

INTRODUCTION

Bronchiolitis is the most common wheezing associated respiratory illness of young children 2 to 18 months of age. It is most frequently caused by respiratory syncytial virus, but other viruses (parainfluenza, influenza, adenovirus) and *Mycoplasma* have also been implicated.

CLINICAL PRESENTATION

Three or 4 days after the onset of upper respiratory symptoms (coryza, sneezing), the infant develops a cough and tachypnea (>40/min), often associated with difficulty feeding and sleeping at night. Fever is variable and is usually low grade. Although wheezing is a fairly constant finding, other signs of respiratory distress may include coarse rhonchi and rales, marked tachypnea, nasal flaring, subcostal and intercostal retractions, and grunting. The illness worsens over the first 3–4 days and then rapidly improves. Frequently, the patient develops otitis media.

DIAGNOSIS

The acute onset of wheezing and respiratory distress in a young infant with a URI is likely to be bronchiolitis.

If the patient has had several episodes of wheezing, a history of BPD, or a strong family history of asthma or atopic diseases, consider the diagnosis of *asthma*. Although a lack of response does not rule out asthma, clinical improvement after a dose of epinephrine (see asthma, p 447) confirms that there is a significant bronchospastic component to the illness and that the patient may benefit from bronchodilators.

Foreign body aspiration can present with wheezing. The patient is usually over 6 months of age, afebrile, and without a URI prodrome. Typically, the wheezing begins after a choking or coughing episode. The diagnosis can be confirmed with lateral decubitus chest x-rays (pp 107–109).

Tachycardia out of proportion to the degree of respiratory distress or fever suggests *cardiac disease*. In the absence of a murmur consider endocardial fibroelastosis or myocarditis.

ER MANAGEMENT

Obtain vital signs and observe the patient's respirations while he is resting, with his shirt off, in his mother's lap. Obtain an ABG and a complete blood count (CBC) if the patient has a respiratory rate >60/min, difficulty drinking, or evidence of significant respiratory distress (grunting, retractions, nasal flaring). A blood culture is indicated for temperature >103°F, grunting, lethargy, or other signs of toxicity.

Hospitalize the infant if he has a $pCO_2 > 40$ torr, or a $pO_2 < 70$ torr in room air, or if he cannot drink or is in respiratory distress. Secure an IV, infuse a maintenance solution, and give supplemental (40%) humidified O_2 via head box or face mask. Persistent hypoxia, worsening hypercarbia, or the development of acidosis ($pH < 7.3$) are indications for intubation and ventilatory assistance in the ER.

Observe the infant with tachypnea (40–60/min), wheezing, but no other signs of respiratory distress. If he eagerly drinks 2–3 ounces of a clear electrolyte solution or juice and the parents feel they can care for the infant, send him home with acetaminophen for fever. Instruct the parents to try a clear liquid diet (not water) if the infant cannot take normal amounts of formula or milk. A cool mist vaporizer may help to moisten the oral cavity and nasal passages and thus provide some relief, but humidification does not treat the underlying disease process. Reevaluate the infant the next day or sooner if he develops more signs of respiratory distress or refuses to drink.

With the moderately symptomatic patient, the decision to send home or to admit is modified by the duration of the illness, the age of the patient, and the degree of parental discomfort. If it is the first day of wheezing, it is more likely to become worse; by the third or fourth day, the infant is probably getting better. Be more cautious with infants <6 months of age who may tire sooner than older patients.

A chest x-ray is indicated for patients who are admitted for respiratory distress, or when the diagnosis of pneumonia is being considered.

Oral aminophylline therapy has not been shown to be helpful in bronchiolitis. Although asthma may occur in patients less than 1 year of age, it is rare under 6 months. Patients older than 6 months who have a history of several wheezing episodes, or BPD, an atopic appearance, or a strong family history of asthma, may respond to epinephrine (0.01 cc/kg subcutaneously [SQ]). If the wheezing improves after a dose of epinephrine, give theophylline (p 457) under close supervision.

INDICATIONS FOR ADMISSION

- Moderate respiratory distress, metabolic acidosis ($pH < 7.35$), or hypoxia ($pO_2 < 70$ torr in room air)
- A "normal" or high pCO_2 (> 40 torr) in a tachypneic infant
- Parents unable to comply with instructions or uncomfortable with the child's level of illness.

REFERENCES

1. Wohl MEB, Chernick V: Am J Dis Child 118: 759, 1978
2. Howard, WA: PIR 1: 239, 1980
3. Outwater, KM, Crone RK: Am J Dis Child 138: 1071, 1984

Hemoptysis

INTRODUCTION

Hemoptysis, the expectoration of blood or blood-tinged sputum, is uncommon in children. Most suspected cases result from blood from the esophagus (vomiting) or oropharynx (URI) mixing with sputum. True cases are usually caused by infections or chronic pulmonary diseases (Table 18-1).

CLINICAL PRESENTATION

Bacterial pneumonia presents with fever, cough, tachypnea, and on pulmonary auscultation, decreased breath sounds or rales. Tuberculosis causes weight loss, fatigue, and cough.

Bronchiectasis causes recurrent pulmonary infections and chronic cough, while cystic fibrosis may have associated chronic diarrhea and failure to thrive.

The aspiration of a foreign body leads to acute respiratory distress, cough, and stridor. If the object remains in the lungs, cough, recurrent pneumonias, and wheezing ensue.

A patient with fractured ribs usually can remember the episode of trauma. On examination there is point tenderness over the fracture site.

An extrinsic mass impinging on the airways presents with subster-

TABLE 18-1. COMMON CAUSES OF HEMOPTYSIS

Infectious (bronchiectasis, airway erosion)
- Bacterial pneumonia
- Tuberculosis
- Coccidioidomycosis
- Cystic fibrosis
- Bronchopulmonary dysplasia

Noninfectious
- Foreign body aspiration
- Fractured rib
- External airway compression (bronchogenic cyst, mediastinal tumor)
- Arteriovenous malformation
- Pulmonary sequestration
- Bleeding diathesis

nal discomfort, cough, and stridor or wheezing. If the mass is a malignancy, there may be weight loss and fatigue.

A patient with a bleeding diathesis may have petechiae, ecchymoses, nose bleeds, hematuria, hematochezia, or hepatosplenomegaly. He or she may be receiving chemotherapy or anticoagulants (heparin, coumadin).

DIAGNOSIS

Palpate the chest wall for point tenderness (fractured rib) or thrill (A-V fistula). Auscultate for rales, decreased breath sounds, or wheezing.

Examine the oropharynx and nasopharynx carefully, looking for a source of bleeding. If none is found obtain anteroposterior (AP) and lateral chest x-rays. Possible findings include an infiltrate (*bacterial pneumonia, tuberculosis*), mediastinal widening (*mediastinal mass*), and localized peripheral densities (*A-V fistula, tumor, bronchogenic cyst*). *Foreign body aspiration* is suggested by unilateral lucency, although often the films are normal.

If a bleeding diathesis is suspected, obtain a CBC with differential, platelet count, prothrombin time (PT) and partial thromboplastin time (PTT), bleeding time, and liver function tests.

ER MANAGEMENT

Admit the patient and consult with a pulmonologist or thoracic surgeon. If the hemoptysis is severe, obtain a spun hematocrit, type and crossmatch, and ABG, and evaluate for a bleeding diathesis (see above). Insert a large bore IV and transfuse 10 cc/kg of packed cells if the hematocrit is less than 25% or the patient has signs of intravascular depletion (orthostatic vital sign changes, tachypnea, congestive heart failure).

The specific management of bacterial pneumonias (p 458), tuberculosis (p 321), foreign body aspiration (p 107), and a bleeding diathesis (p 257) are discussed elsewhere.

INDICATIONS FOR ADMISSION

- Severe hemoptysis
- Hematocrit <25% or signs of intravascular depletion

- Mediastinal mass or peripheral lung density
- Foreign body aspiration
- Suspected tuberculosis

REFERENCES

1. Tom LW, Wersman RA, Handler SD: Ann Othol Rhinol Laryngol 89:419, 1980

Pneumonia

INTRODUCTION

Most pneumonias (90%) are viral and require only supportive care. Bacterial pneumonias, however, can be significant illnesses. They can be viewed as microaspiration syndromes of the oropharyngeal flora, although throat cultures are of *no value* in establishing the diagnosis of bacterial pneumonia. The most common bacterial pathogen is *Streptococcus pneumoniae*. However, for a given patient, consider the most probable flora—depending on age, the prior use of antibiotics, and special disease substrates—and use that as a guide for therapeutic decisions. Etiology is the key to treatment (see Table 18-2).

CLINICAL PRESENTATION

Tachypnea, cough, and fever are the hallmarks of pneumonia. Severe infections may be associated with nasal flaring, intercostal and suprasternal retractions, dyspnea, cyanosis, or apnea. On auscultation, fine end inspiratory rales or altered breath sounds (diminished or increased) are noted. Egophony, dullness to percussion, and diminished breath sounds imply effusion.

Viral pneumonias tend to develop over several days, usually following URI or croup, and are often accompanied by low grade fever. Older children may have associated myalgias or headache.

The onset of a *bacterial* pneumonia is usually more abrupt, with high fever and shaking chills. Localized rales and decreased breath sounds are more likely than with viral pneumonia.

TABLE 18-2. CAUSES OF PNEUMONIA

Age	Agent
<2 wk	Group B *Streptococcus* Coliforms Respiratory syncytial virus *Staphylococcus* *Klebsiella*
2 wk–2 mo	*Chlamydia trachomatis* Respiratory syncytial virus Parainfluenza virus *S. pneumoniae* *H. influenzae*
2 mo–6 yr	Viruses *S. pneumoniae* *H. influenzae*
>6 yr	Viruses *Mycoplasma* *S. pneumoniae*

DIAGNOSIS

Auscultation of fine end inspiratory rales in a child with tachypnea, cough, and fever (variable) suggests pneumonia. More serious signs include grunting respirations, cyanosis, and obtundation. Infrequently, right lower lobe pneumonia can mimic *appendicitis* in a child with fever, and apical pneumonia can cause *meningismus*. The key to the diagnosis is the observation of tachypnea and/or dyspnea.

In young children, especially with right middle lobe pneumonia, auscultation of the chest may reveal no abnormalities. Infants less than 3 months of age may present solely with a cough. This is always abnormal and requires a full evaluation for pneumonia (chest x-ray, CBC, blood culture, ABG).

Chlamydia trachomatis. *Chlamydia trachomatis* is the most common cause of pneumonia in infants between 2 and 3 months of age. Patients are usually afebrile and have a staccato cough, nasal congestion, tachypnea, rales, and occasionally, wheezing. In 50%, there is either a history of or concurrent conjunctivitis. The cough, fine rales, bilateral patchy infiltrates on chest x-ray, and eosinophilia ($>300/mm^3$) help to distinguish *Chlamydia* pneumonia from *bronchiolitis*. The cough of *Chlamydia* pneumonia is occasionally confused with the paroxysmal cough of *pertussis* (see p 313). However, an infant with pertussis has copious nasal secretions, a marked lymphocytosis, and usually no evidence of pneumonia on chest x-ray.

Mycloplasma. *Mycoplasma* is likely in a school-aged child who does not appear terribly sick and who has a history of gradual onset of a nonproductive hacking cough. Wheezing is more common than rales; associated symptoms include headache and myalgias. Commonly, other family members have had a similar illness. Cold agglutinins may be positive: put 5 cc of blood in a lavender top tube and keep it in ice water for a few minutes. Then gently rotate the tube and examine for agglutination.

Congestive Heart Failure. Congestive heart failure (see p 35) can present with diffuse rales, tachypnea, and cough. The infant is likely to have a murmur, while the older child usually has a history of heart disease. Tachycardia and distended neck veins may also be seen.

Metabolic Acidosis. Although the presence of tachypnea suggests pneumonia, if there are no abnormal auscultatory findings, consider metabolic acidosis (see pp 30, 33). Ask about aspirin use, since aspirin overdose can present with fever and tachypnea (hyperpnea). Note also whether there has been any recent weight loss, polydypsia, or polyphagia suggesting diabetes mellitus. Other etiologies include severe gastroenteritis and renal disease.

Obtain a chest x-ray when it may help to make a diagnosis (decreased breath sounds without rales, high fever without a source, cough in an infant <2 months of age), or when the findings may alter the patient's management. A chest x-ray may identify noninfectious causes for rales or wheezing (congenital anomalies of the lungs or vasculature, congestive heart failure). Chest x-rays are also warranted for children with repeated pneumonias in whom aspiration pneumonia, a foreign body, or a sequestered lobe must be considered.

Patients who are sick enough to require hospitalization should also have a chest x-ray. There might be an effusion that can be drained for diagnostic and therapeutic purposes. Effusions are most common in *Staphylococcus*, *Pneumococcus*, and *Haemophilus influenzae* infections. They occur occasionally in tuberculous pneumonia and rarely in viral, *mycoplasma*, and chlamydial infections.

TABLE 18-3. CHEST X-RAY PATTERN AS A GUIDE TO ETIOLOGY

Diffuse pattern
- Viral (95% of cases)
- *Chlamydia* (afebrile infants)
- *Mycoplasma* (school-age children and adolescents)
- *H. influenzae*
- Mycobacteria
- Fungi
- Rickettsia
- *Pneumocystis carinii* (immunosuppressed patients)

Lobar pattern
- *S. pneumoniae* (90%)
- *H. influenzae*
- *Klebsiella* (young infants and debilitated patients)

Pneumonia with effusion
- *S. pneumoniae*
- *H. influenzae*
- Group A *Streptococcus*
- *S. aureus*
- *Mycoplasma* (small and infrequent)
- Tuberculosis (infrequent in U.S.)

The x-ray pattern may suggest the etiology (Table 18-3). A lobar infiltrate is commonly seen in *Pneumococcus* or *H. influenzae pneumonia;* a bilateral interstitial pattern with hyperaeration is consistent with chlamydial and viral infections; pneumatoceles with changing infiltrates suggest *Staphylococcus* pneumonia.

ER MANAGEMENT

General. When pneumonia has been diagnosed, assess the child's mental status, state of hydration, and ability to take fluids. Do not ascribe lethargy, obtundation, or irritability to the pneumonia. If the child has a high fever, see if the mental status improves following aspirin or acetaminophen. Otherwise, perform a lumbar puncture to rule out meningitis.

Give oxygen to all patients with dyspnea; begin with 40% and titrate the percentage by measuring the arterial pO_2.

Place a PPD (0.1 cc, 5 TU) on the forearm and either ascertain that the parents can read (measure) it or schedule a return visit in 48–72 hours to have it interpreted. In most cases this can coincide with a follow-up visit to assess the patient's status (see below).

Infants <6 Months. Admit all patients under 6 months of age. Obtain a CBC, blood culture, ABG, and chest x-ray, and, if the patient appears toxic or is less than 2 months of age, perform a lumbar puncture and obtain serum electrolytes. Secure an IV in patients with fever who appear toxic or are not taking fluids by mouth, and begin treatment with ampicillin, 100 mg/kg/day and chloramphenicol, 75 mg/kg/day. For infants under 2 months of age, use ampicillin and cefotaxime (see p 286).

If *Chlamydia* is suspected, obtain a nasopharyngeal culture and admit the infant for supportive care and the start of antibiotic therapy (erythromycin 40 mg/kg/day PO for 2–3 weeks).

Patients Older Than 6 Months. If a patient over 6 months of age is in moderate respiratory distress (respiratory rate 40–60/min, moderate retractions), obtain an ABG. Admit patients with a $pO_2 < 70$ torr in room air, or a $pCO_2 > 40$ torr.

Patients between 6 months and 6 years of age who are drinking well and do not appear toxic may be sent home with amoxicillin (40 mg/kg/day). Treat patients over 6 years with erythromycin (40 mg/kg/day, to maximum 250 mg qid).

Commonly, a school-age child presents with low grade or no fever, diffuse rales, minimal tachypnea, and no respiratory distress. Since the majority have self-limited viral infections, follow these patients without antibiotic therapy. Either have the child return if the fever goes higher or symptoms worsen, or ask the family to come back in 48 hours for a follow-up examination.

Follow-Up

A child under 2 years of age must be seen in the next 24–48 hours; advise an older patient to return if he or she does not improve over the next 2–3 days. Refer all patients to a primary health care provider for examination at the end of treatment. Follow-up x-rays are not necessary for an uncomplicated pneumonia. A chest radiograph may be helpful for a patient who continues to be febrile for several days, develops worse symptoms, has recurrent episodes of pneumonia, or has a chronic cough without an apparent cause. Chest x-ray abnormalities can persist for 8–12 weeks after the acute illness.

INDICATIONS FOR ADMISSION

- Patients less than 6 months of age
- Dehydration or toxic appearance
- $pO_2 < 70$ torr, $pCO_2 > 40$ torr
- Parents unable to comply with instructions

REFERENCES

1. Wald ER: Pediatr Infect Dis 3: 521–523, 1984
2. Grossman LK, Wald ER, Nair P, et al: J Pediatrics 63: 30–31, 1979

19

Renal Emergencies

Acute Glomerulonephritis

INTRODUCTION

Acute glomerulonephritis (AGN) is a clinical syndrome characterized by one or more of the following: diminished glomerular filtration rate with or without oliguria, azotemia, hypertension, peripheral edema, proteinuria, or hematuria with red blood cell (RBC) casts. Most instances of AGN result from deposition of immune complexes in glomerular structures. The etiologies include infectious agents, including bacteria (group A *Streptococcus, Pneumococcus, Staphylococcus aureus,* etc), viruses (hepatitis B, Epstein–Barr virus [EBV], adenovirus), and parasites (malaria, toxoplasmosis, etc), immune-related diseases (systemic lupus erythematosus, Henoch-Schönlein purpura, Berger disease, subacute bacterial endocarditis [SBE], shunt nephritis) or disorders of undetermined origin (membranous nephropathy, membranoproliferative glomerulonephritis, hemolytic-uremic syndrome).

CLINICAL PRESENTATION AND DIAGNOSIS

In addition to the clinical feature of the underlying disease, the renal symptoms that are the hallmarks of AGN are gross hematuria, edema (particularly periorbital), weight gain, hypertension, and decreased urine output. With increasing degrees of renal failure there are more constitutional symptoms such as abdominal pain, nausea, and vomiting. With mild hypertension, central nervous system (CNS) symptoms such as lethargy, headache, disorientation, and seizures may occur. Circulatory congestion can lead to dyspnea and orthopnea in association with pulmonary rales and pleural effusion.

Postinfectious Glomerulonephritis. Postinfectious glomerulonephritis occurs primarily in school-age children, 1–3 weeks after the primary infection. In the case of group A *Streptococcus,* this may be a sore throat (1–2 weeks before) or impetigo (2–3 weeks prior). For other infections, there may be a upper respiratory infection (URI), a mono-like syndrome, or hepatitis and jaundice. The onset of the AGN is abrupt, with tea-colored urine, periorbital edema, and elevated blood pressure.

Henoch-Schönlein Purpura. Henoch-Schönlein purpura (HSP) also occurs in school-age children who present with one or more of the following: a purpuric rash on the extensor surfaces of the lower extremities, abdominal pain and hematochezia, and arthralgias of the large joints.

Hemolytic-Uremic Syndrome. With the hemolytic-uremic syndrome (HUS), pallor, lethargy, and weakness occur after a gastrointestinal or URI prodrome. A generalized microangiopathy occurs and results in a diffuse colitis with hematochezia or bloody diarrhea and neurologic symptoms (coma, seizures, personality changes).

Other. AGN can be the presentation of *lupus,* although an acute nephrotic syndrome is more common. Usually other manifestations (butterfly rash, polyserositis, arthritis, etc) of the disease are also present. SBE presents with fever, splenomegaly, and a changing murmur; a patient with *shunt nephritis* has, of course, hydrocephalus and a ventriculoatrial or ventriculojugular shunt.

ER MANAGEMENT

If AGN is suspected, obtain a urinalysis, complete blood count (CBC) with differential, platelet count, serum electrolytes, calcium, BUN, creatinine, total protein, albumin, cholesterol, triglycerides, FANA, and complement (C3). Hypocomplementemic forms of AGN include postinfectious, systemic lupus enthematosus (SLE), membranoproliferative diseases, and shunt nephritis.

If the clinical picture is compatible with post-*Streptococcus* AGN, obtain a throat culture and ASLO or streptozyme. If there are any bleeding manifestations, a prothrombin time (PT) and partial thromboplastin time (PTT) are required. These are abnormal in HUS; also the peripheral blood smear shows microangiopathic changes and thrombocytopenia. The clotting studies and platelet count are normal in HSP. Obtain serial blood cultures for patients with fever, murmur, and splenomegaly.

Admit all patients with AGN and have them evaluated by a nephrologist. Management requires meticulous attention to blood pressure, fluid status, potassium level, acid–base balance, and renal function. Treat hypertension promptly and aggressively, especially in poststreptococcal AGN in which hypertensive encephalopathy can occur at a modestly increased blood pressure. In the asymptomatic hypertensive child use hydralazine (0.2 mg/kg IV or 0.5–1.5 mg/kg PO); give diazoxide (5 mg/kg rapid IV push) to patients with any neurologic symptoms (headache, seizures). The management of hypertension is discussed on p 473.

The cornerstone of medical management is fluid and sodium restriction, as discussed for acute renal failure (p 468). Pending evaluation of the glomerular filtration rate (GFR), do not give potassium. Then, if the patient can eat, limit the sodium and potassium to 1 g/day and 0.5 g/day, respectively. Conservative medical therapy is the rule, with hemo- or peritoneal dialysis employed for severe volume overload with congestive heart failure (CHF) or pulmonary edema, life-threatening hyperkalemia (≥7 mEq/L), intractable acidosis, intractable hypocalcemia with seizures, or symptomatic uremia (pleuritis, pericarditis, gastrointestinal (GI) bleeding, encephalopathy).

INDICATION FOR ADMISSION

- Acute glomerulonephritis

REFERENCES

1. Nissenson AR, Baraff LG, Fine RF, et al: Ann Int Med 91: 76–86, 1979
2. Madaro MP, Harrington TJ: N Engl J Med 309: 1299–1302, 1983

Acute Renal Failure

INTRODUCTION

Acute renal failure (ARF) is characterized by a sudden decrease in the GFR, associated with increases in the serum urea nitrogen and creatinine concentrations. Oliguria (≤0.5 cc/kg/hr) is a frequent, but not invariable finding.

ARF can be divided into three pathophysiologic categories (Table 19-1). Prerenal azotemia is a consequence of inadequate kidney perfusion secondary to hypovolemia, hypotension, or hypoxia; postrenal azotemia is secondary to urinary tract obstruction; and nephrotoxins or tubular ischemia can occasionally cause renal azotemia.

CLINICAL PRESENTATION

The clinical presentation can be varied. There may be findings secondary to the renal insufficiency, such as edema, hypertension, nausea and vomiting, hypocalcemic tetany, and neurologic symptoms (coma, seizures). Alternatively, the presentation may reflect the primary pathologic process, such as hypotension and orthostatic vital sign changes (shock), dysuria and fever (pyelonephritis), difficulty voiding (obstruction), lethargy and fever (sepsis), cutaneous burns, bleeding, jaundice (hemoglobinuria), and pallor and bloody diarrhea (hemolytic-uremic syndrome).

TABLE 19-1. CLASSIFICATION OF ACUTE RENAL FAILURE

	Prerenal	Postrenal	Renal
Mechanism	Hypovolemia Hypotension Hypoxia	Obstruction	Nephrotoxin Ischemia
Etiologies	Dehydration Sepsis Anaphylaxis Hemorrhage Burn	Urolithiasis Posterior urethral valves	Acute pyelonephritis Drugs Heavy metals Myoglobinuria Hemoglobinuria Hemolytic-uremic syndrome Acute glomerulonephritis Renal vein thrombosis

TABLE 19-2. LABORATORY FINDINGS IN ACUTE RENAL FAILURE

Diagnosis	SG[a]	Urine Na[b]	BUN/Cr[c]	FENA[d]	U/A[e]
Prerenal azotemia	>1.020	<20 mEq/L	>20	<1%	
Acute glomerulonephritis	>1.020	<20 mEq/L	<20	<1%	RBC casts
Acute tubular necrosis	1.010	>20 mEq/L	<20	1–3%	

[a]SG = urine specific gravity.
[b]Urine Na = urine sodium.
[c]BUN/Cr = ratio of BUN to creatinine.
[d]FENA = fractional excretion of sodium (Una × Pcr)/(Pna × Ucr).
[e]U/A = typical urinalysis finding.

DIAGNOSIS AND ER MANAGEMENT

Make a rapid assessment of the patient's volume status, looking for clinical signs of dehydration (orthostatic vital sign changes, hypotension) or volume overload (edema, rales, cardiac gallop). To help distinguish between the various types of ARF, obtain urine for specific gravity, microscopic examination, and sodium determination, and blood for electrolytes, BUN, and creatinine (Table 19-2).

If urine is unavailable or the urinary findings are inconclusive, and there is no evidence of volume overload, rapidly infuse 15–20 cc/kg of an isotonic solution (normal saline, Ringer's lactate). If the patient remains oliguric and there are no signs of volume overload, repeat the bolus. If there is no diuresis, give intravenous furosemide (2 mg/kg) or mannitol (0.5–1 g/kg). If oliguria persists, the diagnosis of ARF is established; if urine output increases with these measures, the patient has *prerenal insufficiency*.

Renal ARF requires fluid restriction: curtail fluids to insensible losses plus urine output. Insensible losses are estimated as 400 cc/M^2/day, but are higher with fever and burns and less with mechanical ventilation. Sodium should be withheld from intravenous solutions and limited to 0.5–1.0 g/day in the diet. Remove potassium from all IV solutions; dietary restriction (0.5 g/day) is sufficient if $K^+ \leq 6$ mEq/L. A higher potassium requires an immediate electrocardiogram (ECG) to look for peaked T-waves (T-wave ≥ half the R- or S-wave).

In their absence, Kayexalate 1 g/kg dissolved in 4 cc of water, with sorbitol (PO or PR), is sufficient therapy. This dose lowers the serum K^+ by 1 mEq/L. Hyperkalemia accompanied by ECG changes requires more aggressive IV therapy, including glucose (2–4 cc/kg of D25), insulin (0.1 U/kg), calcium chloride (0.1–0.3 cc/kg), and sodium bicarbonate (1–2 mEq/kg).

Absolute indications for dialysis include life-threatening hyperkalemia ($K^+ \geq 7$), intractable acidosis, symptomatic volume overload (CHF, pulmonary edema), and overt uremia (pleuritis, pericarditis, encephalopathy, GI bleeding).

If the patient has *postrenal insufficiency,* immediately consult with a urologist to determine the appropriate therapy. Treat *prerenal azotemia* by maintaining adequate intravascular volume.

INDICATION FOR ADMISSION

- Acute renal failure

REFERENCE

1. Gordillo PG, Velasquez-Jones L: Pediatr Clin North Am 23: 817, 1976

Hematuria

INTRODUCTION

Hematuria is defined as ≥ 5 RBC/high power field of unspun urine, or ≥240,000 RBC per 12-hour urine collection. Up to 5% of school-age children have microscopic hematuria on a single specimen, and 2% have this finding subsequently confirmed. The incidence increases with age and is greater in females. The etiologies of hematuria can be divided into nonrenal and renal causes. Renal bleeding may be nonglomerular or glomerular in origin.

CLINICAL PRESENTATIONS AND DIAGNOSIS

Nonrenal Bleeding. Hematuria arising from nonrenal sources is either microscopic or gross. With lower urinary tract bleeding there is often suprapubic pain and dysuria. A *bacterial urinary tract infection* is accompanied by symptoms of urgency and frequency, as well as pyuria and bacteruria. The hematuria resolves with antibiotic treatment. *Viral cystitis* often occurs in association with upper respiratory symptoms, and is accompanied by fever and suprapubic tenderness. The hematuria resolves within 5–7 days without any specific treatment. Suspect a *foreign body* in an afebrile toddler with dysuria.

Trauma to the urinary tract (see p 215) can cause bright red or microscopic hematuria. *Urolithiasis* can present with microscopic or gross hematuria and intense renal colic. Often the patient has a history of urinary tract abnormalities, infections, or stones.

Nonglomerular Renal Bleeding. This is usually brownish in color, but in contrast to glomerular bleeding, RBC casts are not seen. *Sickle cell* trait is associated with gross or microscopic hematuria without other obvious manifestations of renal disease. *Wilm tumor* must always be considered in a child under 6 years of age who presents with brown or tea-colored urine. Congenital and anatomical abnormalities such as *polycystic kidney, renal hemangioma,* and *hydronephrosis* can also present with hematuria. *Idiopathic hypercalciuria,* in the absence of urolithiasis, is a common cause of nonglomerular hematuria, usually gross.

Glomerular Bleeding. Hallmarks of glomerular bleeding include RBC casts and proteinuria in association with microscopic hematuria. In addition, edema, hypertension, and oliguria can occur. A history of URI or impetigo in the previous 2 weeks (*poststreptococcal glomerulonephritis*) or 1–2 days (*IgA nephropathy*) may be helpful. A family history of deafness and renal disease defines *Alport syndrome* (familial glomerulonephritis). Palpable purpura of the lower extremities, abdominal pain, hematochezia, and arthralgias suggest *Henoch-Schönlein purpura.* Hematuria can be the presenting sign of SLE, or there can be associated findings (butterfly rash, polyserositis, arthritis, hematologic abnormalities). Microscopic hematuria that only occurs with fever or exercise can be seen with *benign hematuria,* a disease that does not progress to renal insufficiency.

ER MANAGEMENT

Hematuria must be confirmed by microscopic examination of the urine, since not all red urine contains blood. Foodstuffs such as beets, red dyes, and drugs such as rifampin, Povan, and Pyridium can give the urine a red tint. Myoglobin and hemoglobin cause a false-positive dipstick determination without RBC in the urine. The two are differentiated by centrifuging a sample of serum—a pink tinge is found with hemoglobin and clear serum is seen with myoglobin.

Traumatic hematuria requires radiographic evaluation (see p 215). In the absence of edema, hypertension, an abdominal mass, or oliguria, the work-up of nontraumatic hematuria can be performed on an outpatient basis. A complete urinalysis and urine culture are performed first—pyuria suggests a urinary infection, which should be treated with antibiotics once it is confirmed by a positive culture. If the culture is negative, additional work-up includes serum electrolytes, BUN, creatinine, complement (C_3,C_4), total protein, albumin, 24-hour urinary protein excretion, creatinine clearance, PPD, and (when applicable) a sickle prep. If these are all negative, an IVP and urinary calcium excretion (abnormal $\geq$ 4 mg/kg/day) are indicated.

Admit any patient with signs of acute glomerulonephritis (edema, hypertension, oliguria, proteinuria in association with microscopic hematuria). In addition to the initial work-up outlined above, further evaluation includes consultation with a nephrologist, and further serology (antinuclear antibodies [ANA], ASLO, VDRL). The management of acute renal failure is detailed elsewhere (p 468).

INDICATIONS FOR ADMISSION

- Acute glomerulonephritis or acute renal failure
- Posttraumatic hematuria with abnormal IVP (renal contusion, laceration, collecting system injury, major vessel injury)

REFERENCES

1. Brewer ED, Benson GS: JAMA 246: 877–880, 1981
2. West CD: J Pediatr 89: 173–182, 1976

Hypertension

INTRODUCTION

Hypertension in the ER can be considered in two categories. In most cases, the blood pressure elevation is mild and is an incidental finding in a patient being evaluated for some other problem, such as asthma, benign head trauma, fever, anxiety, fracture, etc. These cases are not true emergencies and further diagnostic evaluation can usually be deferred until a later, scheduled visit.

Hypertension is an emergency if the patient has symptoms (headache, disorientation, seizures) that can be ascribed to the increase in blood pressure, the blood pressure is dangerously high (systolic over 160 mm Hg, diastolic over 100 mm Hg), or the primary disease demands emergency treatment (increased intracranial pressure, renal failure). In these cases, urgent therapy is required. The detailed diagnostic evaluation can be deferred to the inpatient setting.

CLINICAL PRESENTATION AND DIAGNOSIS

The evaluation of patients with mild hypertension should not be performed in the ER. In the emergency situation, treatment is the priority and determining an etiology can be deferred.

Helpful information, however, includes a history of previous hypertensive episodes, medication use, renal disease, and hematuria. Useful physical examination findings include signs of increased intracranial pressure, differential blood pressure and pulses between upper and lower extremities, abdominal mass, and virilization.

ER MANAGEMENT

The drug of choice for life-threatening hypertension is diazoxide, 5 mg/kg (300 mg maximum), as a rapid intravenous bolus. The onset of action is immediate, duration is several hours, and hypotension rarely occurs, although hyperglycemia is occasionally seen. If the blood pressure remains severely elevated, a second bolus can be given 30 minutes after the first. If the blood pressure responds to diazoxide, admit the patient to an intensive care setting, consult a nephrologist, and start maintenance therapy (vasodilator and a diuretic).

If the hypertension persists, move the patient to an intensive care unit, begin a sodium nitroprusside continuous infusion (1 μg/kg/min), and titrate the dose against the blood pressure.

Prior to admission, obtain a urinalysis, serum electrolytes, BUN and creatinine, chest x-ray, ECG, and, if an adrenal etiology is suspected (virilization, Cushingoid appearance), a serum cortisol and 17-hydroxyprogesterone.

INDICATIONS FOR ADMISSION

- Symptomatic or severe hypertension (systolic over 160 mm Hg, diastolic over 100 mm Hg)
- Hypertension of any degree associated with acute glomerulonephritis

REFERENCES

1. Blumental S, Epps RP, Heavenrich R: Pediatrics (Suppl) 59: 805–810, 1977
2. Loggie JMH, New MI, Robson AM: J Pediatr 94: 685–699, 1979

Proteinuria

INTRODUCTION

Normal urine contains no protein. However, with vigorous exercise, stress, or fever, or when the urine is highly concentrated or alkaline, small amounts of protein may be present. The urine dipstix is very sensitive, detecting protein concentrations as low as 10–15 mg/dl. Therefore, qualitative proteinuria is very prevalent (5–15%) in otherwise normal individuals. Significant proteinuria, defined as 100 mg/M^2/day (4 mg/M^2/hr) of protein excretion, occurs in only 1–2% of these patients. The nephrotic syndrome is defined as proteinuria more than 40 mg/M^2/hr. There are numerous etiologies, although minimal change disease is most common (80%).

CLINICAL PRESENTATION

Most often, proteinuria is an unexpected finding in a child being evaluated for fever, vomiting, or diarrhea. Consider renal disease or the nephrotic syndrome if there is edema, hypertension, oliguria, or associated microscopic hematuria.

DIAGNOSIS AND ER MANAGEMENT

Since very few patients with dipstix proteinuria truly have renal disease, in the absence of the signs and symptoms enumerated above, merely repeat the urinalysis in 1 to 2 weeks. If the protenuria is confirmed, then the initial work-up is a urine culture. Treat a positive culture with an appropriate antibiotic.

If the culture is negative, perform an orthostatic protein excretion test to rule out orthostatic proteinuria: obtain two urine specimens, the first while the patient is still in bed after waking in the morning and the second after 30–60 minutes of moderate activity. If the protein excretion increases with activity, but remains less than 4 mg/M^2/hr, follow the child. Patients with either increases larger than 4 mg/M^2/hr or protein excretion in both specimens and children with associated microscopic hematuria require a more complete work-up. This includes serum electrolytes, BUN, calcium, creatinine and creatinine clearance, cholesterol, total protein and albumin, and complement (C3, C4). If these are all normal, an IVP is indicated.

Obtain the same laboratory examinations for the patient with signs and symptoms of renal disease or the nephrotic syndrome and admit him or her to the hospital. Hypoalbuminemia (<3 g/dl), hyperlipidemia, hyponatremia, and hypocalcemia are other laboratory findings in the nephrotic syndrome.

INDICATION FOR ADMISSION

- Proteinuria in association with signs and symptoms of renal disease or the nephrotic syndrome (edema, hypertension, oliguria, associated microscopic hematuria)

REFERENCES

1. West CD: J Pediatr 89:173–182, 1976
2. McEnery PT, Strife CF: Pediatr Clin North Am 89: 875–894, 1982

Urinary Tract Infections

INTRODUCTION

Urinary tract infections (UTI) occur in 1–3% of infants (predominantly males) and 3–5% of school-age girls. The two most common types of infection are cystitis (infection confined to the bladder) and pyelonephritis (infection involving the renal parenchyma). The most frequent etiologic organism is *Escherichia coli.* Other organisms include *Klebsiella, Pseudomonas, Enterococcus,* and *Staphylococcus epidermidis,* which should not be dismissed as a contaminant if cultured repeatedly. *Proteus* is an important pathogen in uncircumcized boys but is less common in girls.

CLINICAL PRESENTATION

The presentation in infancy is nonspecific and includes poor feeding, vomiting, diarrhea, irritability, jaundice, and seizures. From 1 month to 2 years, fever is more common, and some urologic symptoms (change in voiding pattern, foul-smelling urine) occur. Preschool and school-age children have specific urologic complaints such as frequency, urgency, dysuria, and enuresis. However, even in this age group, less specific symptoms, such as abdominal pain and vomiting can occur. High fever (>103°F), flank (CVA) tenderness, and systemic toxicity may be seen with pyelonephritis.

DIAGNOSIS

The concept of "significant bacteriuria" ($>10^5$ colonies/ml in a culture of a single midstream clean catch urine) is a statistical one indicating an 80% chance of true infection; two consecutive positive cultures increases the likelihood of infection to 95%. A culture with a *pure growth* of less than 10^5 colonies/ml is adequate for diagnosis in a patient with UTI symptoms, and any growth in a culture of urine obtained by suprapubic bladder tap or urethral catheterization is significant.

In the presence of infection, the urinalysis usually has ≥10 white blood cells (WBC)/hpf of spun urine, although in up to 20–30% of culture-proven UTI, pyuria may be absent. In addition, proteinuria and hematuria often occur. White blood cell casts are pathognomonic for pyelonephritis; other laboratory findings include a leukocytosis (WBC $\geq$ 15,000/mm^3) and an elevated sedimentation rate ($\geq$ 30 mm/hr).

Neither symptoms nor a routine urinalysis are sufficient for a definitive diagnosis. The presence of organisms on Gram stain of an unspun urine correlates with a colony count in excess of 10^5/ml, and is presumptive evidence of a UTI, although a properly obtained urine culture remains essential.

Dysuria, frequency, urgency in a patient with suprapubic tenderness and hematuria without pyruia suggest viral cystitis. The same findings in a patient with pyuria but no bacteriuria are compatible with the acute-urethral syndrome (urine culture is negative, see p 239).

ER MANAGEMENT

After the urine cultures are obtained, measure the blood pressure and treat lower tract infections on an outpatient basis with a 10-day course of sulfisoxazole (150 mg/kg/day divided qid), trimethoprim-sulfamethoxazole (8 mg/kg/day of trimethoprim [TMP] divided bid), or amoxicillin (40 mg/kg/day divided tid). Single dose therapy (amoxicillin 3 gm PO) is an alternative for a non-pregnant adolescent female with an uncomplicated lower tract infection. This may be especially useful when compliance with a 10-day oral regimen is not assured.

Since many organisms are ampicillin resistant, admit children with upper tract infections (pyelonephritis) and treat them with IV ampicillin (100 mg/kg/day) and an aminoglycoside (gentamicin, 6 mg/kg/day) until the causative agent is identified and antibacterial sensitivities are determined.

Patients who will be receiving antibiotics because of either strong presumptive evidence of a UTI or another focus of infection (eg, otitis media) must have a bladder tap or a catheter-obtained urine specimen. Two clean catch urine samples may be substituted only if the patient is old enough to perform the midstream collection properly. In these patients, the urinalysis is a useful guide to the adequacy of the specimen: a large number of epithelial cells suggests contamination. A bag urine culture is reliable only when sterile and therefore is adequate only if the patient will not receive antibiotics until the culture report is ready.

Follow-up urine cultures, obtained within 48–72 hours of initiating therapy, should be sterile. Clinical response serves only as a guide to the adequacy of therapy, which must be verified by negative culture results. Because laboratory sensitivity for both sulfisoxazole and ampicillin are unreliable, sterilization of the urine is a more accurate gauge of the adequacy of response when using these drugs. A culture 24–48 hours after the completion of the course of antibiotic therapy is also mandatory to ensure that the infection was eradicated.

Recurrences are common, especially in girls and in infants under 1 year of age. All patients must have follow-up cultures monthly for 3 months, then every 3 months for a year, and then every 6 months for 2 years.

It is important to determine if anatomical or functional uropathology exists. Girls less than 3 years of age and all boys require an IVP or renal ultrasound and a VCU after the first UTI. In addition, radiographic work-up is indicated for all girls with evidence of pyelonephritis. However, a girl older than 3 years with a lower tract infection requires no radiologic work-up until the second episode. Although the IVP or ultrasound may be performed at any time after a UTI is diagnosed, delay the VCU until approximately 6 weeks after the acute infection. A sterile urine culture must be obtained 1–3 days before the VCU is performed.

INDICATIONS FOR ADMISSION

- Upper tract infection (pyelonephritis)
- UTI with fever in a patient at risk for decreased renal function (decreased GFR, single kidney)

REFERENCES

1. Ogra PL, Faden HS: J Pediatr 106: 1023–1029, 1985
2. Selden RV, Friedman J, Kaplan MR: Ped Ann 10: 12–24 1981

20

Trauma

Cardiac Tamponade

INTRODUCTION

Cardiac tamponade is a life-threatening emergency requiring immediate intervention. It most commonly occurs following trauma, but it can also be secondary to infection (*Staphylococcus aureus, Hemophilus influenzae* type B, *Neisseria meningiditis,* and *Streptococcus pneumoniae*), or juvenile rheumatoid arthritis.

CLINICAL PRESENTATION AND DIAGNOSIS

Suspect cardiac tamponade if there are failing vital signs or electromechanical dissociation after blunt or penetrating chest trauma. Shock, associated with tachypnea, clear lungs with equal breath sounds bilaterally, neck vein distention and distant heart sounds suggests the diagnosis. An important finding is pulsus paradoxus, a 10–20 mm Hg drop in the systolic blood pressure on inspiration. The electrocardiogram (ECG) may reveal low voltage and nonspecific ST-T wave changes; the chest x-ray usually reveals a normal sized heart. Insert a central venous pressure line if tamponade is suspected; the pressure should be elevated (>12–15 cm H_2O) if tamponade is present.

The onset of tamponade is usually much slower in patients with nontraumatic etiologies. There may be a history of fever, chest pain or dyspnea. Order a chest x-ray (large heart, straight left heart border) and an echocardiogram if an effusion is suspected and the blood pressure is adequate.

The presentation of a *tension pneumothorax* may resemble tamponade, and, in the trauma patient, they may occur together. Diagnosis of tamponade is confirmed by a poor response to thoracentesis followed by rapid improvement in the vital signs (especially blood pressure) after pericardiocentesis.

Pulsus paradoxus may be noted in patients with severe *asthma* (wheezing, poor air movement) or *congestive heart failure* without a pericardial effusion.

Distended neck veins may be seen in patients with *congestive heart failure* or in *trauma victims* wearing military antishock (MAST) trousers.

Tachypnea and tachycardia occur in patients with *respiratory infections,* particularly when accompanied by fever. A pleural rub, rales, wheezing, or decreased breath sounds suggest the correct diagnosis.

ER MANAGEMENT

If the blood pressure continues to fall during the resuscitation of a trauma victim (multiple trauma, p 488), despite a 40–60 cc/kg fluid challenge, pericardiocentesis is indicated. While aspirating, insert an 18-gauge pericardiocentesis or spinal needle inferior to the xiphoid process at a 45 degree angle to the skin, and direct it toward the left shoulder. Attach an ECG lead to the needle. Free flow of nonpulsatile blood indicates that the pericardium has been entered. A current of injury pattern (ST segment elevation) indicates that the needle is touching the epicardial surface and should be withdrawn slightly. An improvement in the vital signs follows removal of as little as 10–20 cc of blood. However, a negative tap does not rule out tamponade since the blood in the pericardial sac clots rapidly. Immediate thoracic surgery is the definitive treatment.

Rarely is pericardiocentesis indicated in the ER for a patient with effusion on an inflammatory basis. Secure an IV and admit the patient to an intensive care unit for close observation and treatment of the primary illness.

INDICATIONS FOR ADMISSION

- Pericardial tamponade
- Evidence on echocardiography of fluid in the pericardial space

REFERENCE

1. Shabetar R, Fowler ND, Guntheroth WG: Am J Cardiol 26: 481, 1970

Cervical Spine Injuries

INTRODUCTION

Although cervical spine injuries are very rare in children, they may accompany serious head trauma or follow injuries to the top of the head or the back of the neck.

CLINICAL PRESENTATION

Occasionally, a patient with severe head injury has an associated cervical spine injury. Thus, neck injury may be possible in a child who is unconscious or has an altered mental status following head trauma.

In the awake patient, the most common symptom is pain in the posterior neck. Less often, there is weakness or pain along the involved nerve roots.

DIAGNOSIS

See p 393 for the approach to the patient with head trauma.

Often, an awake, alert patient arrives in the ER with his head and neck immobilized. Ask about the presence of pain at the top of the head (C_{2-3}) or back of the neck and paresthesias of the hands, arms, or legs. If none of these are present, carefully remove the neck restraint without moving the patient, and palpate the spinous processes for local tenderness, muscle spasm, or obvious deformity. The first process that can be palpated is C_2, and C_6 and C_7 are the largest. Ask the patient to move his fingers and hands and raise his arms and legs. If there is no tenderness or evidence of trauma and the patient moves his extremities easily, ask him to move his neck gently from side to side and then up and down. Do not attempt to move the patient's neck yourself and insist he stop immediately if any movement causes pain.

Suspect a cervical spine injury in a patient with (1) neck trauma, (2) pain on top of the head, (3) paresthesias or weakness, (4) inability to cooperate with your examination, (5) unresponsiveness after head trauma, (6) injury above the clavicles, or (7) deceleration injury.

ER MANAGEMENT

Immediately immobilize the head and neck of every patient suspected of having a cervical spine injury, if this was not already accomplished in the field. An easy method is to place sandbags or large IV bags on both sides of the patient's head and apply 2–3 strips of adhesive tape across his forehead, securing the ends under the sides of the stretcher. A soft collar is not adequate since it permits too much movement, but in the older child, a hard plastic Philadelphia collar may be used instead of sandbags and tape.

Next, perform a rapid survey of the patient's airway and cardiopulmonary status as outlined on pp 488–489. If intubation is necessary, never delay it because the lateral neck x-ray has not been obtained or interpreted. Apply axial traction to the head, perform the jaw lift maneuver to open the oropharynx, and have an assistant apply slight downward pressure over the trachea to bring the vocal cords into view. Avoid hyperextending or flexing the neck during the process.

Order a cross-table lateral of the cervical spine. All 7 vertebrae must be visualized since C_{6-7} are the most commonly injured. Once that film has been interpreted as normal, the patient may be moved to the x-ray suite for anteroposterior (AP) and oblique views, if he is stable. An open mouth view, which permits visualization of the odontoid (C_2) and the ring of C_1, is mandatory if there was trauma to the top of the head or the upper neck.

When a cervical spine injury is suspected clinically or diagnosed radiographically, call a neurosurgeon immediately to assist in further management (application of Gardiner tongs).

INDICATIONS FOR ADMISSION

- Cervical spine fracture
- Focal neurologic deficit

REFERENCE
1. Babcock JL: Arch Surg 111: 646–651, 1976

Hand Injuries

INTRODUCTION

The injured hand requires a thorough evaluation, as improper management may lead to permanent disability. A systematic approach is essential to avoid overlooking subtle injuries.

CLINICAL PRESENTATION

Lacerations. Hand lacerations (see p 501) may involve the skin only or may be deep and involve underlying structures. Active extension of a digit, by the intrinsic muscles and intertendonous bands distal to the injury, is possible despite partial laceration of the extensor tendon. A dorsal hand laceration associated with pain on extension of the digit against resistance suggests a partial tendon injury.

Bites. Bites (see p 496) are actually a combination of lacerations and crush injuries. Suspect that an irregular laceration over the MCP joint is a human bite sustained by punching another person in the mouth. This is a serious injury, as oral flora can be inoculated into the MCP joint.

Fractures and Dislocations. *Phalangeal fractures* are common, but not serious injuries unless the joint, volar plate, or collateral ligament is involved.

The most commonly fractured bone in the hand is the *scaphoid.* The key finding is tenderness to deep palpation in the snuff box area distal to the radial styloid. Unless an oblique radiograph is obtained, this fracture is easily missed.

An *MCP dislocation* causes fixed digit hyperextension, sometimes associated with a volar laceration through which the metacarpal head can be seen. A *PIP dislocation* presents as an obvious deformity, unless it has already been reduced at the scene by the patient or an onlooker.

Tendon Injuries. Acute radial deviation of the thumb at the MCP joint may tear the *ulnar collateral ligament* (gamekeeper's thumb). Typically, the injury occurs when a skier falls and his or her thumb lands on the ground or ski pole. Tenderness along the ulnar aspect of the thumb MCP joint with laxity of the joint on radial abduction stress (under local anesthesia) are noted.

A *mallet* (baseball) *finger* results from a direct blow to the tip of an extended digit, rupturing the DIP extensor tendon or avulsing it from the base of the distal phalanx. The finger is flexed at the DIP joint, and x-rays may reveal an avulsed bone chip remaining attached to the extensor tendon.

A *boutonniere deformity* involves PIP flexion with DIP hyperextension. The lateral bands of the intrinsic muscles are pulled volar to the PIP axis, so that the PIP ''buttonholes'' through the torn extensor hood.

Nail Bed Injuries. Blunt trauma to the nail often causes a *subungual hematoma,* or bleeding between the nail and the nailbed. A very tender nail with a bluish-black discoloration is seen.

Infections. A *paronychia,* an infection of the soft tissues around the fingernail, usually beings as a hangnail. An exquisitely tender, erythematous swelling along the margin of the nail results. There may be a purulent discharge. A *felon* is a distal pulp space infection that can spread down the flexor tendon sheath. Tense, tender, erythematous swelling of the volar surface of the distal phalnax is seen.

Purulent tenosynovitis, an infection of the tendon sheath, is a surgical emergency. The sheaths of the thumb and fifth finger communicate at the wrist and allow a horseshoe infection to develop. Other sheaths connect the midpalm and distal phalanges. Kanavel's four cardinal signs of tenosynovitis are (1) swelling, (2) slight flexion of the finger, (3) tenderness over the tendon sheath, and (4) exquisite pain on passive finger extension.

Palmar space infections present with tense, tender, erythematous swelling of the palmar surface with pain and decreased mobility of the third and fourth fingers (midpalmar space) or thumb (thenar space). These infections can spread to the flexor tendon sheaths.

Ganglions. These are well-defined, smooth, cystic lesions that are fixed to the deep tissues. They are usually found on the volar or dorsal surface of the wrist or on the palmar surface of the base of a digit.

Amputations. Most amputations involve the distal fingertip only, while loss of the entire nail bed results in a more significant injury. However, children have unusual regenerative ability, so consider re-implantation of virtually any amputation.

DIAGNOSIS

Evaluation begins with a careful history, including hand dominance, tetanus immunization status, and previous hand injuries. Inquire about the mechanism of injury, including the hand position at the time, the elapsed time since the injury, and whether the trauma occurred in a clean or dirty environment.

Next, inspect the hand and evaluate the vascular status. Look for an alteration in the usual resting cascade of the digits, suggestive of a tendon or nerve injury. Check the color and temperature of the injured digit and assess capillary refill (compress the distal fingertip pulp). If there is any suspicion of arterial insufficiency, perform the Allen test by compressing the radial and ulnar arteries at the wrist while the patient opens and closes his hand several times. Upon releasing either artery, the palm and all five fingers should turn pink. The same test can be performed on the radial and ulnar digital arteries.

Prior to anesthetizing the hand, assess sensory function by evaluating two-point discrimination with two points of a paperclip. Apply both points to the radial side of each digit. Then move the points closer together until the patient can no longer distinguish between them. The normal range is 3–5 mm, but use an uninjured digit as a control. Repeat the examination on the ulnar side. In this way, evaluate the median (index fingertip), radial (dorsal web space between the first two fingers), and ulnar (fifth fingertip) sensory nerves.

Motor (tendon and nerve) function testing must be performed in a systematic manner. First, test the extrinsic flexors: thumb IP (flexor pollicis longus), then finger DIP while the PIP is held in extension (flexor digitorum profundus), then finger PIP while the other fingers' PIPs are held extended (flexor digitorum superficialis). Next, have the patient flex his or her wrist against resistance and palpate the three tendons (flexor carpi ulnaris, palmaris longus, and flexor carpi radialis, from medial to lateral) at the base of the wrist. Evaluate the thenar muscles and median nerve function by opposing the pulp of the thumb with that of the other four fingers. Test thumb adduction (adductor policis) and ulnar nerve function by having the patient grasp a piece of paper between the thumb and radial surface of the proximal index finger. Weakness is indicated by Froment's sign, flexion of the IP thumb joint. To test the hypothenar muscles, ask the patient to abduct the fifth finger. The interossei and lumbrical muscles (median nerve) are tested by asking the patient to spread the fingers apart or to flex the digits at the MCP joints while keeping the PIP and DIP joints extended.

ER MANAGEMENT

Manage profuse bleeding with elevation and pressure for 15 minutes. Never use clamps for hemostasis as the nerves travelling with the blood vesels can be damaged.

Palpate for localized bony tenderness or soft tissue swelling and examine for obvious deformities, ecchymoses, and functional deficits. If any of these findings are present over the wrist or hand, obtain x-rays. Radiographs of the fingers are indicated for gross deformities, lacerations in association with crush injuries, or loss of IP joint mobility.

Perform anesthesia only after a satisfactory sensory examination has been completed. If a digital block is required, wait 5 minutes after preparing the skin with povidone-iodine. Use a 25- or 27- gauge needle to inject 2–4 cc of 2% xylocaine (NEVER with epinephrine) into both lateral margins of the digit at the level of the metacarpal head.

Lacerations and Bites. Carefully debride and irrigate these wounds after anesthesia (pp 502–503). Close with 4-0 to 6-0 nylon, using simple sutures that are left in place for 10–14 days. Do not suture *bite wounds* closed, but the edges of large lacerations may be approximated with several loose sutures. Evaluate *MCP human bite injuries* carefully for evidence that the joint capsule has been breeched. Treat wounds that penetrate the capsule with open irrigation in the operating room and either intravenous clindamycin (40 mg/kg/day) or oxacillin (100 mg/kg/day) and penicillin (50,000 units/kg/day). Give prophylactic dicloxacillin (50 mg/kg/day), cephradine (25 mg/kg/day), or erythromycin (40 mg/kg/day) for 7 days to patients with deep lacerations and bite injuries.

Fractures and Dislocations. Refer patients with *intraarticular* and *carpal fractures, MCP dislocations,* or *snuffbox tenderness* to an orthopedist. Treat *phalangeal fractures* that do not involve the joint with splinting or "buddy" taping to the adjacent digit. A *PIP dislocation* can be reduced with traction, buddy taped and splinted after x-rays are obtained to rule out an associated avulsion fracture.

Tendon Injuries. Refer patients with a *gamekeeper's thumb* or *boutonniere* deformity to an orthopedist. Treat a *mallet finger* with a short dorsal splint, ensuring DIP extension with free PIP mobility, for 8 weeks.

Infections. A *paronychia* without pus requires warm soaks q 2–3h, elevation, and dicloxacillin, cephradrine, or erythromycin. If pus is present, lift the edge of the eponychial fold with a number 15 blade. One drop of pus signifies adequate drainage. Warm soaks, elevation, and antibiotics are also necessary. If pus extends under the nail, partial removal of the nail is indicated. Refer *felons* to a hand surgeon for immediate drainage. Admit patients with *purulent tenosynovitis* (culture for gonococcus, see p 418) and *palmar space infections* for intravenous oxacillin (100 mg/kg/day) or clindamycin (40 mg/kg/day), if allergic to penicillin, and immediately consult with a hand surgeon.

Ganglions. Elective surgical removal is indicated if the lesion is painful or very disfiguring.

Amputations. The care of an amputated part includes rinsing it gently in saline, wrapping it in saline-soaked gauze, and placing it in a sealed plastic bag immersed in ice (do not allow direct contact with the ice). Distal fingertip amputations may require wrapping in Xeroform. For more serious injuries obtain a complete blood count (CBC) and type and cross-match, start an intravenous line with maintenance fluids, give IV morphine sulfate (0.1 mg/kg/dose) for pain, and infuse prophylactic oxacillin or cefazolin (100 mg/kg/day). Gently clean the wound and cover it with Xeroform- or saline-soaked gauze, until the patient can be taken to the operating room. Obtain an x-ray if there is suspicion of a crush injury to the distal phalanx.

INDICATIONS FOR ADMISSION

- Purulent tenosynovitis or palmar space infection
- Deep bite wound (especially punch bite wound)

- Intraarticular fracture (>25% articular surface), and MCP dislocation
- Amputation other than distal fingertip
- Tendon laceration which requires open repair

REFERENCES

1. Billmire DA, Neale HW, Stein PT: Surg Clin North Am 64: 683–698, 1984
2. American Society for Surgery of the Hand: The Hand: Examination and Diagnosis. Aurora, Colorado, 1978

Multiple Trauma

INTRODUCTION

Trauma is the leading cause of death in children over 1 year of age. Blunt injuries are most common at all ages, although the incidence of penetrating trauma increases in adolescence. The main factors contributing to morbidity and mortality are hemorrhage, respiratory failure, and central nervous system (CNS) injury. Trauma resuscitation requires an aggressive team approach, with one member serving as team leader who takes responsibility for directing and coordinating the resuscitative effort.

CLINICAL PRESENTATION

The presentation usually depends on the degree of blood loss, respiratory compromise, and CNS damage. However, the trauma victim, particularly after blunt injury, may be in early shock with little or no external evidence (see Shock, p 11).

DIAGNOSIS AND ER MANAGEMENT

The priority is a rapid (30 seconds) initial assessment to identify life-threatening problems that require immediate intervention. Note the patient's general condition and palpate the pulse (carotid, femoral, or brachial), skin, trachea, and chest. Listen to the lungs while watching

TABLE 20-1. MANAGEMENT OPTIONS FOR LIFE-THREATENING CONDITIONS

Finding	Problem	Management
Noisy breathing Stridor	Upper airway obstruction	Chin lift or jaw thrust Intubation
Neck pain or tenderness Head trauma Multiple trauma Deceleration injury	Possible C-spine fracture	Immobilize neck (sandbags) Lateral C-spine x-ray
Asymmetrical breath sounds and hyperresonant percussion note	Possible tension pneumothroax	Insert 16-gauge needle into 2nd ICS in MCL
Penetrating chest wound	Possible sucking chest wound	Apply occlusive dressing Insert chest tube
Penetrating chest wound with muffled heart sounds or distended neck veins	Possible cardiac tamponade	Pericardiocentesis (4th ICS 1 cm lateral to left sternal border or subxiphoid)
Paradoxical chest wall movement	Flail chest	Positive pressure ventilation for respiratory distress
Orthostasis Pale, cool skin	Hypotension or shock	Apply MAST garment Establish two large bore IV, 20 cc/kg crystalloid boluses Transfusion

the chest excursions, measure the blood pressure, and note the response to verbal and painful stimuli.

If life-threatening problems are identified (Table 20-1), the team leader must immediately summon surgical assistance and organize a sequence of therapy, corresponding to the alphabetical order listed below.

A. Airway/C-Spine. As described in the section on cardiopulmonary resuscitation (p 1), establish and maintain a patent airway. Noisy or stridulous breathing suggests airway obstruction, often secondary to the tongue falling against the posterior pharyngeal wall. Perform a chin lift or jaw thrust and insert an oropharyngeal or nasopharyngeal airway. If these measures are unsuccessful, perform orotracheal intubation while axial traction is applied to the head. If severe oral and facial injuries prevent orotracheal intubation, insert a large bore needle with internal catheter through the membrane between the thyroid cartilage (Adam's apple), and cricoid. Attach the catheter to high flow oxygen via a Y-connector, and intermittently insufflate by occluding the open end of the Y.

Severe multiple trauma, significant head or neck trauma, neck pain and tenderness, or a history of a sudden deceleration suggest the possibility of C-spine injury. Maintain neck immobilization (sandbags, rigid cervical collar) until a lateral C-spine x-ray and a careful neurologic examination rule out an injury (p 481). However, do not sacrifice the airway by efforts to maintain neck immobilization; never delay intubation because a radiologist or neurosurgeon has not yet confirmed that the film shows no fracture.

B. Breathing. Provide 100% O_2 to all severe trauma victims, without waiting for the results of blood gas analysis. Immediately intubate all patients who are unconscious, have decreased breath sounds, or have any evidence of respiratory distress after a chin lift or jaw thrust.

Palpate for rib fractures and look for signs of a tension pneumothorax (p 493), including a hyperresonant percussion note, subcutaneous emphysema, tracheal deviation, distended neck veins, and continued respiratory distress after intubation. Immediately insert a 16-gauge needle into the second intercostal space in the midclavicular line on the affected side, without waiting for x-ray confirmation.

Asymmetrical breath sounds associated with a hyperresonant percussion note and subcutaneous emphysema suggest a simple pneumothorax. Asymmetrical breath sounds with a dull percussion note suggests a simple hemothorax. Tube thoracotomy is indicated for both, *after* the airway, breathing, and circulatory priorities have been adequately addressed.

Hypotension after penetrating wounds near the heart suggest the possibility of pericardial tamponade. Distended neck veins and muffled heart sounds are variable findings. Urgent pericardiocentesis (pp 479–481) is indicated and emergency thoracotomy may be required.

Penetrating chest trauma can cause a sucking chest wound. Cover it with an occlusive dressing (vaseline gauze).

A flail chest causes paradoxical chest wall movement after blunt chest trauma. Positive pressure ventilation is required if respiratory distress persists despite supplemental oxygen.

Obtain a chest x-ray (after securing the airway) if there are any of the above abnormalities upon examination of the chest. Possible findings include a simple or tension pneumothorax, rib fractures, lung densities (pulmonary contusion), pleural fluid (hemothorax), mediastinal emphysema, and a widened mediastinum (ruptured aorta).

C. Circulation. Control external bleeding with direct digital or manual pressure, pressure dressings, or pneumatic splints, but do not use tourniquets or clamps. If there are signs of hypovolemia or shock (p 11), immediately apply the MAST trousers. The pediatric size fits most children over 4 years of age.

Secure two large bore IV, one of which must be in an upper extremity. Give 20 cc/kg of isotonic crystalloid (normal saline or Ringer lactate) as an IV bolus after obtaining blood for a CBC, spun hematocrit, type and cross-match, and arterial blood gas (ABG). Monitor the blood pressure carefully, and repeat the bolus every 5–10 minutes, if needed. If 40 cc/kg does not raise the blood pressure, transfuse with 20 cc/kg of packed cells (uncross-matched, type-specific blood can be available in 10 minutes).

Attempt to identify sources of potential or ongoing blood loss. Following a careful physical examination, obtain a chest x-ray to rule out hemothorax; also obtain a pelvic x-ray, since a pelvic fracture is a common cause of retroperitoneal hemorrhage. Obtain urine for a urinalysis. Hematuria may indicate urinary tract injury (p 215). Although this is rarely a life-threatening problem, urgent radiographic evaluation of the urinary tract is indicated.

Abdominal paracentesis is not routinely performed in children with suspected intraabdominal bleeding. Conservative, nonsurgical management of solid organ (liver, spleen, kidney) injury is standard, so that a "positive" peritoneal lavage is not an indication for surgery. Abdominal paracentesis is indicated for the child with unstable vital signs in whom the source of the bleeding is unknown. If available, abdominal CT may be the procedure of choice for identifying injuries and bleeding sites in these patients.

Cardiopulmonary arrest in a trauma victim is an indication for emergency thoracotomy with cross-clamping of the descending aorta, if personnel experienced in the procedure are available.

If life-threatening problems are not identified during the initial 30-

second survey, secure a large bore IV, obtain frequent vital signs, and proceed with the secondary survey.

D. Deficit (Neurologic). Once adequate vital signs are established, efforts can be directed toward the diagnosis and treatment of CNS injuries (pp 393–399).

E. Expose. Expose the patient completely and perform a complete physical examination, looking for associated injuries. Palpate all bones, including the facial bones, and palpate and percuss the teeth. Check the extraocular movements (EOM), corneal clarity, and pupillary regularity and symmetry. Look for signs of a basilar skull fracture (hemotympanum, clear rhino- or otorrhea, infraorbital and retroauricular ecchymoses). The diagnosis and management of ocular (p 408), dental (p 51), orthopedic (p 419), genitourinary (p 215), and soft tissue (p 501) trauma are detailed elsewhere.

F. Foley Catheter. Monitor the urine output closely in unconscious or hypotensive patients by inserting a catheter into the bladder. The sole exception is males with suspected urethral disruption (p 217) suggested by blood at the urethral meatus. These injuries are usually associated with a pelvic fracture, straddle injury, or penetrating wound. Call a urologist immediately.

G. Gastric Emptying. Insert a nasogastric tube and attach it to suction to prevent aspiration and, secondarily, improve ventilation. If there has been facial or frontal head trauma, use an orogastric tube instead.

Almost all multiple trauma victims require at least three x-rays: lateral cervical spine, chest, and pelvis. The only exception is the victim of minor trauma with stable vital signs who is awake, alert, and able to ambulate normally. Obtain a urinalysis and give tetanus prophylaxis (0.5 cc IM of toxoid).

INDICATIONS FOR ADMISSION

- Hypotension or orthostatic vital sign changes
- Respiratory distress or compromise
- Serious head or neck injury
- Suspected intraabdominal injury
- Severe fracture or soft tissue injury

REFERENCES

1. Templeton JM Jr, O'Neill JA Jr: Emerg Clin North Am 2: 899–912, 1984
2. Feins NR: Pediatr Clin North Am 26: 759–771, 1979
3. Advanced Trauma Life Support Student Manual. Amer Coll. of Surgeons: Comm. on Trauma, 1981

Pneumothorax

INTRODUCTION

Pneumothorax can result from blunt or penetrating thoracic trauma. It can also occur in asthmatics, newborns, and, occasionally, in otherwise healthy young persons without trauma.

CLINICAL PRESENTATION

A pneumothorax presents with signs of respiratory distress, including nasal flaring, tachypnea, accessory muscle use, and anxiety or altered mental status. Breath sounds may be decreased or absent on the affected side, and pulsus paradoxicus >10 mm Hg may be noted. The percussion note can be tympanitic (pure pneumothorax), dull (hemothorax), or both (hemopneumothorax).

Signs of a tension pneumothorax include deviation of the trachea to the contralateral side, cyanosis, jugular venous distention, and deterioration of the vital signs, including electromechanical dissociation. Pneumomediastinum can occur with or without pneumothorax.

DIAGNOSIS

Always be suspicious of the possibility of pneumothorax in a trauma victim (see multiple trauma, p 501). Any chest trauma can produce pneumothorax by fracturing ribs or by direct penetrating injury; however, a pneumothorax can occur in the absence of either. Air can leak from the lung, the tracheobronchial tree, esophagus, or through a sucking wound in the chest wall. Suspect a pneumothorax in an asthmatic who is tachypneic without wheezing or in an otherwise healthy child who presents with sudden onset of chest pain and dyspnea. Unless a tension pneumothorax is suspected, obtain a chest x-ray to confirm the diagnosis.

Pleural effusion in the asthmatic with pneumonia can mimic a hemopneumothorax. In *cardiac tamponade,* the breath sounds are adequate, but the heart sounds are diminished and ECG monitoring may reveal low voltage. In *hypovolemic shock,* breath and heart sounds are usually normal. The neck veins are flattened and a prompt response (rise in blood pressure) with fluid resuscitation and application of pneumatic antishock trousers (MAST) confirms the diagnosis of hypovolemia.

ER MANAGEMENT

Immediately give high flow (10 L/min) oxygen and secure a large bore (16-gauge) IV.

Tension pneumothorax must be relieved immediately. Insert a 14- or 16-gauge needle with a Teflon catheter over the top of the third rib in the midclavicular line on the affected side. A rush of air and improvement in the patient's ventilatory status confirm both the diagnosis and adequacy of therapy. Remove the needle, leave the catheter in place, and attach a one-way flutter valve to the end of the catheter. This can be the finger of a surgical glove with the tip end removed. Air will be able to flow out during expiration but the valve will collapse in inspiration. The definitive relief of a hemopneumothorax is a chest tube thoracostomy in the fourth intercostal space over the fifth rib in the anterior axillary line with the tube attached to an underwater seal.

INDICATIONS FOR ADMISSION

- Posttraumatic pneumothorax of any size
- Nontraumatic pneumothorax that is enlarging or is >10% of the lung surface area
- Fractured ribs for 24 hours of observation (relative)

REFERENCE

1. Eichelberger MR, Randolph JR: Surg Clin North Am 61: 1181–1198, 1981

21

Wound Care

Abscesses

INTRODUCTION

A cutaneous abscess is a localized collection of pus that is usually secondary to disruption of the integrity of the skin. The common organisms, therefore, are *Staphylococcus* and *Streptococcus*.

CLINICAL PRESENTATION AND DIAGNOSIS

An abscess presents as a discrete mass with central fluctuance, erythema, warmth, and tenderness, occasionally accompanied by the drainage of pus. This can be differentiated from a *cellulitis,* which may have local swelling, tenderness, warmth, and redness, by the central fluctuance.

ER MANAGEMENT

The definitive treatment for an abscess is incision and surgical drainage. Maintain strict aseptic technique to prevent the spread of infection. Prepare the skin with povidone-iodine (see wound management, p 501) and infiltrate the skin over the point of maximal fluctuance with 1% lidocaine without epinephrine. A regional block (outside of the infected area) may be used instead of wide infiltration of lidocaine, to avoid spread of the infection into the contiguous tissue planes.

Make the incision along the direction of the natural skin lines to prevent excessive scarring. Obtain cultures of the abscess contents and explore the cavity with a blunt instrument (swab, clamp, gloved finger) to break up any loculations. Take care, however, not to injure healthy tissue by excessive probing.

Copiously irrigate the cavity with Betadine and saline (1:1) or bacitracin and saline (50,000 units in 500 cc) and pack it loosely with an iodoform gauze wick. If there is excessive bleeding, pack the cavity tightly for the first 24 hours.

Instruct parents to keep the wound clean and not to change the dressings unless drainage seeps through. The next day, remove the packing, irrigate the wound gently with 2% hydrogen peroxide, and lightly repack it. Repeat this procedure again in 24 hours. Usually by 48 hours the incision remains open without packing while the cavity heals from below. Once the packing has been removed, recommend sitz baths or warm soaks at least twice a day until healing is completed.

Antibiotics (dicloxacillin, 50 mg/kg/day divided q 6h to 500 q 6h, erythromycin or cephradine, 40 mg/kg/day divided q 6h) are indicated if tender lymphadenopathy or fever accompanies the abscess, or if there is a large area of surrounding cellulitis.

Refer breast, perirectal, Bartholin gland, finger tip and hand abscesses, as well as deep abscesses of the neck, to an experienced surgeon.

INDICATIONS FOR ADMISSION

- An abscess associated with lymphangitis, high fever (>102°F), or other signs of toxicity (lethargy, irritability, poor intake)

REFERENCE

1. Hill GJ Jr: Outpatient Surgery, 2nd ed. Philadelphia, Saunders, 1980, pp 146–7, 1137–1140

Bites

INTRODUCTION

Bites account for 1% of all ER visits, and many more victims do not seek medical attention. Dog bites are most frequent (50%), followed by human (25%), cat (15%), and others (rats, mice, squirrel, bats, etc). Controversy exists over closure of the wounds and the use of prophylactic antibiotics, while the possibility of acquiring rabies from wild animals is always a concern.

CLINICAL PRESENTATION AND DIAGNOSIS

Usually, the history of an animal bite injury is readily obtained, so the diagnosis is evident. Suspect that a laceration over the metacarpalphalangeal joints in an adolescent was caused by punching another person in the mouth.

On examination, bites generally are of two types (which may coexist on a given patient)—lacerations or puncture wounds. The latter are of particular concern, as the small break in the skin belies the significant risk of infection.

ER MANAGEMENT

General Measures. Thoroughly clean every bite wound and give the victim tetanus toxoid, unless it is clear that a booster has been given in the preceding 5 years. Then irrigate the wound with 500–1000 cc of bacitracin solution (50,000 units/500 cc). Use either a 16-gauge needle attached to a 500 cc IV bag, around which a blood transfusion cuff is inflated to 300 mm Hg, or a 20–60-cc syringe with a 16-gauge angiocatheter attached. If the procedure is painful, anesthetize the intact skin margins of the wound with 1% lidocaine. Debride devitalized tissues as these wounds may also be crush injuries, and the dead tissue serves as an excellent culture medium.

Suturing bite wounds is associated with a higher infection rate. However, if aggressive debridement and irrigation are performed, face wounds may be closed when cosmetic concerns are of primary importance. The edges of large gaps elsewhere on the body can be loosely approximated with either sutures or Steri-strips. While there is no consensus as to the value of prophylactic antibiotics for these wounds, most surgeons recommend a 3- to 5-day course of an antistaphylococcal antibiotic.

Reexamine all bite wounds within 24–48 hours. Instruct the patient to return sooner for fever, increasing pain, erythema, induration, or purulence at the wound site.

Dog Bites. Infection is most likely in cases of puncture wounds, hand wounds, and when there has been a delay (>24 hours) in seeking medical attention. Give antibiotic prophylaxis for these high-risk wounds, although preinfection wound cultures are of no use. Infection occurring within 24 hours of the injury suggests *Pasturella multocida* as the causative organism. However, the majority of dog bite infections occur after the first day, when *Staphylococcus aureus* and *Streptococcus viridans* are more common. Therefore, appropriate prophylaxis is 5 days of an antistaphyloccocal antibiotic dicloxacillin 50 mg/kg/day, erythromycin or cephradine 40 mg/kg/day with penicillin (50,000 units/kg/day).

Rabies prophylaxis (p 315) is an issue in dog bite management. If the dog has received shots or if the attack was provoked by the patient, there is little concern. Observe the animal involved in an unprovoked attack for signs of rabies. If the dog was a stray for whom no information is available, then the incidence of rabies in the community determines whether immunization is indicated.

Human Bites. These are of two types, true bites and the more serious lacerations that occur when the patient has punched another person in the mouth. In this type of injury, great force is involved, so that there is more tissue damage, increased hemorrhage, and a deeper inoculation of oral flora. Since these wounds are so frequently infected, do not close them and give the patient prophylactic penicillin and dicloxacillin or, if penicillin-allergic, clindamycin (25 mg/kg/day) for 5 days. Obtain an x-ray if there is any suspicion of a metacarpal fracture or osteomyelitis. Untreated "punch" wounds are at risk for infection of the metacarpal-phalangeal capsule with subsequent permanent joint stiffness. Elevate and immobilize all of these hand injuries until any swelling subsides. Admission is advisable if this cannot be guaranteed.

Human bites on sites other than the hands require only the routine measures. In general, however, do not suture these lacerations.

Cat Bites. Infections after cat bites are very common (50%). In addition, because of their grooming habits, cat scratches are also at risk for infection with the cat's oral flora. Since *Pasturella multocida* is the most common organism, give all patients prophylactic penicillin (50,000 units/kg/day) after irrigation and debridement.

Other Animals. In general, the principles of management, including antibiotic prophylaxis, are identical to those for a dog bite. However, some wild animals (bats, raccoons, skunks) are significant reservoirs of rabies. Therefore, the animal should be sacrificed and the brain examined for evidence of rabies, especially if the attack was unprovoked. If the animal is unavailable, consider it to be rabid.

INDICATIONS FOR ADMISSION

- Any infected hand or face wound
- Bite wound cellulitis (except hand and face) unresponsive to oral antibiotics
- Human bite from "punch" trauma that breaches the metacarpal-phalangeal joint capsule, or if proper immobilization and elevation cannot be maintained.

REFERENCES

1. Elenbaas RM, McNabney WK, Robinson WA: Ann Emerg Med 11: 248–251, 1982
2. Malinkowski RW, Strate RG, Perry JF, et al: J Trauma 19: 655–659, 1979
3. Schweich P, Fleisher G: Pediatr Emerg Care 1:51–53, 1985

Foreign Bodies in the Skin

INTRODUCTION AND CLINICAL PRESENTATION

Small fragments of wood or pieces of glass are the most common foreign bodies embedded in the skin. The patient may have fallen on glass fragments or scraped himself on a rough wooden surface. If the wound is fresh, it is usually tender and the foreign body is often seen or palpated just below the surface. If the patient is not seen soon after the injury, the wound may be indurated and tender with or without purulent or serosanguinous drainage.

Fishhooks are frequently caught in the skin. Usually, a barb from a single or multibarbed hook is embedded in the skin, although if a finger or earlobe is involved, the barb may completely penetrate the tissue, emerging from the other side and leaving only the shaft of the hook still embedded.

DIAGNOSIS

Except for fishhooks, obtain an x-ray of the involved soft tissue to ensure that there is only one foreign body and that it is not fragmented. An x-ray is also indicated when the presence of a foreign body cannot be ruled out, eg, an old wound that does not heal, continues to drain serosanguinous or purulent material, or remains tender. Virtually all glass is radioopaque, and wooden splinters can be seen if they have dirt particles on them.

ER MANAGEMENT

Attempt to remove a foreign body only if it is close enough to the surface to be seen or palpated. Clean the skin well with povidone-iodine and allow it to dry. Then infiltrate the skin overlying the proximal half of the object with 1–2% lidocaine. Using a number 11 blade, make a small incision in the skin directly over the middle of the foreign body. This provides the greatest opportunity for finding the fragment in the subcutaneous tissue. Once it is found, extend the incision along the long axis of the object toward the proximal end. Grab the end with a small clamp and slowly pull the fragment out. Then gently palpate with a gloved finger over the wound to try to identify any fragments that may remain.

When the foreign body is very small or cannot be palpated, probing the wound is likely to cause significant tissue injury. If the wound is tender and crusted over, unroof it using the point of an 18-gauge needle. If pus escapes during this procedure, it may carry the foreign body(ies) with it. Continue with warm soaks at home and have the patient return in 48 hours.

When the foreign body cannot be removed, the amount of discomfort caused by the fragment determines further management.If the wound is very painful, consult with a surgeon to plan for exploration in the operating room. If it is not painful, have the patient soak the wound in warm water several times a day until the foreign body migrates closer to the surface.

To remove a fishhook, advance the point until you determine where it will emerge from the skin and infiltrate some 1–2% lidocaine in that area. Then advance the point until the barb exits from the skin, cut the barb off, and pull the shaft of the fishhook back out through the entrance wound. If the fishhook has multiple barbs, separate them with wirecutters and remove each one individually. If the barb is already through the skin, cut it off and pull the shaft back. Lidocaine is not necessary in this latter situation.

Give tetanus toxoid to all patients who are not sure that they have received a booster in the last 5 years or have not completed the primary immunization series. Use 0.5 cc of DT for patients <6 years of age, and 0.5 cc of dT for older patients.

Refer patients with foreign bodies in the face or hand to an experienced surgeon, and consult with a surgeon before attempting to remove a foreign body from the neck, unless it is clearly superficial.

REFERENCE

1. Wolcott MW: Ferguson's Surgery of the Ambulatory Patient, 5th ed. Philadelphia, Lippincott, pp 101–108

Wound Management

INTRODUCTION

Lacerations occur throughout childhood and can often be treated without surgical consultation. Proper wound management requires a systematic approach.

CLINICAL PRESENTATION AND DIAGNOSIS

History. Determine the mechanism of injury, the site where the injury occurred (is the wound likely to be clean or dirty), and the position of the wounded part when it was injured. Also determine the time of injury. Wounds older than *8 hours* are usually too contaminated to suture. Assess the general health of the patient and ask about underlying chronic illnesses (diabetes, vasculitis) since these patients may have delayed wound healing and be at greater risk for developing an infection.

Examination. Determine the extent of the injury and evaluate sensation, general strength, vascular supply, motor function, and range of motion with and without resistance (looking for tendon injuries). This is difficult in the young, uncooperative child, but if an extremity is involved, observe the child moving it normally through a full range of movement before closing the wound. During the assessment, keep the wound edges moist by applying gauze pads moistened with normal saline. For dirty wounds, use a 1:1 solution of 10% povidone-iodine and normal saline.

Radiology. When the history or physical examination suggests the possibility of a foreign body in the wound, obtain an x-ray. Metal fragments and glass can be seen, and wood fragments are visible if they have radioopaque particles of dirt on them. Also order x-rays of crush injuries to rule out a compound fracture.

ER MANAGEMENT

Shaving. In general, shave hairy areas prior to suturing. However, the eyebrow must never be shaved since there is no guarantee how or if the eyebrow will grow back. Use the border of the eyebrow as a guide for the first suture.

Anesthesia. To prepare the wound for anesthesia, apply povidone-iodine solution twice to the skin surrounding the wound, allowing it to dry for approximately 4 minutes between applications. Lidocaine HC1 (Xylocaine), the usual anesthetic agent, is available at 1%, 2%, and 2% with epinephrine. Use 1% lidocaine for local infiltration of wounds, 2% for digital blocks, and 2% with 1:100,000 epinephrine for facial nerve blocks and scalp wounds. Never use lidocaine with epinephrine in an area that has end artery circulation (eg, fingers, hands, feet, nose, and toes), and do not rely on the vasoconstrictive properties of epinephrine for hemostasis. The amount of lidocaine used should never exceed 7 mg/kg. In unquestionably clean wounds, inject the lidocaine through the open wound (less painful), but in wounds likely to be dirty, administer it through the surrounding skin to avoid injecting debris into the deeper tissues. Apply viscous lidocaine to dirty abrasions to reduce the amount of discomfort when the wound is scrubbed to remove imbedded dirt.

Irrigation. After anesthesia has been achieved, clean and irrigate the wound. Use a large (60 cc) syringe attached to a 16-gauge IV catheter tip. It is soft and pliable and does not cause further damage if the patient moves. Avoid high pressure irrigation; injection of solution with the wound contaminants through the surrounding tissue planes may result in a very severe infection. The least toxic solution for irrigation is normal saline, but use copious amounts (500–1000 cc depending on the wound size). An alternative irrigating solution is povidone-iodine solution either diluted 1:1 in normal saline or full strength. Undiluted iodine is caustic to the wound edge; do not use it on the face. Use bacitracin irrigating solution (50,000 units of anhydrous bacitracin in 100–1000 cc of normal saline) for wounds likely to be very dirty (animal bites, wounds filled with particles of dirt and debris). It can also be used to irrigate abscess cavities just prior to insertion of the packing.

Exploration. Examine every wound for foreign substances and any associated trauma that may have been missed in the earlier examination. Remove fragments of hair, pieces of clothing, other debris, and blood clots which may camouflage other injuries and be a source of infection.

Suturing. For skin closure, nonabsorbable suture material is indicated, the least reactive of which is monofilament nylon. For typical outpatient wounds, deep sutures must be absorbable. Synthetics (Dexon) are less reactive than naturally occurring substances (gut). The appropriate suture size for different areas is given in Table 21-1. In

TABLE 21-1. SUGGESTED SUTURE SIZE

Scalp	3–0 ±1 size. Consider wounds at the hairline to be facial
Face, orbit	6–0
Neck—ventral	5–0, 6–0
—dorsal	4–0, 5–0
Arms, legs, trunk	4–0 ±1
Hands—dorsum	5–0, 6–0
—palmar	5–0 ±1
—fingers	5–0, 6–0
—fingertips	6–0
Feet—dorsum	4–0, 5–0
—plantar	3–0
—toes	5–0, 6–0
DEEP (absorbable)	
—hemostasis	4–0, 5–0
—deep closure	4–0 ±1, the more superficial the subcutaneous suture, the smaller the size

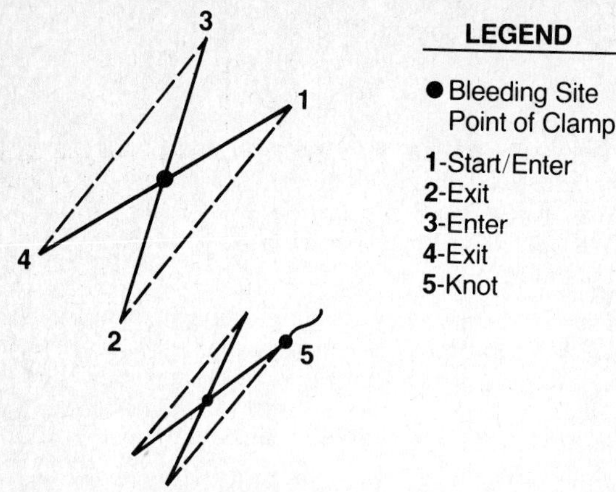

Figure 21-1. Figure-of-eight suture.

areas such as joints, where there is an increase in tension, choose the next heavier size.

Hemostasis may be accomplished with a simple ligature, a loop of absorbable suture either around the bleeder or tied in a small figure of eight (Fig. 21-1). Never use a hemostat clamp blindly, as a tendon, tendon sheath, or nerve may be clamped and destroyed.

Close *deep wounds* in two layers to prevent a dead air space (Fig. 21-2). When using deep sutures, bury the knot (Fig. 21-3), except where it will cause friction (ie, facia, tendon sheaths), and cut the ends fairly short.

Most wounds can be closed with simple interrupted sutures (Fig. 21-4). The skin edges must be everted and touching. Inverted edges result in poor healing but can be avoided by insuring that the suture is at equal depth on both sides of the wound, that the depth is greater than the width (B > C), and that the width at the bottom of the suture (C) is greater than at the top (A). Evenly space the sutures so that the tension is shared between several sutures rather than there being excessive stress on one.

A vertical mattress (Fig. 21-5) is a good method of closing a wound where there are problems with wound edge eversion, tension on the wound edge, or when a wound is deep but does not require a two-

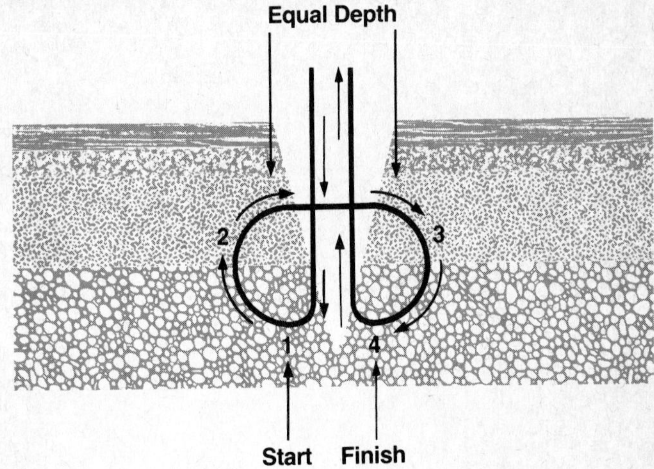

Figure 21-2. Suture for a deep wound.

layer closure. The area inside the suture has all the tension, leaving the wound edges with none. The suture must be of equal depth on both sides of the wound to prevent a stepping scar.

Employ a horizontal mattress (Fig. 21-6) when there are problems

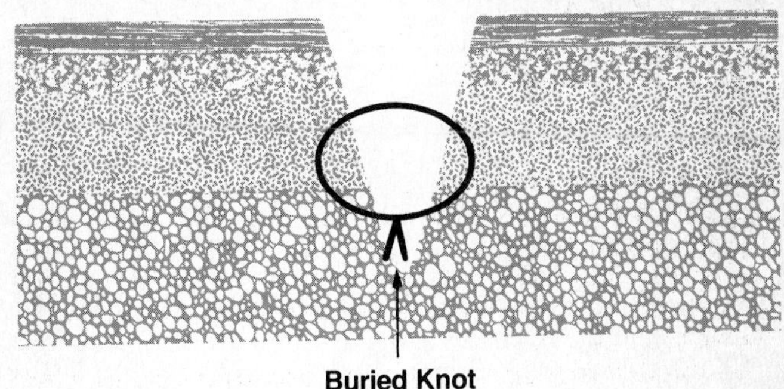

Figure 21-3. Suture for a deep wound—burying the ends.

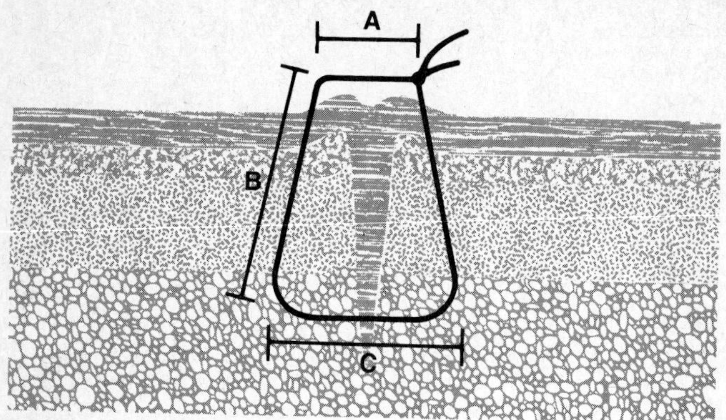

Figure 21-4. Interrupted suture.

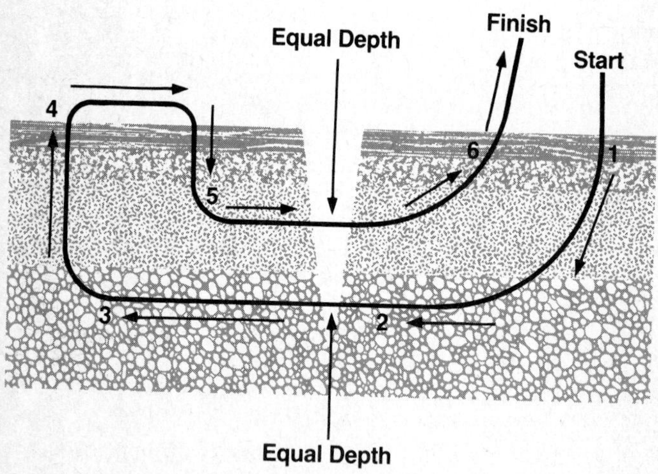

Figure 21-5. Vertical mattress suture.

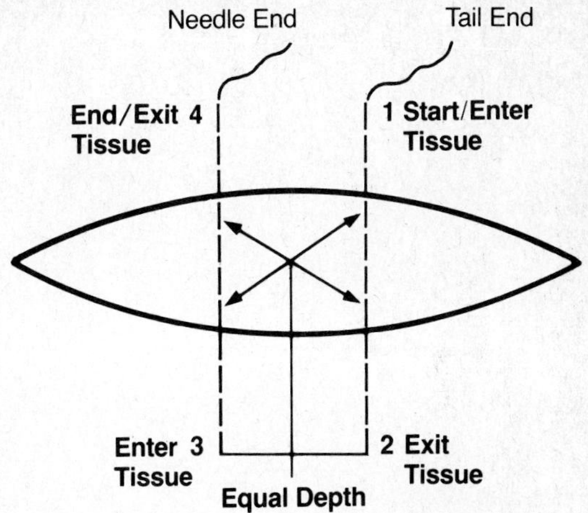

Figure 21-6. Horizontal mattress suture.

with wound edge eversion; do not use one where there will be any tension or to eliminate a two-layer closure. Note that each horizontal mattress takes the space of two sutures, so that this is a fast way to close a wound.

The half-horizontal mattress is the best way to handle any sharp corner (Figs. 21-7A, 21-7B) and can be used for a "v," "y," "t," stellate or "z" type of wound (Figs. 21-7C through 21-7F).

In wounds involving the lip, the first suture must bring together the edges of the vermillion border. Otherwise, a very noticeable scar results.

Referral. Refer complex wounds, in which underlying structural injury is a possibility, to a surgeon. Among these are deep lacerations of the wrist or hand, chest, abdomen, perineum, or anterior neck. Ear and eyelid wounds should also be referred.

Tetanus. Give all patients tetanus toxoid (0.5 cc of DT < 6 years old, dT > 6 years old), unless the wound is a clean one and documented tetanus prophylaxis has been given within the past 5 years.

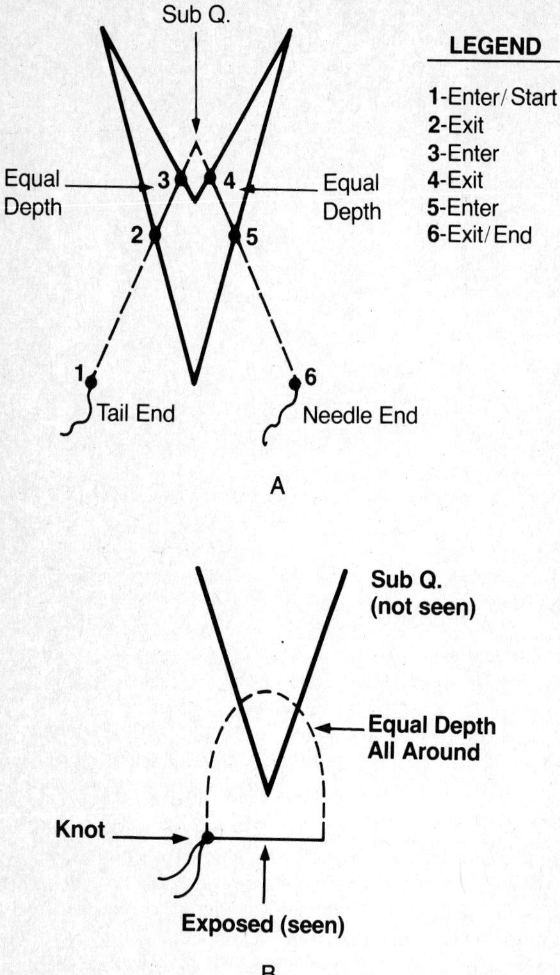

Figure 21-7A through F. Half horizontal mattress sutures.

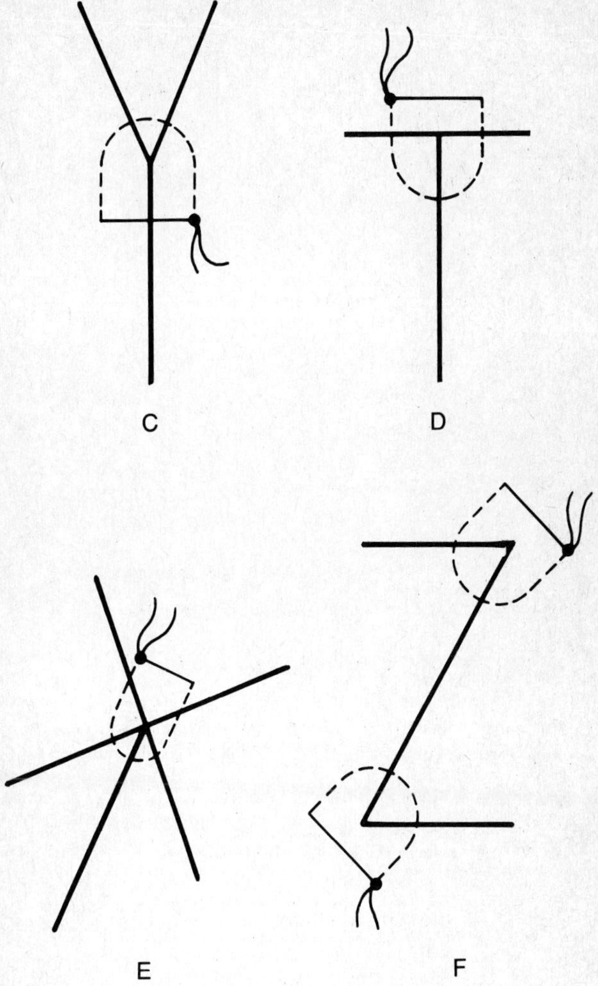

Figure 21-7. Continued

TABLE 21-2. TIMETABLE FOR REMOVING SUTURES

Scalp	10 days ± 2
Face	5 days
Orbit	3 days
Neck—dorsum	9 days ± 1
—ventral	5 days
Trunk, arms, legs	9 days ± 1
Hands	8 days ± 1
Fingertips	7 days
Feet—dorsum, toes	8 days ± 1
—plantar	10 days ± 2

If packing has been inserted, reevaluate the wound in 24 hours and remove the packing at that time.

Other Measures. *Immobilize* wounds in areas of great mobility (across joints on the hand) using a thick wrapping of gauze for 2 days, until healing is underway. Patients should avoid getting the wound wet for the first 24 hours. After that, it can be cleaned gently and allowed to air dry.

Antibiotics (dicloxacillin, cephalosporin) are indicated for:

1. Wounds on the feet, and deep wounds on the hands
2. All dirty wounds
3. Certain bite wounds (see p 496)

Give the parents dry bandages to apply in case the original dressing becomes wet and instruct them to bring the child back if they see any signs of infection (fever, erythema and induration, or purulence).

Suture Removal. Remove sutures according to Table 21-2. When sutures are removed, cut them just below the knot and pull them out. This prevents pulling contaminated material through the tissue. After sutures are removed, Steri-strips may be applied to the wound to give additional strength for a few days without the risk of infection or foreign body reaction.

REFERENCES

1. Dushoff I: Emerg Medicine 5:21–43, 1973
2. Tandberg D: JAMA 248: 1872–1874, 1982

Index

References to figures are indicated by an italic *f*. References to tables are indicated by an italic *t*.